Oral and Maxillofacial Surgery

AN OBJECTIVE-BASED TEXTBOOK

SECOND EDITION

Commissioning Editor: Michael Parkinson
Development Editor: Clive Hewat
Project Manager: Elouise Ball
Design Direction: Erik Bigland
Illustration Manager: Bruce Hogarth
Illustrator: Ian Ramsden

Oral and Maxillofacial Surgery

AN OBJECTIVE-BASED TEXTBOOK

SECOND EDITION

Edited by

Jonathan Pedlar BDS PhD FDSRCS (Eng)
Senior Lecturer in Oral Surgery, Leeds Dental Institute, Leeds, UK

John W. Frame PhD MSc BDS FDSRCS (Eng & Ed)
Emeritus Professor of Oral Surgery, The University of Birmingham, School of Dentistry, Birmingham, UK

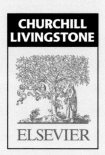

CHURCHILL LIVINGSTONE

ELSEVIER

EDINBURGH LONDON NEW YORK OXFORD PHILADELPHIA ST LOUIS SYDNEY TORONTO 2007

CHURCHILL LIVINGSTONE
ELSEVIER

CHURCHILL LIVINGSTONE
An imprint of Elsevier Limited

First published 2001
Reprinted 2003
Second edition 2007
  Reprinted 2008

ISBN: 9780443100734

British Library Cataloguing in Publication Data
A catalogue record for this book is available from the British Library

Library of Congress Cataloging in Publication Data
A catalog record for this book is available from the Library of Congress

Note
Knowledge and best practice in this field are constantly changing. As new research and experience broaden our knowledge, changes in practice, treatment and drug therapy may become necessary or appropriate. Readers are advised to check the most current information provided (i) on procedures featured or (ii) by the manufacturer of each product to be administered, to verify the recommended dose or formula, the method and duration of administration, and contraindications. It is the responsibility of the practitioner, relying on their own experience and knowledge of the patient, to make diagnoses, to determine dosages and the best treatment for each individual patient, and to take all appropriate safety precautions. To the fullest extent of the law, neither the Publisher nor the Authors assumes any liability for any injury and/or damage to persons or property arising out or related to any use of the material contained in this book.

The Publisher

Contents

Preface to the first edition   vii
Preface to the second edition   viii
Contributors   ix

1. Why and how you should read this book   1
   J. Pedlar

2. Diagnosis: the process and the result   4
   J. Pedlar

3. Control of pain and anxiety: selection of and preparation for sedation or anaesthesia   12
   J. Pedlar

4. Extraction of teeth   24
   J. Pedlar

5. Removal of unerupted teeth   45
   G. R. Ogden

6. Surgical endodontics   67
   I. R. Matthew

7. Spreading infection   83
   J. Pedlar

8. Oral lesions: differential diagnosis and biopsy techniques   100
   C. G. Cowan
   J. Marley

9. Cysts   115
   J. Marley
   C. G. Cowan

10. Malignant disease of the oral cavity   127
    J. D. Langdon

11. Surgical aids to prosthodontics, including osseointegrated implants   145
    I. R. Matthew

12. Surgical aids to orthodontics and surgery for dentofacial deformity 166
    C. M. Hill
    D. W. Thomas

13. Maxillofacial trauma 183
    J. P. Shepherd

14. Salivary gland disease 199
    J. D. Langdon

15. The maxillary antrum 215
    K. H. Taylor

16. Facial pain and temporomandibular disorders 228
    J. Pedlar

17. Surgery of the temporomandibular joint 242
    J. Pedlar

18. Surgery for the compromised patient 253
    J. P. Rood

    Appendix A 261
      Suggested surgical kit
      Suggested additional instruments for apicectomy

    Appendix B 262
      Answers to self-assessment

    Index 272

Preface to the First Edition

This book is directed at dentists in training. It should provide a basic theory background, to assist the development of skills in diagnosis, treatment planning, active surgical care and postoperative management. We hope it will also aid personal development, by pointing toward further reading and stimulating the desire to read more deeply. We have endeavoured to bring together a variety of authors all of whom have extensive experience in undergraduate and postgraduate education in Oral and Maxillofacial Surgery to form a team, which represents a mainstream view in UK dental schools.

We are very grateful to all the authors for the time and effort they have contributed, over and above their normal work in their departments, for their responses to our requests for amendments and for their tolerance of our editorial interference. Undoubtedly, their families, as well as ours, will have taken back seats for prolonged periods during this work. To them we apologise and hope they will forgive us on the grounds that the book, in the end, is worth it. Our secretaries too have given their efforts unstintingly. Ms Janice Urquhart at Harcourt Brace has been, throughout, patient, supportive and optimistic; there must have been times that she thought this book would never materialise.

In addition, we would like specifically to thank Professor Ken-Ichiro Murakami for access to the photographs of the arthroscopic views of the TMJ and to Mr P N Hirchmann for the two radiographs for Chapter 16. There are those also, who have made significant input to the text itself, even though their names do not appear formally as authors: Dr A Aiken for Chapter 4 and Mr J D Fenwick, consultant Otorhinolaryngologist, who kindly reviewed Chapter 16 and made many helpful suggestions.

We also thank the departments of medical and dental illustration and of radiology around the United Kingdom who have made a major contribution to illustration of this text and Mr Ian Ramsden who has expertly redrawn and polished the artwork. The department of medical and dental illustration at Leeds University has taken a particularly heavy burden and has consistently, cheerfully and speedily produced high-quality photographic illustrations for us. We are indebted also to the universities and hospital trusts of the authors' host institutions for permission to use their material.

J. P., J. W. F. 2001

Preface to the Second Edition

We are delighted to produce this second edition following the success of the first and the warm tributes and reviews which it received. This allows us to take into account the inevitable advances in knowledge, technique and terminology that occur over a period of just a few years, but even from shortly after publication of the first edition we were aware of issues where improvements were necessary.

Thanks to advances in printing it has become much easier to use colour illustrations and we have thus, where possible, replaced black and white clinical photographs with colour ones. The chapters covering pathological conditions of the oral mucosa and bone, along with biopsy as an investigative tool, have been completely reshaped. We have introduced a brief overview of cleft lip and palate. We have also extended the self-assessment questions into the chapters on diagnosis and medically compromised patients and rationalized the introductory chapters.

Readers will also find new succinct sections on osteonecrosis of the jaws, associated with bisphosphonate medication, and on infection with methicillin-resistant *Staphylococcus aureus*, the former because it has recently become recognized as a serious complication of tooth removal and the latter because it has become more important in the minds of politicians and the public since the first edition was produced.

We remain indebted to our authors and those who have made contributions in the form of illustration, secretarial support, advice or permissions and to colleagues at Elsevier who, as previously, have remained patient and supportive.

J. P., J. W. F. 2007

Contributors

C. Gerry Cowan BDS FDSRCS FFDRCSI
Head of Division of Oral Surgery, Oral Medicine,
Oral Pathology and Consultant in Oral and Maxillofacial
Surgery, School of Dentistry, Queen's University, Belfast, UK

John W. Frame PHD MSc BDS FDSRCS (Eng & Ed)
Professor of Oral Surgery, University of Birmingham, School of
Dentistry, Birmingham, UK

C. Michael Hill MDSc FDSRCS (Ed) BDS FDSRCS (Eng) MSc
Consultant in Oral and Maxillofacial Surgery, University of
Wales College of Medicine, Department of Oral Surgery,
Medicine and Pathology, Dental School, Cardiff, UK

John D. Langdon MB BS MDS FDSRCS FRCS FMedSci
Professor of Oral and Maxillofacial Surgery, Guy's, King's and
St Thomas' School of Dentistry, London, UK

John J. Marley BSc BDS PhD FDSRCS(OS) (Eng) FFDRCSI
Senior Lecturer and Consultant in Oral and Maxillofacial
Surgery, School of Dentistry, Queen's University, Belfast, UK

Ian R. Matthew PhD MDentSc BDS FDSRCS (Eng & Ed)
Assistant Professor of Oral Surgery, University of British
Columbia, Faculty of Dentistry, Vancouver, Canada

Graham R. Ogden BDS MDSc PhD FDS RCPS
Professor of Oral and Maxillofacial Surgery, University of
Dundee, Dental School, Dundee, UK

Jonathan Pedlar BDS PhD FDSRCS (Eng)
Senior Lecturer in Oral Surgery, Leeds Dental Institute, Leeds, UK

J. Philip Rood MDS MSc MB BS FDSRCS FRCS
Professor and Consultant in Oral and Maxillofacial Surgery,
Guy's, King's and St Thomas' School of Dentistry, London, UK

Jonathan P. Shepherd DDSc PhD BDS MSc FDSRCS (Eng)
FDSRCS (Edin)
Head of Department and Professor of Oral and Maxillofacial
Surgery, University of Wales College of Medicine, Department
of Oral Surgery, Medicine and Pathology, Dental School,
Cardiff, UK

Kathryn H. Taylor BSc BDS FDSRCS
Lecturer in Oral and Maxillofacial Surgery, Leeds Dental
Institute, Leeds, UK

David W. Thomas PhD MScD FDSRCS
Professor and Consultant in Oral and Maxillofacial Surgery,
University of Wales College of Medicine,
Department of Oral Surgery, Medicine and Pathology, Dental
School, Cardiff, UK

1 Why and how you should read this book

J. Pedlar

Surgery is a very practical subject and requires 'hands-on' experience to develop the skills required to practise it successfully. However, it also requires extensive theoretical knowledge to back up the manual skills. This makes it possible for surgeons to:

- reach a reliable diagnosis
- select cases for treatment
- determine the urgency of treatment
- determine who has the skill to perform the treatment
- identify the best environment for treatment
- advise the patient on options, success rates, complications, etc.
- perform treatments within their skill level and know how to extend their limits
- evaluate their own surgical performance
- recognize when treatment has not gone according to plan and take appropriate action.

This book is directed at dentists in training. It should provide you with a basic theory background to assist you in developing your skills, point you towards further reading and stimulate your desire to read more deeply. It is not expected that you will merely 'cram' your way through it, regard yourself as trained and launch immediately into major surgery.

You may have certain expectations of a textbook. Does this text give answers to exam questions? Yes, we hope it will help you to pass any dental school exams in oral surgery; yes, we hope it will help you pass your finals; yes, we hope it will help if you are preparing for postgraduate exams. But **no**, these are not the reasons we have written the book. It has been produced with the intent of developing particular abilities which will make you a more competent dentist. If you are looking for a magical key that you can use to unlock the hardened hearts of your examiners without having to develop an understanding of your subject, this book is probably *not* for you.

Because the book is firmly directed at developing skills, chapters start with lists of objectives that we attempt to address within the chapter. Each of these objectives has direct relevance to the work a young practitioner may be expected to undertake. We have not stipulated a precise career level at which this book would become important, nor when it would cease to be of value, partly because undergraduate courses will continue to vary in the timing of various components and partly because the skills required to practise in either a primary care or a hospital setting vary from practice to practice and over a period of time.

It should be clear exactly what skills are being addressed in each part of the book. **Think hard about skills objectives before reading each chapter.**

Should you read the chapters in the order they are presented? No, not necessarily. We have tended to put toward the beginning of the book those subjects often taught early in an oral surgery course, but the chapters are independent of each other and can be read in any order. However, the beginning of each chapter contains a brief statement of the assumed knowledge that you should have before reading the chapter. The 'assumption' is ours, but if you do not have a command of the stated areas you will gain far less from that chapter. It is in your interest to develop your skills in a sensible and logical order, recognizing areas of weakness (even if they have already been taught on your course), and addressing them before attempting to move on.

Should you read the whole book before starting oral surgery? Almost certainly, no. If your course extends over months to years, you are probably best served by reading small chunks regularly, preferably in parallel with lectures and small group learning, or in relation to specific patients you have seen. Likewise, do not leave it all till the night before finals: you may pass the examination but will be unlikely to retain any useful skills for more than a few weeks afterward.

Should you take the tests at the end of each chapter? Although we do not wish to be prescriptive as to how our readers should learn (and some students do not find this sort of exercise enjoyable), learning is a process that benefits from reflection on the degree to which understanding has been achieved. We believe that these tests will help you and, like the text itself, they are directed at specific learning objectives. Try them, or at least some of them, and see for yourself.

How should you use the references? To cover all the relevant fact and opinion related to oral surgery would take a book the size of an encyclopaedia. This book must be brief to enable you to get to grips with the content. At times authors must simplify subjects just to get them in, and in these areas your understanding will be limited if you read only what is between these covers. The articles and books referred to offer you a little more background, a little more detail and in some places controversy. Read as many of them as you can and by all means add to the list with references you have found or that have been suggested to you by your tutors. Try to get a feel for the fact and science that underly the didactic content of the book: do not just accept it as 'the truth'.

In most areas of medicine and dentistry there are issues which are taught dogmatically, without there being a clear scientific basis. Such subjects are very likely to be addressed differently in different schools. Examples from the oral surgery field are whether patients should be brought back for a follow-up appointment after minor surgery, or if steroids should be used to reduce swelling after third molar surgery. Where you find in this book dogmatic statements that are at odds with what is taught in your school, do not feel that either the book or your teachers are necessarily wrong, but ask your tutors for clarification on the basis and significance of the difference of opinion. There is room for honourable difference of opinion between clinicians (particularly where there are few hard data) that must be respected. Such differences can also often be very stimulating topics for research.

The term 'surgery' is derived from the Greek *chir* (meaning hand) and *ergos* (meaning work). So surgery might be almost any work done with the hands; however, usage is generally restricted to practical *therapies*, such as those involving cutting, repairing and dressing living tissues. Surgery has a long history of management of wounds and infections, but, since the advent of sound aseptic principles, there has been a dramatic increase in the application of surgery to improving function and aesthetics under a wider range of conditions. The term 'oral' pertains to the mouth but, even in the 1950s and 1960s, those who particularly developed oral surgery as a branch of dental surgery in the UK did not restrict themselves solely to diseases of, or operating within, the mouth.

There has been increasing specialization within dentistry and the rest of medicine over many decades; the development of dentistry itself could be seen as a specialization within medicine. The advantage of specialization is increased skill amongst practitioners in that area of practice; the disadvantage is loss of some general and widely applicable abilities. It is unavoidable that boundaries will be set to specialities and that specialists will practise within limits, but there has long been a reluctance to define limits too precisely. Attempts to set rigid limits to any speciality would be likely to stifle development and enterprise, and could not satisfactorily account for variation in interest and ability amongst its practitioners. So, although oral surgery could be said to be an area of practice within dentistry, its limits are not well defined and it spreads somewhat towards other aspects of surgery. 'Maxillofacial surgery' is a term that implies a greater scope of surgical interest (hospital consultants in the speciality are appointed as consultants in oral and maxillofacial surgery); 'craniofacial surgery', on the other hand, is a more specific term relating to the small specialized area dealing with disorders that affect both the cranial and the facial skeleton.

The general dental practitioner is required to undertake surgical treatments beyond the tooth and its supporting ligament as well as to diagnose a range of disorders that may benefit from a surgical solution or may have to be distinguished from those that require surgery. There is also an important distinction to be drawn between those conditions a dentist should treat in the practice and those better treated by a specialist or in a hospital setting. Further distinction must be made between what is common practice in one country and what is not accepted in another. Some of these differences are cultural and some historical.

Oral surgery, for the purpose of this book, is taken to include:

- the removal of teeth, by whatever means
- surgery to eliminate infection of oral origin
- management of pathological conditions of the oral mucosa and bone
- traumatic injuries, usually excluding injuries purely to the crowns of teeth
- disorders of the masticatory apparatus and structures adjacent to the mouth, particularly when teeth or dental treatment influence those structures

- surgery to assist conservative treatment of oral or dental disorders
- diagnosis of disorders that require surgical treatment and those that do not.

It specifically excludes surgery to the crown of the tooth.

Note that diagnosis is not, by any means, specifically a part of oral surgery. Rather, it is included in the subject often, because it is during courses on oral surgery and oral medicine that undergraduates are exposed to frequent need for diagnosis of disorders extending beyond the teeth, and requiring a range of skills very different from those that they have become used to using.

Consideration was given to the inclusion in this book of chapters on medical emergencies, local anaesthesia, sterilization and infection control, radiological diagnosis and therapeutics (in general). These issues, though often taught by oral surgeons, are not essentially oral surgery, being of relevance to all dentistry. There are also good textbooks on these specific subjects. The areas of temporomandibular disorders, temporomandibular joint surgery and the surgical management of the medically (and otherwise) compromised individual seemed worthy of inclusion.

We hope that we have achieved our objectives in terms of providing you with a basic theory background to assist you in developing your skills, pointing you towards further reading and stimulating your desire to read more deeply. Having read the book, or a substantial part of it, consider how valuable (or otherwise) it has been to you. If you have any comments to make, however critical, please write to us—we would like to know.

2 Diagnosis: the process and the result

J. Pedlar

- Diagnosis, the key to understanding and treating disease, is a systematic process by which we uncover the identity of a patient's problem, leading to reliable predictions of its behaviour and possible therapy.
- The process is a detective story in which the information obtained is matched with patterns of known disease.
- A standard framework is used to record findings and acts as a checklist and an aid to communication between colleagues.
- Special investigations may be required to lead you to a definitive diagnosis, which must relate directly to the reason for attendance.
- A treatment plan should be based on the diagnosis and agreed with the patient.
- The diagnosis or identity of a disease is used:
  — to predict its behaviour or natural history
  — to plan treatment
  — to support the patient in understanding their condition
  — to link similar cases for research purposes
  — to enable communication between professionals.

- human disease and pathology in general, and how they pertain to dentistry
- anatomy of the face, jaws and the planes and tissue spaces of the neck
- common disease processes of the mouth and associated structures.

If you think that you are not competent in these areas, revise them before reading this chapter or cross-check with relevant texts as you read.

INTENDED LEARNING OUTCOMES

At the end of this chapter you should be able to:

1. Elicit from a patient by interview the information needed to guide the diagnostic process
2. Approach extra- and intra-oral examination in a structured manner
3. List the essential points of the signs and symptoms of a pain, a lump or swelling and an ulcer
4. Relate additional investigations to the differential diagnosis
5. Explain how a treatment plan and the patient's consent relate to diagnosis.

ASSUMED KNOWLEDGE

It is assumed that at this stage you will have knowledge/competencies in the following areas:

INTRODUCTION

In courses in oral surgery and oral medicine undergraduates come face to face with disorders, which they need to unravel, using a range of interview and examination techniques, before treatment planning. It is worth thinking in some detail about how to get the maximum benefit from the process and the best understanding of the result. A comprehensive evaluation of a patient's problem involves history taking and physical examination.

Over many years a standard method of performing and recording the history and examination has evolved. This is useful, both for communication with colleagues and for structuring clinical practice. Because this examination is a significant event for most patients, the examiner must display a professional attitude in order to develop the patient's trust. Ensuring the patient's cooperation is an important part of achieving the correct diagnosis.

The scene must be set carefully, and the examination carried out in privacy with a chaperone if necessary. The clinician should exhibit appropriate body language to encourage the patient's confidence. For example, sitting face to face at the same level as the patient is more reassuring than standing over a patient reclined in a dental chair.

The written medical notes are a record of the course of the patient's care and may have to be submitted in evidence in a case of litigation. Therefore, use of humorous remarks and unusual abbreviations is inappropriate in the notes.

Diagnosis may reflect a clinical picture, histological features, tissues involved, microbial cause, or other perceived mechanisms of disease and is not drawn from a unified taxonomic system. It is common to find variation in disease naming because of dispute over the nature of a condition or the particular impact that one name or another may have on those using it. Names of some disorders may also change under the influence of national or international organizations. For example, some previously common diagnoses such as 'dropsy' or 'scrofula' have disappeared as medicine has advanced.

You should not think of diagnosis as absolute, for you are not uncovering a predetermined truth. Rather you are measuring, comparing and estimating to move towards a functional grasp of your patient's problem.

THE PROCESS

A systematic approach helps. Many clinicians begin with a conversation with the patient and work stepwise through examination until eventually they reach a diagnosis. In theory, this ensures that all questions that might be asked are asked, and that no points are missed.

We will start by describing how you can make the best of this style, but will follow up with additional material that more accurately reflects what experienced practitioners actually do.

RECORD KEEPING

The following sections are divided according to commonly used subdivisions in a patient record. The concept of this progression and the written record certainly help to keep one's thoughts in a logical order.

Demographic details

The patient's full name, address, date of birth, gender, ethnic origin and marital status should be recorded. Include the sources of information used in ascertaining the history. These may include the patient, relations and friends, an interpreter and any referral letters.

Presenting complaint

This is usually written as an abbreviation: C.O. ('complaining of'). If you wish to write the complaint in the patient's own words, ensure you put it in inverted commas—for example, 'I've been in agony for ages with neuralgia'. Complaints can be multiple and should be dealt with one at a time.

History of presenting complaint

This is usually written as H.P.C. Record the history chronologically, beginning with the onset and detailing the progress of the complaint to the present day.

In oral surgery the common complaints are of pain, swelling or lump, or ulcer. Allow the patient to tell the story in her or his own way and do not ask leading questions. Main points to cover include:

- What was the first thing that was noticed?
- Are there any other symptoms?
- What is the main trouble today?
- Does anything worsen or improve the symptoms?

● Does the complaint incapacitate the patient (i.e. does it stop the patient from sleeping, working, eating, carrying out normal activities)?

It is important to note recurrence of problems. For example, wisdom tooth infections may settle spontaneously, but tend to recur at intervals of weeks to months, whereas malignant tumours tend to be relentlessly progressive.

Past medical history

This is often written as P.M.H. A medical history is essential in order to assess the fitness of the patient for any potential procedure. The history will also help to warn you of any emergencies that could arise and any possible contribution to the diagnosis of the presenting complaint.

The medical history should be reviewed systematically.

In physical medicine it is common, after initial open questions about the patient's general health, to ask questions in relation to each body system in turn: cardiovascular, respiratory, CNS, gastrointestinal tract (including the liver), genitourinary tract (including the kidneys), etc. It is essential also to ask specific questions about drug therapy, allergies and abnormal bleeding.

Another possible scheme is:

*A*naemia
*B*leeding disorders
*C*ardiorespiratory disorders
*D*rug treatment and allergies
*E*ndocrine disease
*F*its and faints
*G*astrointestinal disorders
*H*ospital admissions and attendance

Features of pain worth noting in the history

- Character
- Severity
- Site
- Radiation (spread)
- Onset
- Duration
- Periodicity
- Aggravating factors
- Relieving factors
- Associated phenomena

---

*I*nfections
*J*aundice or liver disease
*K*idney disease
*L*ikelihood of pregnancy, or pregnancy itself.

However, any system that ensures that all relevant questions are asked is satisfactory. It is equally important to follow up any positive responses to determine the full extent and implications of the condition. The patient's general medical practitioner may provide additional necessary information or examine the patient afresh if appropriate.

It is important to record negative as well as positive findings in a patient's dental history.

If a general anaesthetic or intravenous sedation might be considered, the American Society of Anesthesiologists Classification of Physical Status is useful (see Ch. 3, p. 19, Table 3.1).

Social history

Occupation, home circumstances and travelling arrangements should be reviewed so they can be used to help formulate the details of the treatment plan. For example, planning third molar surgery as an outpatient, for a parent with small children, with a one-hour journey to the surgery by public transport, returning to an empty house would be unsympathetic and unwise as the patient would have difficulty in dealing with postoperative complications such as haemorrhage or fainting.

Smoking and alcohol consumption should also be considered under this heading.

Past dental history

If the patient is new to your practice then you should note details of previous attendance and treatment. This would include the name and address of their previous practitioner, frequency of attendance and any problems relevant to the presenting complaint. The reason for discontinuing attendance at that practice should also be noted.

EXAMINATION

There are two ways of approaching the examination. You may look at the site of complaint first and subsequently carry out extraoral and intraoral examination. Alternatively you may do a systematic extraoral examination followed by a systematic intraoral examination, which will encompass the area of complaint. The patient might expect you to examine the site of complaint first and may be puzzled if your routine does not allow this.

The author favours extraoral examination followed by intraoral examination because, if a system is adhered to time after time, then no area is neglected in the enthusiasm of looking at the site of complaint. A colleague appointed to oversee primary oral health care receiving casual patients diagnosed nine new primary squamous cell carcinomas in the first six months, probably because of adherence to this system.

Be systematic in examination; start by inspecting the area of concern, then if appropriate, palpate it. In a full medical examination you might proceed to auscultation and percussion.

Extraoral examination

The general appearance of the patient should be considered. Do they look ill or well; are they anxious? Look for obvious upper respiratory tract infection. Note the skin complexion and mucosal colour for signs of anaemia or jaundice. Assess the body in general and the head and neck for signs of deformity or asymmetry. In trauma cases look carefully for lacerations and abrasions.

Look systematically at, or for:

- lymph nodes: these should be palpated for enlargement or change in texture
- trismus: defined as limitation of mouth opening of musculoskeletal origin, trismus can be partial or complete. Normal mouth opening is at least 40 mm
- rima oris (oral entrance): a small mouth opening can make surgery difficult. Limitation could be due to scarring or the patient may naturally have a small mouth
- swellings or deformity.

Intraoral examination

The size of the oral cavity and the distensibility of the soft tissues should be noted. The soft tissues should then be examined in sequence, and this sequence should always be used by that clinician, so no area is omitted. A suggested sequence is:

- buccal sulci (upper and lower)
- floor of the mouth
- tongue (dorsal and ventral surfaces)
- palate (hard and soft)
- oropharynx
- gingivae.

Next, the teeth may be examined and charted using a conventional system to identify the number present and their distribution; noting dentures, crowns, bridges, implants, partial eruption of teeth and coronal disease. The periodontal condition should be noted.

The surgical or problem area should now be examined. Redness or swelling or inflammation should be noted, as should any discharge of pus. Look specifically for ulceration, erosion or keratosis of mucosal surfaces and for any lumps or deformity.

Consider which teeth may be involved in the disease process and whether any are in abnormal position.

DIFFERENTIAL DIAGNOSIS

When many diagnoses might explain the signs and symptoms of the chief complaint, a *differential diagnosis* is made. This is a list of possible diagnoses written in order of probability. It is unhelpful to arrange special tests unless there is a list of different possible diagnoses that must be distinguished.

Features worth noting during history and examination of a lump or swelling

- Duration
- Change in size
- Any possible cause
- Exact anatomical site
- Associated lymph nodes
- Single or multiple
- Shape
- Size
- Colour
- Definition of periphery
- Consistency
- Warmth
- Tenderness
- Attachment to skin
- Attachment to deeper structures
- Fluctuance
- Inflammation
- Pulsation
- General well-being of the patient

Features worth noting on examination of an ulcer

- Anatomical location
- Single or multiple
- Size
- Shape
- Base
- Edge
- Adjacent tissues
- Discharge
- Is it painful?
- General condition of the patient

Differential diagnosis initially involves the consideration and comparison of groups of diseases, but ultimately of perhaps two or three individual conditions with various clinical and pathological features in common. Whole groups of conditions, and then individual diseases, can be eliminated because certain features are unlike those of the patient's illness. Ultimately a single condition is chosen on a 'best-fit' basis.

A diagnosis, therefore, involves the recognition of a specific pattern in the available data. Even in straightforward cases, alternative diagnoses should be considered, although they may rapidly be dismissed if they are clearly incorrect. This way any feature that may be inconsistent with the obvious solution and which suggests the possibility of some alternative explanation is not overlooked.

Dealing successfully with the variability of the disease and of the patient in whom it manifests is part of the intellectual pleasure to be gained from surgical practice. Here lies the value of clinical experience. No clinician has seen it all, but the more he or she has seen, the more likely he or she is to have seen a patient with a condition similar to the one being examined.

FURTHER INVESTIGATION

Often the history and clinical examination are not sufficient to clarify the diagnosis and enable a sound treatment plan to be drawn up. Further investigation might involve a wide range of measures, such as:

- radiography and other imaging
- vitality tests

- haematological investigations
- microbial culture
- temperature, pulse, respiratory rate, blood pressure, weight
- urinalysis
- biopsy—incisional or excisional.

These investigations are key to reaching a sound diagnosis, but you should resist the common temptation to make the diagnosis solely on the basis of a radiograph (or any other individual investigation). This risks undervaluing clinical information.

DEFINITIVE DIAGNOSIS AND TREATMENT PLAN

The outcome of the history and examination should be a definitive diagnosis and a treatment plan, both of which should be recorded fully. The diagnosis can be multiple, in which case the treatment plan should relate to each complaint.

Before any treatment is carried out, it must be explained to the patient, other options discussed and possible complications explained.

Consent

All patients must be fully informed before any decision concerning treatment is made and no treatment should be performed without a patient's full consent. Surgery is regarded as an assault on the body. Adults may give consent to such a process, but cannot be regarded as having consented if they do not fully understand the implications.

What a patient should be told should be influenced by what a reasonable patient could be expected to want to know. This is difficult to judge, so it is proper to offer more rather than less information. For example, surgery for an impacted wisdom tooth has potential complications of pain, swelling,

---

For a patient to give consent to a procedure, they must know:

- The implication of not having treatment
- What treatments are available
- All possible serious adverse effects of each treatment
- The more likely but less serious effects

> **To give informed consent, a patient must be:**
>
> - Over 16 years of age
> - Mentally competent to understand and judge the implications of the decision
> - Allowed to make the decision, without pressure of time and away from the environment in which treatment will be performed

trismus, altered sensibility of the lip and/or tongue. Patients should also be advised as to the likelihood of incidence, the approximate extent and probable duration of each of the problems.

The UK Department of Health provides extensive advice on consent on its website (DoH 2005). For patients under 16 years of age it is generally accepted that a parent or legal guardian will give consent on the child's behalf. However, it is important to remember that a minor may withhold consent, if they are able to understand the issues involved: this must also be respected. For adults who are not competent to give consent it is appropriate to involve close family members or legal guardians *and* another non-involved individual, such as the medical practitioner, in determining whether the patient would consent to the procedure if they were able. Note: this is a rather different concept from the patient actually agreeing to the procedure!

The process of obtaining consent should include making a written record of the advice given to the patient and may require their signature to indicate consent, but the essential processes are the giving of information, the response to the patient's additional enquiries and their indication of a willingness to proceed.

Consent may be withdrawn at any time. The patient's wishes *must* be respected.

WHAT DO THE EXPERTS DO?

The process of diagnosis, as described earlier, tends to gather a great deal of information, much of which is not directly relevant to the specific condition from which the patient suffers. The process is complete, but inefficient.

Diagnosis for the expert is often a combination of:

- open gathering of data
- recognition of patterns in signs and symptoms
- focusing on specific features
- progressive narrowing of the search (or occasionally broadening it).

Formation of questions in taking the history is in the form of a dialogue. It is an iterative process in which the result of one question or finding may reduce the search field or suggest a further question. The examination is also guided by the findings during the history and may prompt further questions. There is also a strong component of the 'hypothetico-deductive' reasoning recommended for scientific endeavour, by which a likely diagnosis (or list of diagnoses) is tested against the results found thus far. If the proposed diagnosis is not excluded, further evidence may be sought to support or refute the proposal. For example, if a patient volunteered that pain was centred in a particular tooth, was worsened by cold stimulation and had been present for a few days, the practitioner might ask specifically about any observed swelling or about pain in the tooth on pressure, to exclude periapical inflammation. It would still be necessary to examine lymph nodes and the oral mucosa as routine screening, but not because malignancy is anticipated as the cause of the pain. Failure to find caries or a large restoration in the tooth indicated by the patient would make you redouble your efforts to find a cause of pulpitis in an adjacent or opposing tooth.

What is not so clear is how, and to what degree, experienced clinicians place weight on particular clues, such as the change in a disease process over time. Some of this can be learned from books, some by asking more experienced colleagues, but sadly some must come from personal experience.

TOOLS AND TRICKS

It still seems that, to arrive at a diagnosis and a treatment plan, you are going to have to remember the whole of medicine and dentistry all at one time, but fortunately the process can be eased somewhat by *aides-mémoire* and guidelines.

Surgical sieve

A surgical sieve is an *aide-mémoire* which cross-references disease processes and tissues involved.

Disease processes may be listed as:

- traumatic (physical, chemical, thermal, irradiation)
- inflammatory
- infective (bacterial, viral, fungal and possibly protozoal)
- immunological
- neoplastic
  — benign
  — malignant
- congenital and developmental
- degenerative
- nutritional
- metabolic
- idiopathic (of unknown cause).

Some lists will also include 'vascular' (e.g. stroke), 'haematological' (e.g. anaemias) or 'cystic' (particularly in relation to the jaws), all of which tend to cut across the other categories. However, as this is only an aid to memory, you may include whatever categories you find helpful.

The anatomical classification might include:

- surface or glandular epithelium
- connective tissue
- muscle
- nerves
- vessels
- lymphatics
- joints
- bone
- tooth (enamel, dentine, pulp, cementum, periodontal ligament, structures from tooth development).

You may find it helpful to think which tissue plane is involved as well as the tissue type.

In this process you aim to link together knowledge of anatomy, physiology, pathology and human disease. But remember: a surgical sieve is not an end in itself. It is merely a tool to help you think about the range of possible diagnoses.

Decisional support systems

These may take the form of written texts or computer-based, interactive schemes. The latter have been shown markedly to improve the diagnostic accuracy of junior surgeons dealing with acute abdominal pain. Simple algorithms of the type 'If A is true then branch right, then if B is true branch right again, etc.' do not work well because there is rarely sufficient information at all of the required steps. However, systems that allow for missing data and place weighting on particular factors, shown by research to be indicative of specific conditions, can be very powerful.

At present, little of this sort of system is available for clinical decision-making in dentistry. Clinical guidelines on treatment planning, based on published evidence of efficacy, are, however, now becoming available for much of the subject.

Albatrosses and sparrows

It is said that 'common things occur commonly'. This means that you should take some note of the likelihood of particular diagnoses before deciding what is wrong with your patient; however, you must do so with care. Toothache as pain referred from myocardial ischaemia is exceptionally unusual, but in a patient with pain in the left lower jaw which is worse on exercise and with no local dental disease in the upper or lower jaw on that side, it should be

Summary

- A standard framework should be followed to elicit information from the patient and record the findings.
- A definitive diagnosis should be drawn from a list of alternatives, on the basis of which offers the best fit to the factors elicited in the history and examination, and consistent with the results of further tests.
- Tools such as *aides-mémoire* and decisional support systems can make diagnosis more efficient and accurate, while clinical guidelines can help match treatment more closely to the diagnosis made.
- Diagnosis is a process of measuring, comparing and estimating, and enables a functional grasp to be made of the patient's problem.

considered. If, on the other hand (as is much more likely), the pain becomes worse with local thermal stimulation and the lower first molar shows extensive caries, pulpitis should be considered. Similarly, just because oral carcinoma is rare in people under 40 years of age, you should not ignore the possible diagnosis in a 25-year-old patient.

If you are struggling with a diagnosis, it is more likely that your patient's disorder is an unusual form of something common than an entirely new disease.

FURTHER READING

UK Department of Health (DoH). Consent key documents. [Online]. 2005 [cited 2005 September].

Available from: URL:http://www.dh.gov.uk/PolicyAndGuidance/HealthAndSocialCareTopics/Consent/ConsentGeneralInformation/fs/en

SELF-ASSESSMENT

1. A patient attends with a history of a lump on the partially edentulous, left mandibular alveolus, posterior to the last standing tooth (first premolar). It has been growing slowly for 12 months and over 2 months has occasionally been traumatized when eating. What clinical features of this lump will you seek at clinical examination?

2. What is a 'differential diagnosis' and what is its value?

Answers on page 262.

3 Control of pain and anxiety: selection of and preparation for sedation or anaesthesia

J. Pedlar

- Any surgical procedure would generally be extremely painful if no countermeasures were taken.
- Many people (possibly 25% of the UK population) find severe anxiety a major barrier to dental treatment, particularly surgical treatment.
- General anaesthetics have been used in the past to overcome problems of potential pain or anxiety, but their administration imposes risks and inconvenience that make them unacceptable for routine use in general dental practice.
- Thus, selection and preparation of the patient for measures to control pain and anxiety is an important part of dental practice.
- Patients have a right to expect adequate and appropriate control of pain and anxiety.

ASSUMED KNOWLEDGE

It is assumed that at this stage you will have at least some knowledge/competencies in the following areas:

- basic techniques of local anaesthesia (local analgesia)
- drugs used for the relief of pain and anxiety, including conscious sedation
- the basic principles of general anaesthesia

- principles of behavioural management.

If you think that you are not competent in these areas, revise them before reading this chapter or cross-check with relevant texts as you read.

INTENDED LEARNING OUTCOMES

At the end of this chapter you should be able to:

1. Select a means of pain control suited to a particular patient
2. Select a means of anxiety control
3. Prepare a patient for the use of sedation or general anaesthesia
4. Anticipate and avoid significant problems with any of these methods.

THE PURPOSE OF THIS CHAPTER

It is not possible to cover in detail, in this book, all the issues concerned with control of pain and anxiety in oral surgery. There are, however, other texts which do deal thoroughly with these matters. Nonetheless there are several issues of direct relevance to the practice of oral and maxillofacial surgery, which are worth covering here.

We would not wish pain and anxiety control to appear separate from surgical treatment planning: it is a central issue. This chapter therefore attempts to summarize important points of surgical relevance that should make the treatment less upsetting for both patient and dentist.

PAIN

What pain is

Pain is a defence reaction that tends to be associated with actual or perceived injury. A key feature of pain is that it conditions avoidance. It must be unpleasant to be effective. Not all pain, however, is the same. The distinction between the sharp pain of a needle prick and the ache of overworked muscles is all too obvious and the separation of these two examples into fast, type 1, or acute pain and slow, type 2 or more chronic pain is fairly easy. It is also of considerable therapeutic advantage because the latter responds well to analgesics, but the former does not. However, there are almost as many types or descriptions of pain as there are conditions that cause it. Colicky abdominal pain, the throbbing pain of an abscess and the dull ache of myofascial pain are remarkably different in nature.

Pain may result from a range of stimuli: penetrating injury, pressure, heat, electrical stimulation, inflammation, muscular fatigue, etc. Almost any tissue (excluding dental enamel) may be the source.

This chapter is concerned with pain associated fairly closely with surgery. This includes the pain that would be associated with the surgery if no measures (such as local anaesthesia) were taken to prevent it *and* the pain so often experienced after surgery, which is more associated with inflammation.

Although we have said that pain is a defence reaction, there is little evidence that it is in any other way beneficial and for that reason we should do all that we can to prevent it during and after any surgery.

It is important to remember that only one individual is in a position to define pain: the patient. Therefore when a patient says that they have pain, they *have*—it is of no practical benefit to debate with them whether their experience is pressure, movement or whatever! It is wise to remember also that pain requires consciousness to be experienced, and that it is influenced by emotional state, tiredness and anticipation. Local sensitization of the peripheral nerves by inflammatory mediators considerably increases pain experience and can cause difficulty in controlling the pain of patients who have been

in pain for several days. This is probably one of the commonest reasons for failure of local anaesthesia in such patients.

How to recognize pain

Your patient will tell you when they are in pain. However, there are some situations where a patient has difficulty in communicating or might not wish to worry you about their pain. Some will even think it is 'normal' to experience pain during a surgical procedure.

Pain tends to elicit certain reactions, which can be noted. Bodily movement, tensing of the body, wide opening or screwing shut of the eyes, dilation of the pupils, skin pallor and sweating are all readily recognizable. Noises (ranging from grunts to screams) can be illustrative—and may require immediate action.

ANXIETY

What anxiety is

Anxiety is also a defence reaction, ranging from disquiet, through apprehension and anxiety, to fear and downright terror. Like pain, we must accept that anxiety is a factor that may need to be measured, rather than simply noted as present. Anxiety is the anticipation of an unpleasant event that conditions avoidance.

Some anxiety or fear is clearly advantageous. For example, finding oneself at the edge of a cliff or having misjudged the speed of an oncoming car makes one move swiftly to reduce the danger (many people will also go out of their way to cause anxiety by bungee jumping or fairground rides). But anxiety associated with dental treatment is often unhelpful because it not only causes great suffering but also creates barriers to dental care. It is the dental practitioner's obligation to aim to minimize their patients' suffering—and that includes their anxiety.

Some anxiety may even be frankly damaging. For example, in a patient with moderate to severe ischaemic heart disease, the increase in work done by the heart as a result of the fear might not be matched by an increase in coronary blood flow. This can precipitate angina or worse.

Where fear of a particular thing, event or concept

is unreasonably excessive it may be described as a phobia. The distinction between what is a somewhat exaggerated concern about dental treatment and what is a true phobia is rather blurred.

How to recognize anxiety

The patient's description is again of great value, and many people will openly discuss their concerns about dental treatment. However, embarrassment or loss of face can be experienced (particularly amongst men) by admitting to fear, particularly when the patient feels that their fear may be irrational. There is therefore an underreporting of anxiety and considerable variation in the weight that individuals place on their own fear. For this reason it is important that you actively look for and assess the level of anxiety.

Clues can be found in body language: posture and facial expression. Overt signs of sympathetic nervous system activity such as pallor and sweating may be diagnostic. Behaviour such as failing to attend or cancelling appointments, aggressive behaviour or tearful episodes may also be clues. If you need more evidence, the patient's pulse and blood pressure would show considerable increases.

LOCAL ANAESTHESIA

Why use local anaesthetics?

Local anaesthetics have become the most widely used form of pain relief in dentistry. A variety of techniques and drugs are available and can be varied depending on the patient's medical and dental history

and the pharmacology of the agent.

The drugs are safe to use. Tens of millions of cartridges of local anaesthetics are administered by dentists in the UK each year. The mortality rate associated with dental treatment that does not involve general anaesthesia is about one case per annum and even amongst such cases local anaesthesia is rarely regarded as causative of the death. Few drug systems in medicine have such a good safety record.

The drugs are effective. In almost all dental applications it is possible to completely abolish pain during the procedure and, with care, pain on admin-istration of the drug can be kept to an acceptable level.

Reducing pain on administration

The application of lidocaine or benzocaine in the form of a paste, gel or spray to the oral mucosa can result in loss of sensibility to a depth of a few millimetres in a few minutes. This can abolish the pain of needle penetration and, for superficial injections, dramatically reduce the discomfort on injection. This can also have a major impact on the anticipation of pain in those particularly frightened by injections.

The use of topical local anaesthetics does have disadvantages, however. By spreading widely around the mouth they can induce numbness in a much wider area than would otherwise be necessary. Also, they cannot penetrate to the depth at which the inferior alveolar nerve block or greater palatine nerve block injections are given.

For procedures involving the skin topical lidocaine is of no value. However, EMLA cream does penetrate deeply enough to be effective. It should be left on the skin for at least one hour before the procedure. Amethocaine gel can also be effective on skin, and possibly over a time period shorter than that of EMLA, but is more likely to cause skin irritation.

Pain of injection can also be reduced by injecting slowly, distracting the patient and perhaps by stimulating nearby tissues (such as by compressing the cheek between finger and thumb) to activate the central neurological 'gate mechanism'. Rapid penetration of the mucosa by the needle results in far less discomfort than that experienced on slow pressure. This is made easier in lax tissues by tensing the mucosa before needle penetration.

Summary: pain and anxiety

- Both are defence reactions.
- Both interfere with surgical treatment and may be damaging.
- Acute surgical pain and postoperative inflammatory pain are distinct.
- How to recognize pain: patient tells you, movement, eyes, pallor and sweating.
- Anxiety consists of a range of responses.
- How to recognize anxiety: patient may not tell you, body language, increased activity of the sympathetic system, failed appointments, aggressive behaviour.

Extent of anaesthesia required

In preparing for surgical procedures you should plan carefully the area of anaesthesia. If a mucoperiosteal flap is to be raised, the extent of anaesthesia required must include the area at the centre of the surgery, the whole of the distribution of the flap itself and all the areas of mucosa through which a suture needle will eventually pass. Where surgery is to involve more than one quadrant you should consider exactly how much local anaesthetic will be required; for example, if you were attempting to extract three molar teeth in each quadrant in one session, it may not be possible to achieve satisfactory anaesthesia without exceeding the recommended maximum dose.

Failure

Failure to achieve satisfactory pain relief for surgical procedures at the first attempt is not uncommon. Failure may be associated with pain and local inflammation, which result in local neural sensitization (see p. 13). This is a difficult problem in a patient who is particularly anxious about dental treatment and who puts off attending until their pain is unbearable. There may also be a relationship between failure and severe anxiety, which is a common problem in the latter type of patient.

Failure is more common with regional block anaesthesia, probably for anatomical reasons. Although anatomical landmarks provide a guide, no two patients are the same shape and variation should be expected. If you experience repeated failures in regional block anaesthesia you should revise the anatomical guidance in textbooks and consider the accuracy with which you are following recommendations. Rarely, there may be failure due to aberrant innervation. How

to manage local anaesthetic failure is described well by Meechan (1999).

NON-PHARMACOLOGICAL CONTROL OF ANXIETY

A great deal can be done to reduce anxiety without medication. Seen from the opposite perspective, there are a number of things that might make things worse: uncertainty, worries about pain, worries about being unable to control the situation. The attitude of the whole dental team to the patient can make a major contribution to the comfort of the patient.

Openness and honesty are very important. You do not need to describe unpleasant things in graphic detail, but advising your patient that he or she will feel pressure and hear noises, but should suffer no pain, is reassuring and still permits alternative outcomes.

Long periods of silence are worrying; try to maintain a flow of conversation. Avoid repeated questions as they prompt the patient into action (this can interfere with treatment) and questions such as 'Are you all right?' signal to the patient that you think they might not be. It may be helpful to find a topic of conversation that in some way interests the patient. Distraction by conversation, background music, surgery decor can all contribute to a reduced level of anxiety. It may be helpful to talk through a pleasant scenario for the patient during treatment. They might be asked to imagine that they are on the beach in the sun, it is warm and they are resting on soft sand.

Flexibility in your approach—for instance, at the patient's request performing only one or two extractions at a time, when several are required— can also give the patient a considerable feeling of control. Timing can also be important. For a new and nervous patient it is better to start treatment with less frightening procedures.

Hypnosis is thought of as a more formal psychological technique, which at its best gives the patient full control over whether they suffer pain or any other adverse effect. However, distraction is probably the most minor form of hypnosis. The depth that can be achieved is dependent upon the patient, the environment, the skill of the dentist and the amount of time and effort employed.

Management of failed local anaesthesia

- Check anatomical landmarks
- Repeat injection
- Consider alternate or additional technique
- Settle pain and inflammation and try again about a week later
- Consider whether anxiety may be contributory

SEDATION

What it is

'Conscious sedation' is defined as 'A technique in which the use of a drug or drugs produces a state of depression of the central nervous system enabling treatment to be carried out, but during which verbal contact with the patient is maintained throughout the period of sedation.' The drugs and techniques 'should carry a margin of safety wide enough to render loss of consciousness unlikely.' In the UK 'any technique resulting in the loss of consciousness is defined as general anaesthesia' and thus 'deep sedation' is considered in this category (DoH 2003).

It is anticipated with current sedation methods that there will be considerable relief of anxiety as part of the mechanism that 'enables treatment'. However, unlike general anaesthesia (GA), no currently available sedation technique offers on its own sufficient pain control to permit surgical treatments to be carried out. For that reason a local anaesthetic is also required.

Sedation may be achieved with drugs given by mouth, inhalation or intravenous injection.

It is not possible in this book to review in detail all aspects of sedation for dental purposes and the reader is referred to texts specifically designed for that purpose (e.g. Girdler and Hill 1998, Meechan et al. 1998). However, it is worth considering what is desirable in sedation in order to help select an appropriate technique.

The aim must be to exercise maximum control over the perceived problem (often anxiety) in terms of onset, duration and depth, with a minimum of adverse effects. The latter might include the potential for problems with the cardiovascular or respiratory systems, loss of cooperation by the patient, requirement for venepuncture, the use of a mask, the requirement for altered activities after treatment. Clearly, at present, sedation techniques fall a long way short of being perfectly acceptable and absolutely controllable. For that reason it is usually necessary to tailor the technique chosen to the patient, the treatment to be performed and the particular skills of the team providing the treatment.

Oral, inhalational or intravenous sedation?

Oral sedation

Oral sedation with a drug such as temazepam has the advantages of being safe, highly acceptable to patients and easy to administer. Unfortunately, the effect relies on the patient following instructions, there is a long latent period before the drug takes effect and absorption is unpredictable. Therefore the dose required is unpredictable and, in the interests of safety a lower dose than needed is generally given. Oral sedation can be very successful in the individual who requires relatively little support and in those for whom mask and injections may be unacceptable.

Inhalational sedation

Inhalational sedation commonly uses a mixture of nitrous oxide and oxygen, although much work has been done to develop techniques using other anaesthetic gases. There are great advantages to nitrous oxide sedation. The depth of sedation is controllable, from the deepest to the lightest points, over a period of minutes, because of the rate at which the gas is cleared by respiration. This also means that within 15 minutes of the end of sedation almost all of the sedative effect is gone. With purpose-designed relative analgesia machines the risks due to oversedation can be brought close to zero. finally, nitrous oxide has some analgesic effect, which can contribute to the overall pain relief.

The disadvantages are few. However, the mask limits access to the mouth, and nasal administration requires that the patient breathe through his nose. Some risk is believed to be associated with high concentration of nitrous oxide in the surgery, which means that the environment must be adapted for treatment, such as using active scavenging devices and good ventilation. It may also be that the maximum depth of sedation achievable without the patient becoming disorientated is still not as great as can be achieved by intravenous sedation.

Intravenous sedation

Intravenous sedation is of rapid onset (up to 2 minutes after injection of the drug, e.g. midazolam) and the required dose is usually readily titrated against the patient's needs. The level of sedation achievable whilst maintaining cooperation and verbal contact is somewhat deeper than can be achieved with inhalational sedation. There is no mask; therefore access is marginally better and there is no requirement for continued nasal breathing. However, the use of intravenous sedation in children is not widely accepted and can be associated with unexpected reactions. Also, recovery from sedation with midazolam usually takes about an hour. During recovery the patient must be accompanied and monitored; this usually requires separate recovery facilities other than the dental chair. Although it is possible to reverse midazolam sedation with the antagonist flumazenil, this is not regarded as ideal routine practice as the latter drug has a shorter half-life.

Advantages

Conscious sedation offers a lower mortality risk than GA, but quantifying that risk for sedation in dentistry is not accurate. The figure is believed to be of the order of one in a million. It also has the distinct advantage, in theory, of maintaining active reflexes to protect the upper airway. The patient is able to cooperate in the treatment. In addition, the patient can be offered the opportunity of reduced levels of sedation for future treatment; this may allow some patients who are terrified of dental treatment to move towards more conventional provision of care. Sedation does not require the presence of an anaesthetist and therefore makes the dental treatment more convenient to arrange.

Preparation of patient

There is some dispute as to whether it is necessary to starve the patient fully, as for GA. It is true that reduction in reflex activity is slight, but sedation can be used very successfully to suppress the gag reflex, to permit dental treatment. Regurgitation of gastric contents seems to be particularly rare with moderate sedation and the risk of aspiration must be seen as very small. Nevertheless, most authorities recommend that the patient avoids a heavy meal before treatment, and a period of full starvation of 2 hours is a reasonable precaution.

In almost all other respects preparation is as for GA. All advice to the patient, detailed discussion and a written record of consent should take place preoperatively. There should be a responsible, fit escort and the patient should avoid demanding activity of the hands or brain for 24 hours (for inhalational sedation it may be reasonable to shorten that period considerably). The procedure should be delayed in the presence of acute medical conditions.

Detailed recommendations on both the preparation of the patient for and discharge of the patient after sedation may be found in the document 'Conscious sedation in the provision of dental care' (DoH 2003) as well as in standard textbooks on the subject.

Airway protection

The airway can still be at risk during sedation, partly because the patient is so relaxed and partly because of a reduction in efficiency of reflexes. For this reason some operators place a pack over the back of the tongue for extraction work. There do not appear to be real problems with the reflexes with inhalational sedation.

It is wise to avoid large quantities of water for irrigation and maintain suction throughout the procedure.

Model instructions to patients

Figure 3.1 is an example of the sort of instructions that may be given to the patient at the time of booking a sedation appointment.

GENERAL ANAESTHESIA

Advantages

General anaesthesia has been used widely for the control of pain in dentistry since the end of the nineteenth century. Indeed, a great deal of the early development of GA was carried out by dentists for dental work, particularly in the UK. By eliminating pain, anxiety and other emotional responses to surgery, the technique has an obvious attraction. It is

---

Summary of sedation

- Sedation is a drug-induced, altered state of consciousness.
- Sedation may be oral, inhalational or intravenous.
- Local anaesthesia is still required.
- An appropriately trained dentist and dental nurse may administer sedation without an anaesthetist.
- Morbidity and mortality are lower than with general anaesthesia.
- Patient selection and preparation must still be thorough.

Sweet, Lovett and Jentell Dental Practice

2, Thake St

Anytown

0123 456 7890

APPOINTMENT FOR TREATMENT UNDER INTRAVENOUS SEDATION

Appointment for _____ (name)

Your appointment is on _____ at _____

These instructions are important! If you do not follow them your treatment will not be performed at this appointment.

You must:

- be accompanied by a responsible, fit adult who will attend with you, escort you home (by car or taxi) and stay with you overnight

- you may have a light, fat-free meal up to 2 hours before treatment

- continue to take your normal tablets or medicines (with a sip of water if necessary) unless specifically instructed by our staff not to do so.

You must NOT:

- drive, return to work, operate machinery, cook, look after small children, drink alcohol, make important decisions or do anything that requires careful use of the hands or brain for 24 hours after the procedure

- permit children to return to school, play unsupervised or ride bicycles for 24 hours after the procedure

- be left alone in the house for 24 hours after the procedure.

Please contact the practice if you are uncertain about any of the above, or if you are unwell shortly before the appointment.

Fig. 3.1 Instructions for a patient undergoing sedation.

possible rapidly to render a patient non-responsive, permitting the dentist to concentrate wholly on the surgical task in hand. It can also eliminate muscular activity and reflex responses such as tremors or retching that can make some dental manipulations difficult. And, better still, the patient usually has no recollection of any of the events that have taken place.

Problems

There is however, a down-side to GA: there is a risk of mortality or morbidity with every general anaesthetic given. Patients need to be assessed on an individual basis, taking into account the range of techniques available for behavioural management, pain and anxiety control. GA should be prescribed only when absolutely essential.

The administration of GA requires many additional measures to maximize safety: an anaesthetist must be present; additional equipment is required, measures must be taken to secure integrity of the airway, preparatory measures are needed and patients less fit to undergo the procedure are excluded.

GA deprives the patient of the ability to cooperate and prevents consultation during the procedure. The loss of muscle tone means that action must be taken to keep the mouth open. Additional procedures may also be required to prevent other injury during anaesthesia, such as taping the eyes shut.

An additional point, of some importance, is that, for the patient undergoing treatment under GA because of anxiety, there is no easy mechanism for them to progress towards treatment by a less risky method: they are either awake or asleep.

Indications

There are no absolute indications for the use of general anaesthesia, but there are circumstances in which it is often the preferred approach to control of pain and anxiety:

- repeated failure of local anaesthesia
- extensive surgery that would require an excessive dose of local anaesthetic drug or where satisfactory pain relief by local anaesthesia alone would be unlikely
- surgery that would be extremely unpleasant if the patient were conscious, such as surgery to the soft palate
- a patient who is unable to remain still while conscious (such as with Parkinson's disease)
- extreme anxiety in a patient who feels unable to tolerate treatment under local anaesthesia even with sedation.

The referring practitioner has an obligation to discuss alternative methods of control of pain and anxiety with a patient and assure themselves that the patient requires, and is fit for anaesthesia, prior to referral.

Equipment, drugs, competencies

The equipment, the drugs and the techniques of anaesthesia have become progressively more sophisticated over the past century and now require considerable training and expertise to operate to maximum safety. Thus an expert anaesthetist is needed to deliver the anaesthesia, and he or she must be supported by staff specifically trained for the purpose. It is now mandatory in the UK that GA for dental purposes be provided in a hospital setting (GDC 2005).

Fitness

The risk associated with GA is dependent on a number of factors. These must be taken into account if a patient is to benefit from GA. A useful simple measure of fitness for anaesthesia is that recommended by the American Society of Anesthesiologists (ASA 1963) (Table 3.1).

Dental treatment on people in classes IV and V is rarely appropriate and would almost never justify general anaesthesia.

Morbid obesity is a special problem with GA. It can result in hypertension, difficulties in airway management, poor ventilation even in the intubated patient, chest infection, deep venous thrombosis, increased doses of anaesthetic drugs and consequent delayed recovery. In addition, moving the overweight, unconscious person is much more difficult. Obesity may be defined as a body mass index (BMI) exceeding 30 (BMI is calculated as weight (kg) divided by height (m) squared).

Age is not of itself a contraindication to GA, but the very young pose particular anaesthetic problems that may be better dealt with by paediatric anaesthetists in a suitably equipped setting. Elderly people are not only prone to diseases that contraindicate GA but may not tolerate the rigours of GA well, even if fit.

Pregnancy is a contraindication to GA because of risks to the fetus and, in the later stages, risks to the mother associated with the enlarged uterus exerting pressure on the chest and the abdominal veins.

A range of temporary disorders, typified by colds, influenza and sore throats increases risks associated with GA. An individual who is currently undergoing medical investigation, but for whom a diagnosis is not yet available, may also be at risk when undergoing GA. Such risks can usually be avoided by deferring the planned procedure.

Some disorders require a degree of preparation before the GA. For example, a person with type 1 diabetes may require administration of glucose (and insulin) by infusion.

Table 3.1 ASA measures of fitness for anaesthesia	
I	The patient has no organic, physiological, biochemical or psychiatric disturbance. The pathological process for which surgery is to be performed is localized and does not entail a systemic disturbance. Examples: a fit patient with an inguinal hernia, a fibroid uterus in an otherwise healthy woman, a cyst of the jaw.
II	Mild to moderate systemic disturbance caused either by the condition to be treated surgically or by other pathophysiological processes. Examples: slightly limiting organic heart disease, diet-controlled diabetes, mild hypertension or anaemia.
III	Limitation of lifestyle. Severe systemic disturbance or disease from whatever cause, even though it may not be possible to define the degree of disability with finality. Examples: angina pectoris, healed myocardial infarction, severe diabetes with vascular complications, moderate to severe degrees of pulmonary insufficiency.
IV	Severe systemic disorders that are already life threatening, not always correctable by operation. Examples: patients with organic heart disease showing marked signs of cardiac insufficiency, persistent angina, active myocarditis, advanced degrees of pulmonary, hepatic, renal or endocrine insufficiency.
V	The moribund patient who has little chance of survival but is submitted to operation in desperation. Examples: the burst abdominal aneurysm with profound circulatory collapse, major cerebral trauma with rapidly increasing intracranial pressure, massive pulmonary embolus. Most of these patients require operation as a resuscitative measure with little, if any, anaesthesia.

Investigation

There are a number of situations in which a potential medical disorder cannot be evaluated entirely from the patient's history and for which further investigation would be wise. The examples given here are in no way a complete list of potential investigations, but should serve to indicate the importance of considering medical risk beyond that which the patient alone can describe.

- When considering GA for an individual with diuretic-controlled hypertension, the blood pressure and the plasma electrolytes should be measured.
- For a patient with chronic obstructive pulmonary disease it would be wise not only to examine the chest carefully but also to order a PA radiograph of the chest and to arrange tests of lung function.
- Investigation may also be advised in the case of people with no known ailment but who may be in an at-risk group. For example, estimation of the blood haemoglobin concentration would be indicated in those at risk of anaemia, such as young women.
- Testing for sickle disease is routine for those whose families derived from areas such as Africa, the Caribbean, the Indian

subcontinent and northern Greece and Turkey where the gene is prevalent. Once such a test has been performed and the patient knows the result, it should not be necessary to repeat it.

For any patient or situation where the best course of action is uncertain the practitioner should discuss the patient with the anaesthetist who would perform the anaesthetic. On occasion, the anaesthetist may wish to see the patient before making a decision to continue.

Feeding

If there is a significant amount of food within the stomach there is a risk that, during anaesthesia, reflux of gastric contents will occur. As loss of consciousness is associated with loss of cough and swallowing reflexes, there is a concomitant risk of aspiration of gastric contents into the lungs. Gastric contents are extremely damaging to the lining of the respiratory tract and can cause a bronchiolitis, pneumonia and adult respiratory distress syndrome. Solid material could also obstruct part of the airway. The risk of aspiration is believed to increase with increased volume of stomach contents.

It is therefore normal practice to require a patient to refrain from eating or drinking for a period before undergoing GA, commonly for at least 6 hours before GA. That period may be shortened for a small, controlled quantity of clear liquid, particularly in children. The emptying of the stomach is greatly delayed by fatty foods, anxiety or trauma. For hospital inpatients it is possible to control these variables, but that is less easy for outpatients. It is also worth remembering that patients may put greater emphasis on their own comfort than on following what they consider to be arbitrary rules given them by doctors or dentists.

Escort

After an outpatient procedure under GA the patient may be permitted to go home when they are steady on their feet and thinking clearly, but the anaesthetic drugs should be regarded as still influencing their system for at least a few hours. In order to ensure their safety, if they are to go home, they must be accompanied by a responsible and fit adult. They should refrain from driving for 24 hours, and thus the mode of transport must be planned in advance.

Consent

Consent must be obtained before any procedure, but it is doubly important before GA or sedation that the whole procedure is discussed thoroughly because the patient cannot be consulted during the procedure. Also, because GA can be a frightening experience, it is important that consent is obtained away from the environment in which treatment is to take place. Written consent is required.

Recovery and discharge

During the recovery phase following GA, the patient must be monitored continuously by the anaesthetist, or other trained individual who is directly responsible to the anaesthetist. Adequate recovery facilities must be available and the patient should be appropriately protected. The anaesthetist decides when the patient is fit for discharge home, and a check must be made that there is an accompanying responsible adult.

Importance of the mode of anaesthesia to the surgery

The mode of administration and maintenance of anaesthesia is determined by the anaesthetist in consultation with the surgeon.

The placement of a naso-endotracheal tube and having the patient supine gives good access and ample operating time, but intubation is not without its problems (e.g. injury to the nasal mucosa with bleeding into the pharynx). Orotracheal intubation may give better access to the anterior maxilla.

The laryngeal mask (a device that connects an anaesthetic tube to an inflatable mask which seals the airway just above the larynx) works reasonably well for oral surgical procedures. The tube enters the patient through the mouth, inevitably obstructing access to some degree, but the device is associated with less damage to the lining of the nose and larynx than formal intubation and the airway is secure enough to permit most minor oral surgical procedures without difficulty.

There are some situations in which control of the airway must be managed via nasal intubation, notably operation on fractures affecting the jaws or on the temporomandibular joint, where being able to place the teeth in occlusion during operation is essential.

Inpatient or outpatient (day stay)?

For GA where the patient is expected to return home the same day:

- they must be fit (ASA I or II)
- they must not be significantly overweight for their height (BMI less than approx. 30)
- the procedure must reasonably be expected to take less than 30 minutes
- a responsible fit adult must be able to take the patient home by car or taxi and stay with them overnight
- they should not live so far from the place of treatment that it would take more than about 30 minutes to travel
- they should not fall outside reasonable age limits (e.g. 2–65 years, depending upon facilities).

In all other circumstances, if a patient is to undergo GA it must be as an inpatient.

WHAT IF NONE OF THESE WILL DO?

Occasionally the practitioner is faced with a patient who is unfit for GA, even on an inpatient basis,

---

Summary of general anaesthesia

- GA prevents all pain and anxiety during treatment because of loss of consciousness.
- Risk of morbidity and mortality makes it necessary to select and prepare patients carefully.
- An anaesthetist must administer the anaesthetic.
- The General Dental Council has given clear and specific guidance on the circumstances surrounding GA for dental purposes.

---

but who will not tolerate treatment under local anaesthesia, with or without sedation. It is right in this situation to attempt to balance the risks and potential suffering for each option.

Sometimes there may be advantage in deferring treatment until after a medical event that might be expected to be followed by an improvement in fitness (for instance a woman in the last trimester of pregnancy or a patient about to undergo a coronary artery bypass graft).

Rarely the decision will be made that the risks associated with treatment, which the patient can accept, outweigh the benefits in terms of reduced suffering or potential future suffering. In those circumstances that particular treatment should not be offered: a final decision on such a course of action may be better taken by a hospital specialist.

ANALGESICS

At the beginning of the chapter it was noted that pain may predictably occur during *and* after a surgical procedure. There are several approaches to postsurgical pain.

Standard local anaesthetics (such as lidocaine with epinephrine) will give pain relief for several hours. It appears that local anaesthetic drugs may reduce the local neural sensitization of surgery and thus reduce pain considerably even after the drug itself has worn off. Longer-acting local anaesthetics such as bupivacaine (with epinephrine) may be used for pain relief after surgical procedures and may give relief for 8 hours or more. However, the numbness associated with these drugs is itself found to be unpleasant by some patients.

Analgesic drugs, such as ibuprofen, paracetamol or opioids are effective against postoperative pain. The author's first choice is ibuprofen on grounds that it is effective, generally safe, cheap, available over the counter and is a rational choice because of its anti-inflammatory effect. However this drug should be avoided in those who have:

- asthma
- allergy to aspirin
- upper gastrointestinal tract ulceration
- systemic corticosteroids
- or who are pregnant.

Many arguments are raised for and against alternatives and it can be very confusing for the young practitioner to choose with confidence. Probably more important than details of precisely which drug to choose is that one does actually prescribe or recommend an analgesic! It is also rational to give the analgesic drug early. Particularly antiinflammatory medication is better at preventing pain than stopping it. When analgesia is given before a painful event this may be called 'pre-emptive' analgesia. The choice may also reasonably be affected by the patient's preference.

Corticosteroids also reduce pain and some surgeons routinely give a drug such as dexamethasone for surgical patients. The drugs reduce swelling simultaneously. There is little evidence of damage caused by use of steroids in this way, but the evidence that steroids add significantly to the benefits of the use of analgesics and local anaesthetics is variable.

FURTHER READING

American Society of Anesthesiologists (1963) New classification of physical status. *Anesthesiology* 24: 111.

Cannell H. (1996) Evidence for the safety margins of lignocaine local anaesthetics for per-oral use. *British Dental Journal* 181: 243–249.

Cawson R. A., Curson I., Whittington I. (1983) The hazards of dental local anaesthetics. *British Dental Journal* 154: 253–258.

Coplans M. P., Curson I. (1982) Deaths associated with dentistry. *British Dental Journal* 153: 357–362.

General Dental Council (GDC) (2005) *Standards for dental professionals*. GDC, London.

Girdler N., Hill C. M. (1998) *Sedation in dentistry*. Wright, Oxford, UK.

Meechan J. G. (1999) How to overcome failed local anaesthesia. *British Dental Journal* 186: 15–20.

Meechan J. G., Robb N. D., Seymour R. A. (1998) *Pain and anxiety control for the conscious dental patient*. Oxford University Press, Oxford, UK.

UK Department of Health (DoH) (2003) *Conscious sedation in the provision of dental care. Report of an expert group on sedation for dentistry*. DoH, London.

SELF-ASSESSMENT

1. Why is general anaesthesia on a day-stay basis not ideal for the insulin-dependent diabetic?
2. A patient is to have a tooth removed and requests general anaesthesia. The patient is 5 ft 2 in. (1.57 m) tall and weighs 16 st 4 lb (104 kg) but is otherwise fit. What advice should you give her?
3. A lower third molar is to be removed using local anaesthesia and intravenous sedation. What can be done to reduce the risk to the airway during the procedure?
4. What activities should you advise a patient *not* to undertake after intravenous sedation? When should that advice be given?
5. A patient describes himself as terrified of dental treatment, and particularly the use of needles. What forms of anxiety control might you suggest for a routine extraction?
6. What analgesic is suitable for a patient to take when she has had a lower third molar surgically removed under local anaesthesia?

Answers on page 262.

4 Extraction of teeth

J. Pedlar

- Removal of a tooth is a surgical procedure, which may be accomplished with forceps, elevators or a transalveolar approach.
- Extraction is irreversible and occasionally associated with complications. It should be employed only when all alternatives have been excluded.
- However, on occasion, teeth must be extracted and extraction is part of the function of the dental practitioner.
- Extractions may pose various problems and it is wise to anticipate difficulty and prepare for it.

ASSUMED KNOWLEDGE

It is assumed that at this stage you will have knowledge/competencies in the following areas:

- anatomy (including radiographic features) of structures surrounding the teeth (including the periodontal ligament)
- root morphology (including common variations)
- the relationships of roots to the maxillary antrum, inferior alveolar nerve and mental foramen.

If you think that you are not well equipped in these areas, revise them before reading this chapter or cross-check with texts on those subjects as you read.

INTENDED LEARNING OUTCOMES

At the end of this chapter you should be able to:

1. Select forceps or elevator suitable for extracting a particular tooth and hold them in an efficient and safe position in the hand
2. Position yourself and the patient for extraction and use your supporting hand effectively for a given extraction
3. Describe the directions of displacement of teeth during extraction
4. List and justify postoperative instructions to be given after tooth extraction
5. Distinguish, on the basis of clinical and radiographic features, those teeth likely to be difficult to remove with forceps from the more straightforward cases
6. Design a mucoperiosteal flap and plan the bone and tooth removal and wound closure in the event that completion of extraction with forceps or elevators alone is not possible
7. Anticipate difficulties with and complications of extraction, avoid them where possible and treat those that occur.

CLINICAL AND RADIOGRAPHIC ASSESSMENT

Not all extractions are straightforward; sometimes teeth fracture or there is risk of damage to adjacent structures during the process. It is important to attempt to evaluate, before the extraction, the likely degree of difficulty and the chances of adverse events. This maximizes the chance of things going according to plan.

History

A patient may give a history of previous difficult extractions, anxiety or wound healing problems. They may describe medical factors interfering with their fitness to undergo the procedure under local or general anaesthesia, such as severe ischaemic heart disease. Valvular heart disease and anticoagulation therapy require special precautions. Some medical factors indicate risks of local problems (e.g. leukaemia and risk of infection, or osteogenesis imperfecta and risk of fracture).

Clinical examination and radiographic assessment

Look for signs of limited access, as occurs with severe temporomandibular joint disease, burn scars around the lips or a restricted view due to abnormal tooth position or crowding. Teeth so displaced from the arch that forceps cannot be applied in the conventional way may be more difficult to remove. Incompletely erupted teeth require a transalveolar approach.

Increasing age is associated with more dense, inelastic bone, a greater risk of ankylosis and brittle teeth due to secondary dentine deposition. These increase the difficulty of tooth extraction.

A bulky alveolus and severe attrition (particularly of posterior teeth) are associated with difficult extractions. Cervical abrasion cavities, extensive restoration and clinically evident fractures all predispose to fracture during extraction. Extensive caries, especially at the site of application of the forceps beaks, also makes fracture more likely.

Radiographs may show extensive caries, large restorations, root-filled teeth (all of which may make fracture more likely) and also demonstrate bulbosity, curvature and other abnormalities of the root not visible clinically. The loss of bone due to periodontal disease, or increased density, influences ease of extraction. Also, if the tooth is likely to be in close relation to the inferior alveolar nerve or maxillary antrum it is important to assess that relation in advance.

Should you take a radiograph for every tooth to be extracted? No. But radiographs *are* indicated in the following circumstances:

- where necessary to confirm the diagnosis or ensure an adequate treatment plan
- where it is likely, on the basis of the clinical features, that the extraction will be difficult
- where the patient has a history of difficult extractions
- where a mucoperiosteal flap will be raised to gain access
- presence of apical infection
- root-filled teeth
- heavily restored teeth
- lone upper molars
- all third molars
- all partly erupted or impacted teeth
- if sedation or a general anaesthetic is to be used (and where it is therefore not possible to take radiographs in the middle of the procedure)
- if difficulty is experienced during extraction.

Check that the extraction is appropriate

The consent of the patient *must* be obtained before any procedure, and it is usual to record this consent in writing. It is not possible for a patient to consent to a procedure unless they know what is being proposed and its likely implications. For this reason careful assessment, as outlined earlier, is essential. A clear diagnosis must be made.

Teeth may be taken out for a number of reasons:

- they are beyond restoration because of caries, periodontal disease, fracture, tooth surface loss, pulpal necrosis or apical infection not amenable to endodontics *and* liable to cause symptoms
- they constitute a significant risk of distant infection
- teeth are partly erupted and causing symptoms
- they are traumatizing mucosa
- the tooth is excessive for the size of arch (crowding) or its position cannot be corrected by orthodontics

- they interfere with satisfactory construction of a prosthesis
- associated disease is treatable only if the tooth is removed.

Teeth should not be extracted unless, following appropriate clinical and radiographic investigation, a satisfactory diagnosis and treatment plan have been reached and agreed with the patient.

EXTRACTION FORCEPS: HOW THEY WORK AND HOW TO SELECT THEM

The application of fingers alone would not produce sufficient controlled force to remove teeth. Forceps enable the practitioner to grasp a tooth firmly and apply leverage to it in any direction.

The design of forceps has remained remarkably constant over many years: it is difficult to improve on the basic shapes. All forceps consist of two blades and handles joined at a hinge. The inner aspects of the blades are concave to fit the root accurately; they should not touch the crown of the tooth. The blades have sharp edges to cut periodontal ligament fibres and are wedge-shaped to dilate the socket. The blades are applied to the buccal and lingual aspects of the root. There are many designs, but for the purpose of this book we will restrict discussion to those most commonly used.

Forceps for upper teeth

Forceps for extracting upper anterior teeth are of a simple design (Fig. 4.1). The handles are straight and 12–14 cm long, joined at a hinge to the beaks, which are 2–3 cm long. The handles are contoured on their outer surface to allow a good grip. The beaks are both concave on their inner aspect (Fig. 4.2), shaped to fit around the root of the tooth

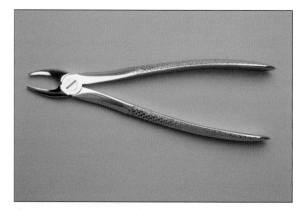

Fig. 4.1 Upper straight forceps (no. 29).

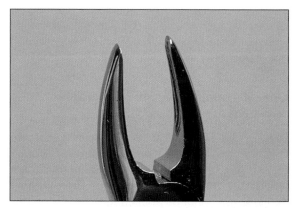

Fig. 4.2 Beaks of upper straights.

as closely as possible (Fig. 4.3) when the forceps are applied in the long axis of the tooth. The beaks are applied labially and palatally. All extraction forceps can be seen as modifications of this basic design.

These forceps can be applied to the long axis of anterior teeth, gaining access by the patient opening their mouth fairly widely (Fig. 4.4). However, if one were to attempt to use these forceps on an upper first premolar, there is a risk of traumatizing the lower lip. Forceps for use in the upper jaw further back than the canine have a curve in the beak (Fig. 4.5), which keeps them above the lip when they are in the long axis of the tooth. The beaks of these forceps are also concave on their inner aspect to fit the root of upper premolars.

These forceps could be used to extract posterior teeth, but for teeth with multiple roots, forceps are available with beaks specifically designed to fit complex root forms (Fig. 4.6). In principle, the more closely the beaks are adapted to the roots, the

Summary of assessment

- Assure yourself, and the patient, that extraction is appropriate.
- Check for medical and psychological factors affecting the patient's fitness for the procedure.
- Look for clinical and radiographic features suggestive of difficulty.
- Look for clinical and radiographic features suggesting an increased risk of tooth fracture.

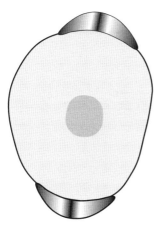 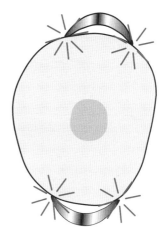

Close-fitting forcep blades
spread the load evenly

Poorly fitting forcep blades
concentrate force at the
point of contact

Fig. 4.3 Fit of the beaks of upper straights around a tooth root. If the blades fit closely around the root, the load will be evenly distributed (left). If there is a poor fit, the load will be concentrated at the points of contact (right).

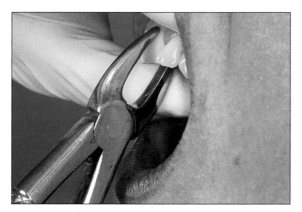

Fig. 4.4 Application of upper straight forceps to an incisor.

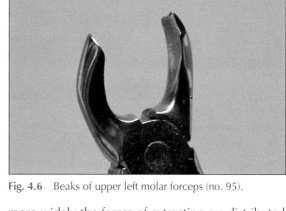

Fig. 4.6 Beaks of upper left molar forceps (no. 95).

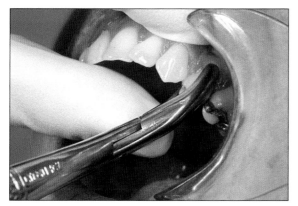

Fig. 4.5 Application of upper premolar forceps (no. 76). Note the curve in the beak.

more widely the forces of extraction are distributed and the lower the likelihood of tooth fracture. The buccal beak has a point to fit into the bifurcation, with concavities on either side to fit around the buccal roots and a broader concave palatal beak. Because of this distinction between buccal and palatal beaks, there must be separate designs for left and right sides of the mouth.

For all upper extractions it is necessary to push firmly in the long axis of the tooth during extraction (see p. 32). For this reason many forceps for upper posterior teeth have a curve at the end of the handle ('Read pattern') so that they fit in the palm of the hand (Fig. 4.7). This inevitably means that such forceps must have separate designs for right- and left-handed operators (Fig. 4.8).

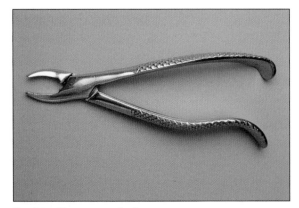

Fig. 4.7 Upper premolar forceps. Note the curve in the 'Read pattern' handles.

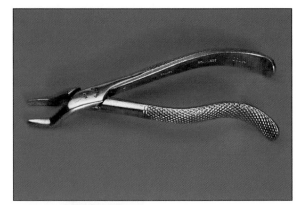

Fig. 4.9 'Bayonet' forceps (no. 101) for upper third molars.

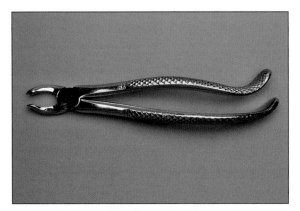

Fig. 4.8 Upper left molar forceps for left-handed use. Compare the handle shape with that in Fig. 4.7.

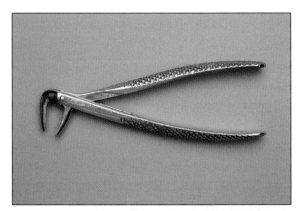

Fig. 4.10 Forceps for lower premolars and incisors (no. 74).

Access for extraction of teeth far back in the mouth can be difficult. A further variation involves a step in the beaks of the forceps (Fig. 4.9), which enables you to put the beaks on the upper third molar whilst avoiding the lower lip.

Forceps for lower teeth

If you were to attempt to apply upper anterior forceps to a lower anterior tooth you would have difficulty in getting past the nose and upper alveolus. In the UK it is usual to overcome the problem by using forceps with a right-angled bend in them; this permits the handles to come straight out of the mouth when the beaks are in the long axis of the tooth (Fig. 4.10). The beaks of these simple forceps are similar to those used on upper anteriors. Such forceps can be used effectively on all lower teeth, from second premolar to second premolar.

Just as with the forceps for upper teeth, beak design has been modified for multiple-rooted teeth. Full molar forceps have a point and two adjacent concave facets on both buccal and lingual beaks (Fig. 4.11).

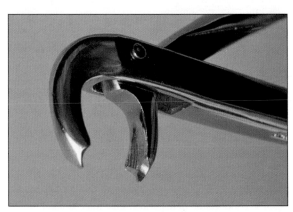

Fig. 4.11 Beaks of lower molar forceps (no. 73).

Other variations

The upper and lower premolar-style forceps are available with narrower beaks for teeth with very small roots, such as lower incisors, or for single retained roots of multi-rooted teeth. They are designated with the suffix 'N' (for narrow) on their catalogue number. The narrow variant of the upper straight forceps is designated 'S' (for small), but there is a broad, short variant for canines also denoted 'S'.

Smaller versions of forceps are available for use on deciduous teeth, which some operators like to use to access lower third molars where vertical space is at a premium.

Forceps designed to actively lift multi-rooted teeth out of their sockets by forcing pointed blades beneath the bifurcation ('cowhorns') do not allow the tooth to be firmly grasped and carry a small risk of fracturing the jaw by forcing roots apart if the tooth does not move. Similar forceps have been designed with beaks to cut or fracture a molar tooth ('eagle beaks'). The potential risk associated with the use of these instruments makes them unsuitable for beginners: they should be used, only with great care, by the experienced operator.

Practitioners in the USA use forceps, the handles of which enter the mouth from the front, to extract lower teeth. This results in a very different extraction movement.

HOW TO HOLD FORCEPS TO BEST EFFECT

During all extractions it is necessary to push the forceps firmly towards the apex of the tooth. For maxillary teeth this is achieved by pushing on the end of the handle. In order to maintain that position, the end of the handle must rest centrally in the palm of the hand, with the wrist held straight (Fig. 4.12). The first three fingers are placed around the handles and initially the little finger is placed between the handles to help hold them apart. The little finger can be brought around the handle once the forceps are thoroughly applied. The thumb is braced on the handle but not placed around it—that could produce too great a compressive force and tends to misalign the instrument in the hand. The thumb should not be placed between the handles as this also misaligns the instrument and tooth breakage during extraction risks injury to the thumb.

For mandibular extraction the position of the forceps is very similar (Fig. 4.13), but it is not necessary to push in the long axis of the forceps, so rigid adherence to keeping the end of the handle in the palm is less important. Nevertheless, the further

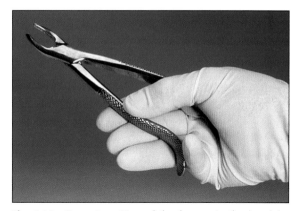

Fig. 4.12 Correct position of the forceps in the hand for upper extractions.

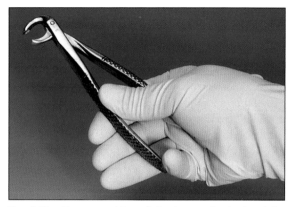

Fig. 4.13 Correct position of the forceps in the hand for lower extractions.

Summary of forceps

- Forceps beaks should fit roots as closely as possible.
- Forceps used in the upper jaw are variants of the straight design.
- Forceps for use in the lower jaw have blades at a right angle to the handles.
- Upper posterior forceps have a bend in the beak and handle to avoid the lower lip, and a curve at the end of the handle to fit the palm of the hand.
- Forceps with a curved end to the handle are therefore either right- or left-handed.

the hand is from the hinge and beaks, the greater will be the leverage applied, and the lower the amount of interference of the hand with the patient's face.

HOW TO POSITION YOURSELF AND YOUR PATIENT

The positioning outlined below is intended for extraction in a patient who is sitting up or partly supine and for an operator who is standing. It is perfectly possible to extract teeth low-seated, in the fully supine patient, but novices should start as shown here and modify the techniques for low-seated work later if they desire. The description assumes a right-handed operator, but a mirror image of the technique can be employed by left-handers.

Extraction of maxillary teeth

The positioning is determined by the need to push in the long axis of the tooth. The operator stands in front and to the right of the patient (Fig. 4.14). The operator's legs should be spaced so that it is possible to push hard with the right leg which should be to the rear and straight. The left leg should be forward and slightly bent. Both feet should be close to the chair and pointed towards the patient's head. The back should be kept straight. The patient should be tipped back by about 30° so that the surgeon can see directly into the mouth. The height of the chair should be adjusted so that the tooth to be extracted is about at the height of the operator's elbow. The patient's head is tipped just far enough to their right that access to the tooth is comfortable.

Extraction of mandibular teeth

For teeth in the lower left quadrant, the operator stands much as for maxillary extractions (Fig. 4.15), but the patient can be placed a few inches lower. When the operator's back is straight and the forceps are applied to the tooth, both of the operator's wrists should be in a comfortable neutral position. This will be helped if the patient turns slightly toward the operator.

For teeth in the lower right quadrant the operator stands behind the patient (Fig. 4.16) but beside the head, usually on the patient's right (occasionally,

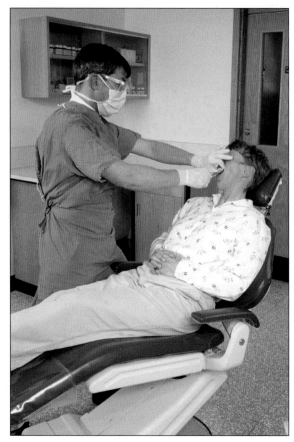

Fig. 4.14 Position of operator for extraction of maxillary teeth.

depending on the angulation of the tooth, it is more comfortable to stand on the other side). The chair can be tipped further back than for the maxillary teeth (maybe as much as 45°) and its height can be a little lower than when standing in front for the left side. There is little advantage in spreading the legs widely; for this extraction one is pushing down.

The supporting hand

The left hand is used to support the jaw and stabilize it during extraction. It also holds soft tissue out of the way to permit good vision. For maxillary teeth, the index finger and thumb are placed either side of the alveolus adjacent to the tooth to be extracted (Fig. 4.17). This usually requires the elbow to be up in the air. The remaining fingers are either kept straight or bunched tightly, so that they do not rest hard against the face or eyes.

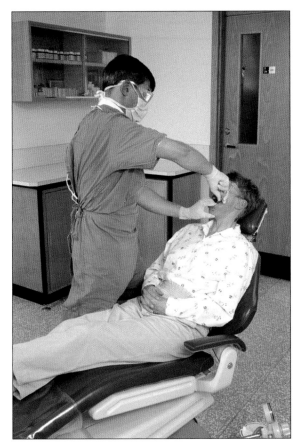

Fig. 4.15 Position of operator for extraction of teeth from the left mandible.

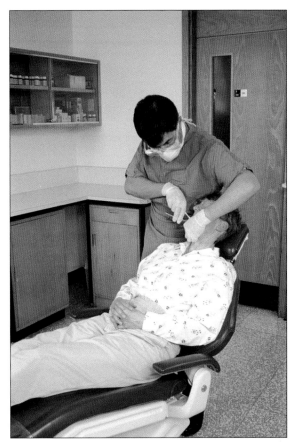

Fig. 4.16 Position of operator for extraction of teeth from the right mandible.

For extractions in the mandible two fingers and the thumb are used (Fig. 4.18). For the lower left this means placing the index and second fingers either side of the alveolus in the mouth and the thumb beneath the mandible outside the mouth to lift up. For the lower right use the index finger and thumb inside the mouth and the second finger beneath the jaw, supporting it.

It is important in all these manoeuvres to ensure that no soft tissues are trapped against the teeth, because this could cause pain or injury.

HOW TO REMOVE THE TOOTH WITH MINIMUM EFFORT

An extraction can be described as comprising two movements: the forceps are applied along the root of the tooth with apical pressure, then the blades are

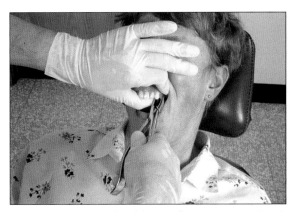

Fig. 4.17 Supporting hand for maxillary extractions (thumb and index finger).

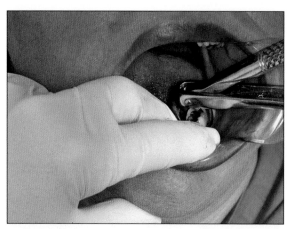

Fig. 4.18 Supporting hand for mandibular extractions (thumb and two fingers).

Summary of positioning

For maxillary extractions:

- keep the end of the handle in the palm of the hand
- fingers come across the handles with the little finger between
- keep the wrist straight
- stand on the right, up close, upright, legs well spaced
- chair tipped back by 30°–35°
- tooth should be at height of elbow
- use finger and thumb to support the tooth and alveolus.

For mandibular extractions:

- keep the hand well out along the handles
- left: position as uppers but chair lower
- right: stand behind, to the side, with chair lower and back by 40°–45°
- use two fingers and thumb to hold mandible.

---

closed while maintaining the apical pressure; the second movement loosens or displaces the tooth.

A tooth is held in place by the periodontal ligament, and if that is disrupted the tooth is readily removed, *provided that the shape of the surrounding bone does not prevent it*. Some teeth generally have conical or near-conical roots. For these teeth, rotation around their long axis breaks the ligament and they can be lifted out.

Maxillary central incisor

The action to remove a maxillary central incisor is to push in the long axis of the tooth, gently turning the forceps around the root, but not gripping it, until the forceps blades are well up the root. Then the tooth is grasped firmly (still pushing hard in its long axis) and turned around its long axis until the forceps blades almost touch the adjacent teeth. The tooth is turned in the opposite direction again until the blades almost touch the adjacent tooth. At this point the tooth can be gently delivered down through the socket. *Do not pull on teeth.* It is likely that some teeth will break if you do—and even if you are successful in removing the tooth, there is a chance you will damage one in the opposing arch.

Maxillary incisors and canines, mandibular premolars and canines

This rotatory action can also be applied to maxillary incisors, canines, mandibular premolars and canines. However, some care should be exercised with maxillary lateral incisors and mandibular canines, which sometimes have marked flattening of their root and may resist this movement. The approach can be extended to mandibular or maxillary third molars if they have conical roots and often also to mandibular second molars.

Mandibular incisors

Mandibular incisors usually have roots too flattened to permit this rotatory movement. For these teeth apply the forceps as described above, getting as far towards the apex as possible before grasping the tooth. Still pushing toward the apex, steadily lean the tooth toward the labial side until it just moves (about 5°). Then tip it lingually to the same degree, a little more labially and so on. Some such teeth are removed readily towards the labial side, some go more readily lingually and some respond better to some rotatory movement for delivery. Beware! Lower incisors are very close together.

Maxillary premolars

About half of maxillary first premolars have two spindly roots. These teeth should be treated similarly to lower incisors, with progressive buccolingual displacement, but once significant movement has occurred the tooth should be delivered down through the socket, not displaced a great distance to either side and certainly *not rotated*. Maxillary second premolars are also occasionally two-rooted and are readily removed the same way as the first premolar.

Maxillary molars

Maxillary molars are often best displaced buccally (again whilst pushing hard in the long axis of the tooth). With any multi-rooted tooth, if a root breaks it is likely to be the root on the side to which the tooth is moved. Fractured buccal roots of the maxillary molar are more accessible than palatal ones. The bone on the buccal side is also thinner and more malleable than that on the palatal side. In addition, displacement toward the palatal side usually brings the forceps rapidly into contact with the lower lip, which can be crushed.

Mandibular molars

Mandibular molars can also be displaced directly to the buccal side. However, often the bone does not yield readily, leading to a very difficult extraction or a significant risk of tooth fracture. If the forceps handles are moved bodily in a 'round and round' (or 'figure-of-eight') motion (Fig. 4.19), while maintaining the relationship of the beaks to the tooth, a tooth can often be wriggled up through the socket, like taking a post out of a hole in the ground. In theory this movement must include a component of mesiodistal rocking of the tooth, which in turn must put pressure on the adjacent teeth. However, the author has not witnessed any damage done in this way.

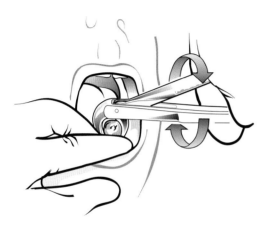

Fig. 4.19 'Round and round' movement to extract a mandibular molar.

Modifying techniques

No two extractions are the same (any more than any two people are), so it is necessary to adapt skills, considering what you are attempting to achieve and any problems that may arise. With experience you will become better at feeling the direction a tooth 'wants' to go. This feeling is better picked up if the tooth displacement movements are slow and deliberate. The method of tooth extraction should be modified to take account of this feel. It should also be modified if the 'standard' displacement would seriously risk tooth fracture. An example of this would be a maxillary molar with extensive palatal caries. Displacing this tooth buccally tends to allow the palatal beak to slip into the carious cavity, so such a tooth should be displaced palatally, taking great care of the lower lip! In general, displace the tooth toward the carious side.

Summary of extraction movement

- Conical rooted teeth: rotate around long axis of tooth
- Upper premolars: buccolingual movement, displace downwards through socket
- Lower incisors: buccolingual then rotation, buccal or lingual displacement
- Upper molars: move buccally only
- Lower molars: buccolingual, round–and–round, buccal, or lingual only (if that is what the tooth 'wants' to do)
- Feel what the tooth 'wants' to do

WHAT IS REQUIRED AFTER THE EXTRACTION?

Bodily displacement of a tooth commonly results in outward bending (or fracturing) of alveolar bone. It is important that this bone is squeezed back into place with finger pressure after the extraction.

It is usual to place a rolled-up gauze swab over the extraction socket for a few minutes, to reduce the degree of postoperative bleeding and help to keep blood localized rather than allowing the mouth to fill up. Bleeding should have stopped in 10 minutes.

Post-operative instructions should include the advice listed in the following.

There is little published evidence that the general measures (such as hot salt-water mouthwashes) outlined above make much difference to healing, but they are commonly recommended throughout Britain. Each dental hospital tends to have its own guidance.

It is essential to check that bleeding has stopped before the patient leaves. The gauze should be removed from the mouth and the wound examined under a good light.

An entry should be made in the patient's record, indicating:

- what surgery was performed
- what drugs were given and in what doses
- any difficulties encountered
- any unusual findings or actions taken
- advice given to the patient.

THE FRACTURED TOOTH

It is not uncommon for a tooth to fracture during extraction. This may be noted from the crack heard at the time or because part is evidently missing on removal. A fractured surface is sharp edged. If there is any doubt as to how much of the tooth has fractured, a radiograph should be taken.

Because you have judged that it is appropriate to take the tooth out, it is generally appropriate to complete the extraction when part has fractured, and not simply to abandon the procedure.

However, it may be appropriate to leave part of a tooth root *in situ* (at least at that time) if:

- there is a considerable risk to adjacent structures (such as the maxillary antrum, the inferior alveolar nerve, the adjacent tooth) consequent on root removal
- the patient declines further surgery.

There are also some additional provisos:

- the fragment should not exceed one-third of the root
- it should not have been displaced from the socket
- there should not be apical infection
- there should not be a significant risk of distant infection (e.g. endocarditis)
- if it is not planned to remove the fragment in the longer term, the patient must be informed and should be reviewed after about a month to ensure no infection has developed
- if the root is to be removed at a future date, arrangements should be made as soon as possible.

By choice, if the remaining piece is accessible, it should still be removed with forceps. If that is not possible, remove the root with elevators (see below).

If satisfactory access for an elevator is not available it may be made via the mucosa (a transalveolar approach, sometimes called a 'minor surgical' or a 'flap procedure').

ELEVATORS

Elevators are single-bladed instruments used as levers or wedges, placed between tooth and bone and turned around their long axis to dislodge the tooth or root. They cannot grasp the tooth and frequently can only move the tooth in one direction (away from the point of application).

There are two main classes (Fig. 4.20): *straight elevators* including the Coupland's chisel (or gouge), which comes in three sizes, and the smaller straight Warwick James; *angled elevators* including the right and left curved Warwick James and the Cryer's elevators.

Principles

Because an elevator is used as a lever, it applies force both to the tooth to which it is applied and to the fulcrum (bone) against which it rests. If that fulcrum is another tooth that tooth could be dislodged. The elevator must rest *only* on the tooth to be removed, unless all the teeth that might be damaged are to be removed at the same sitting.

The instrument is held in the palm of the hand, with the index finger along the axis (Fig. 4.21). It is essential to maintain sound support for an elevator throughout its use. A finger rest is obtained on an adjacent tooth, alveolus or other solid structure. Without such a rest, considerable damage may be done if the instrument slips.

Elevators should be used *only* by rotation around their long axis. The force applied at the tip of the elevator is dependent on the force (torque) applied by the hand holding it and the ratio of the diameters of the handle and tip. The approximate ratios of handle to tip diameter are 2 for the Cryer's, 6 for the straight Warwick James and 7 for the medium Coupland's elevators.

For an elevator 15 cm in length, applying force to the tooth by moving the handle bodily further increases the force applied about tenfold. This makes it readily possible to apply excessive force to the jaws.

Situations in which elevators may be very effective

When one root of a lower first molar fractures a little below bone level, it is likely to be inaccessible to forceps (Fig. 4.22). A Cryer's elevator placed into the empty root socket and turned will lift the root out. It is important not to place the elevator too far down

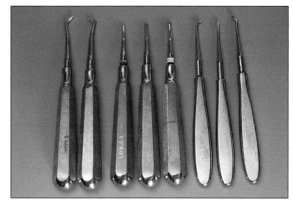

Fig. 4.20 A selection of straight and angled elevators. From left to right: a pair of Cryer's elevators, Coupland's chisels numbers 1, 2 and 3, left curved, straight and right curved Warwick James elevators.

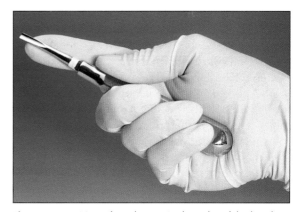

Fig. 4.21 Position of an elevator in the palm of the hand. Note the index finger along the length of the instrument.

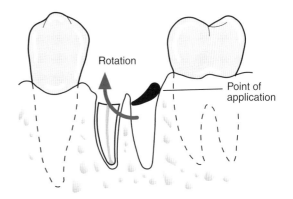

Rotation

Point of application

Fig. 4.22 Removal of the single retained root of a lower molar by applying the Cryer's elevator through the empty root socket.

the socket as it merely jams. It must not rest against the adjacent tooth. If the root is still not accessible it is possible to remove about 0.25 mm of the crest of the interseptal bone at a time with the elevator, until the elevator rests on the root. The root then lifts up as the elevator is rotated.

When a root of a lower premolar has fractured, if a flap is raised and some bone removed it is possible to make a small groove in the root and use the Cryer's elevator to remove it (Fig. 4.23).

For removal of retained roots of upper or lower molar teeth, grooves are made in the bone mesially, distally and in the bifurcation, after raising a muco-periosteal flap, and a Coupland's elevator is placed in from the buccal side to elevate each root in turn (Fig. 4.24).

A small Coupland's or a straight Warwick James elevator is also suitable for elevating a distoangular maxillary third molar downwards and backwards (Fig. 4.25). The curved Warwick James was designed for the purpose but it tends to move the tooth directly backwards, which may increase the risk of a fractured tuberosity.

The curved Warwick James is, however, ideal for elevation of the fractured roots of a deciduous molar (Fig. 4.26). The point is placed between the roots retained and over the crown of its successor. This markedly reduces the risk of displacing the unerupted tooth, which would be caused by placement of an elevator mesially or distally.

Many surgeons like to start all maxillary extractions by separating the buccal plate of bone from the tooth

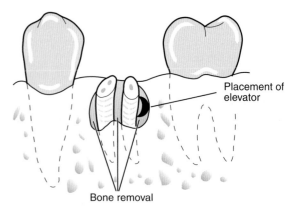

Fig. 4.24 Removal of retained roots of a lower molar. Bone has been removed mesially, distally and between the roots. A Coupland's elevator is placed between bone and root.

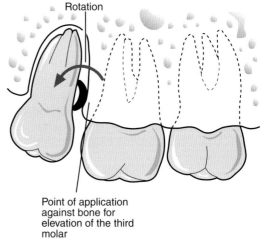

Fig. 4.25 Removal of a maxillary third molar. The Coupland's is placed concave face towards the tooth, but resting on bone.

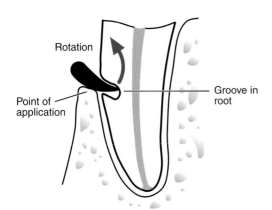

Fig. 4.23 Removal of a mandibular premolar root with an angled elevator after removal of some buccal bone and placement of a groove in the buccal aspect of the root.

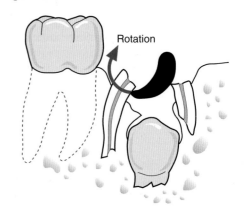

Fig. 4.26 Removal of deciduous molar roots with a curved Warwick James elevator.

with a Coupland's elevator. This can be a good way of developing the skill of handling elevators and reduces extraction forces.

The above list is only a selection of many possible uses, but elevators are not the solution to all problems. For instance, should a root of a maxillary molar fracture but be inaccessible to forceps, an elevator placed up through the socket has a very high chance of pushing the root into the maxillary antrum. Such a root is better approached surgically.

LUXATORS

Luxators look like the Coupland's elevator, but they are not designed to be used like one. The blade is much finer and much sharper than a conventional elevator and to some degree flexible. The intended use is to incise the periodontal ligament, in order to allow removal of the tooth with little or no force and no bone damage. They have not been widely adopted. (See also comment on the Periotome, Ch. 11, p. 151.)

THE TRANSALVEOLAR APPROACH

If it is not possible to remove a tooth (or root) directly from within the socket (what might be called an intra-alveolar approach), access is made through the side of the alveolus (a transalveolar approach).

The need to cover the operative site after tooth removal is satisfied by raising a flap of mucoperiosteum to expose the tooth site at the beginning of the operation, retaining its vitality and replacing it at the end of the procedure. This reduces pain and the time taken for healing. Mucoperiosteal flaps, however, are not only raised to give access in routine tooth extraction: identical techniques are used for access to bone for any dentoalveolar disease.

Flap design

There are several principles underlying the design of a mucoperiosteal flap. The flap must:

1. Give adequate access to the site of interest
2. Be designed to maintain a good blood supply
3. Be amenable to repair with its margin on sound bone
4. Not risk damage to adjacent structures.

The principles may be seen well in relation to one of the most common procedures: the surgical removal of the retained roots of a lower first molar.

In general, if the flap is extended from one tooth behind the tooth concerned to one tooth in front, including the most anterior interdental papilla on the flap (do not bisect the interdental papilla), it will be adequate in length (Fig. 4.27). If mucoperiosteum were separated away from the bone on a convex surface the attached gingiva would tear, so a 'relieving incision' is made extending down into the sulcus. In this case the relieving incision would extend down from the interspace between the two premolar teeth. This would breach principle 4 as the incision would run dangerously close to the mental nerve, so the flap is extended one tooth further forward. The interdental papilla between the canine and first premolar is included in the flap, which makes repair easier. This flap design is sometimes called 'two sided'. The blood supply is not dependent on particular named 'axial' vessels and consequently is determined in part by the width of the base of the flap. A broad flap also gives good access.

A second relieving incision may be placed posteriorly (Fig. 4.28). This does increase the access gained with relatively small flaps, but can make repositioning and suturing the flap more difficult. This 'three-sided' flap can be of value on the very convex anterior maxilla (for example, for surgical endodontics).

Most surgical removal of roots is performed from the buccal aspect of the ridge as this is more accessible, but on occasion it is necessary to raise a flap on the palatal or lingual side. Here there is no

'Two-sided flap'

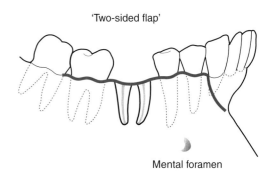

Mental foramen

Fig. 4.27 A standard flap design for access to the roots of a lower first molar. This 'two-sided' flap has been extended anteriorly to include the mental nerve.

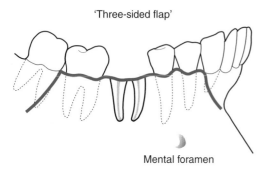

'Three-sided flap'

Mental foramen

Fig. 4.28 A 'three-sided' flap.

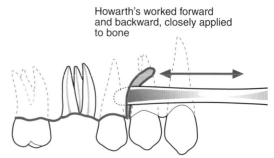

Howarth's worked forward and backward, closely applied to bone

Fig. 4.29 The Howarth's or other periosteal elevator is worked forwards and backwards, firmly applied to bone, to gain access to the subperiosteal plane.

need for a relieving incision as the flap is displaced from a concave surface.

Surgical procedure

The scalpel is held in a pen grip, with a finger rest on a sound support. Incisions are made full thickness through mucosa and periosteum to bone and extended by cutting with the bow of the blade. A suitable list of instruments is given in Appendix A.

The gingival margin incision is made holding the scalpel in the long axis of the tooth, at the posterior extent of the flap and drawing the blade around the tooth in the gingival crevice. The sharp edge of the scalpel must be kept immediately against the tooth surface to prevent inadvertent laceration of the gingiva. Then the scalpel is turned so that the bow of the blade rests on the gingival margin just in front of the canine/premolar papilla and is drawn downwards and slightly forwards, curving into the sulcus, cutting full depth to bone. This should be extended to about the level of the apices of the teeth.

Start by turning out the interdental papillae using an instrument such as a curved Warwick James elevator, or by separating the flap from bone in the relieving incision. The most difficult part to raise is often at the mucogingival junction; this is better done last. A periosteal elevator or Howarth's raspatory is applied firmly to the bone surface, pushed beneath the edge of the periosteum (Fig. 4.29) and worked backwards and forwards until a definite pocket at the correct plane has been made. This is extended backwards, close to the gingival margin, turning the flap outwards. It is essential to raise the flap to expose all of the area of interest (usually beyond the

apices of the tooth to be removed). Although people talk of 'raising' or 'lifting' a flap, lifting movements tend to allow the dissection to occur superficial to periosteum.

Once reflected, the flap is held out of the way or 'retracted' with an instrument such as a Lack's tongue retractor or a rake retractor. The instrument must not pull so hard as to tear the flap, or strip periosteum beyond the area required and should be kept still once it is in position.

Removal of bone to reach the roots is most commonly performed with a bur (a round tungsten carbide-tipped surgical bur is suitable), although under general anaesthesia some surgeons prefer to use a chisel. During drilling it is important that the bone is cooled with running saline, which also washes debris away from the operative site. Avoid excessive pressure and blunt burs. Also beware overheating of the drill due to worn bearings; this can result in a severe burn to the lip. Bone removal must gain access to the roots for their removal (as in Fig. 4.24). Space must be made to place an elevator next to the root and into which to displace the root. In this situation remove bone buccally to see the roots and the bifurcation; remove it distally and mesially to place elevators, and between the roots to make space into which to displace roots. This also permits division of the tooth. Divide the tooth, starting from the bifurcation and cutting occlusally. Sometimes it is not necessary to run the bur all the way through to the lingual side (which risks some damage to lingual mucosa); the roots can be split apart if the cut goes two-thirds of the way. It is wise to use the root surface to guide the bone removal; it is easy to lose your way if you come out buccally away from the tooth. Equally it is not helpful to tunnel down the side of the tooth with a bone cut only the width of the bur; that does not permit adequate vision.

An elevator such as a Coupland's chisel is placed between the roots and turned around its long axis to split the roots. That may also permit the turning out of one root towards the buccal side and occlusally. The Coupland's chisel is now placed on the other side of the remaining root and turned to elevate it out. Having removed the roots, smooth off grossly sharp bone, or that which has been leant on hard and devitalized and irrigate the wound with saline.

Reposition the flap and retain it with sutures. Rapidly resorbing synthetic sutures, such as polygalactin, are suitable for use in the mouth. Black silk is still a useful material when it is essential that sutures remain in place for a week or more (such as closure of an oroantral communication) or where precise tensioning is important (such as for control of postextraction haemorrhage). Sutures are placed both in the relieving incision and interdentally.

Suturing

Most wounds can be closed satisfactorily in the mouth with interrupted sutures.

The needle is held at the end of the needle holders (Fig. 4.30), at right angles to the needle holders and about one-third of the way from the hub to the tip of the needle. The edge of the flap is turned outwards with toothed dissecting forceps and the needle is placed through the flap 1–2 mm from the edge, perpendicular to the mucosal surface. The needle is then grasped on the other side of the mucosa and turned around its curvature to pull it through. The mucosa on the other side of the wound is then turned out and the needle is passed out through it, again perpendicular to the surface.

The needle is held between finger and thumb and the suture is pulled through the tissue until the free end is about 10 cm long, gathering up excess suture

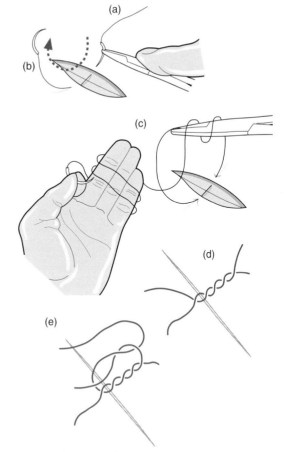

Fig. 4.30 Placement of suture.
(a) A 'bite' of tissue is taken with the needle held one-third of the way from the hub to the tip, at right angles to the needle holders.
(b) A second bite is taken, the same size as and opposite to the first.
(c) The needle is held between finger and thumb, excess length is wound around the fingers, two loops are made around the needle holders and the short end of the suture is grasped with the needle holders.
(d) The knot is slid off the holders and tightened to produce a double overhand knot closing to one side of the wound.
(e) A further knot is made with a single loop around the needle holders in the opposite direction. When slid off and tightened this creates the surgeon's knot.

Three problems to be avoided in transalveolar tooth removal

- Inadequate anaesthesia
- Too small a flap
- Insufficient bone removal

by winding it around the fingers. The needle is held in the left hand and two loops are made around the needle holders held in the right. The loose end of the suture is held in the needle holders and the loops are slid off the needle holders over it. The needle holders (still holding the free end of the suture) are held close to where the suture comes through the mucosa and the needle end of the suture is firmly pulled to tighten the knot. Beware not to rest the suture on the lip as the suture is pulled: it can cut tissues like cheesewire. Now a further single loop, in the opposite direction, is made around the needle holders from the long end of the suture and again the free end of the suture is grasped, the loop slid off and the knot tightened. The ends are now cut, leaving about 5–8 mm beyond the knot.

If significant bone has been removed, or if the patient is at particular risk of infection, it is usual to prescribe an antibiotic such as metronidazole (200 mg three times daily for 5 days), as well as an analgesic such as ibuprofen (600 mg three times daily for 3 days). It is not necessary to review the patient unless problems are anticipated, but it is essential that the patient knows how to contact the surgeon in the event of problems.

COMPLICATIONS OF EXTRACTION: RECOGNITION, AVOIDANCE AND TREATMENT

A complication is any event that would not normally occur and which might increase the patient's suffering. The range of potential complications is vast. It includes adverse events occurring locally, nearby or at distant sites, some things that occur immediately and others that occur a little later or are greatly delayed, some are rare and some frequent, some are serious and some inconsequential. There is considerable variation in the degree to which complications are predictable or preventable. The implications of adverse events are also determined in part by the patient's expectations, the reason for surgery and the manner in which the event is managed once it is recognized.

What should you do when something does go wrong?

- recognize it and accept it
- be honest and open
- be objective, factually accurate, but sensitive
- investigate as necessary
- make the earliest reasonable efforts at correction

- involve experts early if necessary
- tell your defence organization if it could become a legal matter.

In Table 4.1 is an illustrative list of some complications of tooth extraction, divided according to the time and site of occurrence.

Some complications are sufficiently common and amenable to treatment to justify further description.

Dry socket

Dry socket (alveolar osteitis, alveolitis sicca dolorosa, infected socket) occurs after about 3% of routine extractions. It is recognized by pain at the site of extraction, often aching or throbbing in nature but remarkably constant in severity (including during the night), starting within a day or so of a tooth extraction. The pain is often resistant to common analgesics. Examination reveals a socket partly or totally devoid of blood clot with exposed, rough, painful bone (Fig. 4.31). Greyish remnants of clot may be present. The surrounding mucosa and the whole alveolus may be red, swollen and tender. Inflammation

Table 4.1 Complications of tooth extraction

	Local	Regional/distant
Immediate	Fractured crown, root, alveolus, tuberosity, mandible, adjacent tooth Tear of gingiva, alveolar mucosa Oroantral communication; fractured instrument	Crushed or burnt lip; injury to inferior dental or lingual nerves; lacerated tongue or palate Swallowed or inhaled instrument or tooth
Delayed	Dry socket; local infection Delayed or secondary haemorrhage Osteonecrosis	Spreading infection Myofascial pain dysfunction Injection track haematoma
Late	Alveolar atrophy	Osteomyelitis; actinomycosis

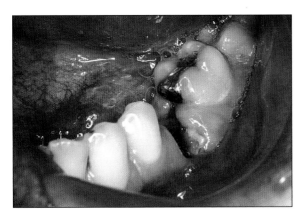

Fig. 4.31 Dry socket.

spreads through the alveolus mesiodistally, resulting in tenderness of the adjacent teeth to pressure. Occasionally a patient will believe that the wrong tooth has been extracted because of the pain in the adjacent tooth. Be aware that misdiagnosis can occur. The mouth smells and tastes foul (a smell of anaerobic bacterial activity or rotting meat). There may be a local lymphadenitis, but severe systemic response in the form of fever is rare.

If no treatment were provided the condition would eventually resolve spontaneously, but it may take up to 4 weeks and during that time the pain would persist. Similar pain is experienced whenever an area of bone is left exposed in the mouth and usually settles when the exposed (and non-vital) bone is either eventually covered by granulation tissue or is separated from the underlying bone and sequestrated. A few untreated cases of dry socket may progress to infection that spreads through the bone marrow (osteomyelitis).

There is obviously a bacterial component to this condition. Its incidence may be reduced by the prophylactic administration of metronidazole, or by the irrigation of the gingival crevice with chlorhexidine before extraction. It should be noted, however, that routine prophylactic administration of antibiotics before extraction is not justified. There are similarities to acute ulcerative gingivitis in the high spring and autumn prevalence, frequency in smokers and possible relationship to female sex hormones. However, some aspects of the condition's behaviour are not so obviously infective in nature.

The condition is most prevalent in patients in their fourth decade. It is more common after extractions of posterior and difficult teeth and seen more often in the lower jaw than the upper. Dry socket is more likely to occur after extractions under local anaesthesia than under general anaesthesia and is less frequent after multiple extractions.

It is probable that the condition represents the outcome of a mixture of disease processes in which trauma, local fibrinolysis and bacterial clot degradation all play a part. Some patients are particularly prone to dry socket, without any other evident medical problem.

Investigation need not be extensive; the condition can usually be diagnosed confidently on clinical grounds. A radiograph is valuable, both as a baseline against which to check bone change, should there not be a rapid resolution, and to assure the dentist and patient that no root has been left behind.

Treatment of the condition is primarily symptomatic. The socket should be irrigated with warm saline to remove the debris. A variety of antiseptic dressings is available to cover the exposed bone. A proprietary, eugenol-containing, soft, fibrous paste can be tucked into the coronal part of the socket to cover the bone. It can be left *in situ* and is usually shed spontaneously from the socket over a few days. Pain relief is usually very effective within hours. If relief is not achieved in a reasonable time, repeat irrigation and dressing of the wound is usually effective. Alternative dressings (each of which must be removed about a week later) include Whitehead's varnish on ribbon gauze, Bismuth Iodoform and Paraffin Paste on gauze (which may have lidocaine (lignocaine) paste added to it). Zinc oxide and eugenol cements are not recommended as they tend to adhere strongly to the bone.

Summary of dry socket

- There is pain and exposed bone after a recent extraction
- There are infective and traumatic components
- Rinse out debris and irrigate with saline
- Dress with a sedative material

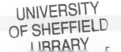

Osteonecrosis of the jaw (ONJ)

It has become apparent since about 2002 that patients taking bisphosphonate drugs (such as zoledronate, alendronate and pamidronate), which reduce bone resorption, are at risk of developing osteonecrosis, particularly after tooth extraction. The condition is recognized as failure to heal, exposure of dead bone (Fig. 4.32) and, often, associated infection. The condition persists with bone remaining exposed and failing to sequester for many months or years. Stopping use of the drug does not appear to make much difference to the outcome, probably because the half-life of the drugs, in the bone, is of the order of months to years. Tooth extraction should, if possible, be avoided in patients taking these drugs.

Postextraction haemorrhage

After a routine extraction it is expected that bleeding will cease after no more than 10 minutes. If bleeding continues, the area should be inspected for signs of mucosal tearing or other evident cause for continued haemorrhage. In the absence of any such sign, a further period of 10 minutes with firm pressure on the wound should be tried. Every effort should be made to determine whether the bleeding is arising from mucosa or bone.

If tears in the mucosa are found they should be sutured. They can be remarkably difficult to find if they have occurred posteriorly, especially lingual to a lower third molar or posteriorly to a maxillary third molar. Suturing can be effectively performed with a variety of materials, but black silk permits the knot to be precisely tensioned.

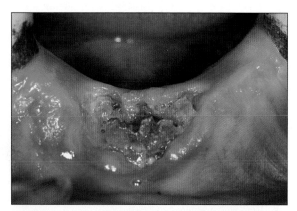

Fig. 4.32 Osteonecrosis of the jaw secondary to extraction of lower anterior teeth in a patient taking a bisphosphonate drug.

If bleeding continues, the next action is to suture the mucosa over the socket, not in an attempt to approximate the mucosal edges but to pull the gingival margin tightly down onto the bone edge of the socket. This restricts the blood supply to the gingiva, from which the bleeding frequently originates. A suture taking bites of tissue from all four corners of the socket, pulled together as a figure of eight, works well.

If suturing alone is not successful, a resorbable haemostatic agent (e.g. oxidized cellulose, fibrin foam, gelatin foam, collagen granules, alginate fibres) is placed in the socket and the wound resutured. Usually a bleeding socket responds to these measures. However, if bleeding continues consideration should be given to the possibility of factors other than a purely local minor problem.

Bleeding, of almost any cause, can be arrested by packing the socket with gauze soaked in an antiseptic such as Whitehead's varnish. This material slowly sets to a firm consistency over hours to days and is well tolerated against bone. It does not become foul for a matter of weeks, so can be left in place for some time if necessary. Because of its consistency the dressing can be compressed into the socket and secured readily with sutures. However, it should be removed, normally at about one week.

In transalveolar (surgical) removal of teeth vigorous bleeding can occur from a defined point in the bone. Such bleeds are often best dealt with by pushing a small quantity of bone wax (a malleable wax commercially available for this purpose) into the bleeding point. This material is not resorbable and tends to become infected if used in large quantities; it should thus be used sparingly. Alternatively, adjacent bone may be crushed into the bleeding point with artery forceps.

Significant arterial or venous bleeds from soft tissue are best dealt with by ligation. A pair of artery forceps is clipped over the bleeding point, leaving the tips showing, then a suture (such as polyglycolic acid) is tied around the forceps and slipped over the end and tightened.

Smaller bleeding points can be dealt with by diathermy or even by clipping the vessel temporarily without a suture.

Tests of bleeding and clotting function

If bleeding continues despite reasonable attempts to stop it, or if it restarts within 3 days, bleeding and clotting function tests should be performed. These include the international normalized ratio (INR) (for the extrinsic part of the coagulation cascade), activated partial thromboplastin time (APTT) (for the intrinsic part) and a platelet count, which may be done as part of a full blood count that will also include haemoglobin estimation. Any further investigations that might be indicated as a result of these tests may be better performed in a haematology unit.

Antiplatelet drugs, anticoagulants and patients with a known bleeding tendency

It is not usual to ask patients about to have extractions to stop taking drugs they are taking to reduce platelet activity such as aspirin or clopidogrel. The incidence of abnormal bleeding in such individuals is low. Patients on warfarin therapy, however, require very careful management. It is now recommended (UK Medicines Information 2004) that provided the INR is 4.0 or less on the day of extraction, treatment may proceed but the sockets should be dressed with a resorbable haemostatic agent such as oxidized cellulose and sutured. Clinical trials have shown few serious bleeding complications with this approach. However, this line is not accepted for general practice use throughout the UK and practitioners should familiarize themselves with local policy before carrying out extractions in this way in general dental practice.

Patients with a known blood-clotting disorder will be under the care of the regional haemophilia centre. Such units are generally extremely helpful in preparation and after care of the patient for dental purposes, but they must be consulted early in the planning process. Patients may require both factor replacement and antifibrinolytic medication.

Fractured alveolus

Most extractions result in delivery of the tooth, intact, with no other tissue apart from some periodontal ligament. However, bone can fracture in a number of circumstances.

A small piece of buccal plate of bone is sometimes removed with the tooth. Provided that it is small, and that the mucosa is not torn in removing it, this is of little consequence. Sharp edges of bone beneath mucosa may need to be smoothed.

A maxillary molar standing alone, or associated with a large maxillary antrum, is particularly prone to fracture of the tuberosity. The tuberosity is also vulnerable to a fully erupted maxillary third molar being elevated backwards (see comments about effects of large elevators). In such circumstances, if the bone fragment is small and the antrum will not be left exposed, it may be best to dissect the bone out with the tooth then close the wound. For large fragments, however, the extraction should be abandoned and the fractured piece should be splinted (other temporary means of pain control may be required) and the tooth surgically removed about 4 weeks later, once the bone has healed.

Fractures may also occur if an instrument is forced between teeth or between roots that do not displace out of their sockets, or if undue force is used in any extraction. It is difficult to measure exactly what constitutes excessive force other than by its adverse effects. However, it is very difficult for most dentists extracting most teeth to apply sufficient force in the correct direction to actually do damage. The human body is remarkably resistant to steadily applied force. It is important to be prepared to stop if it appears that reasonable force is not achieving the goal.

Fracture of bone at tooth extraction is more likely if:

- Greater force is used or if force is applied in directions not likely to displace teeth
- Force is applied suddenly
- The bone is thinner or more is removed
- The bone is brittle (e.g. in osteogenesis imperfecta or Paget's disease)
- The root is large
- The root form makes the tooth resistant to extraction
- There is a true ankylosis

FURTHER READING

MacGregor A. J. (1968) Aetiology of dry socket. *British Journal of Oral Surgery* 6: 49–58.

MacGregor A. J. (1969) Factors affecting the fracture of teeth during extraction. *British Journal of Oral Surgery* 7: 55–62.

Meechan J. G., MacGregor I. D., Rogers S. N., Hobson R. S., Bate J. P., Dennison M. (1988) The effect of smoking on immediate post-extraction socket filling with blood and on the incidence of painful socket. *British Journal of Oral Surgery* 26: 402–409.

Rood J. P., Murgatroyd J. (1979) Metronidazole in the prevention of dry socket. *British Journal of Oral Surgery* 17: 62–70.

UK Medicines Information. Surgical management of the primary care dental patient on warfarin. [Online]. 2004 [cited]; Available at: URL:http://www.ukmi.nhs.uk/med_info/documents/Dental_Patient_on_Warfarin.pdf

SELF-ASSESSMENT

1. Describe the beak and handle design for forceps intended for a left-handed person to remove the left maxillary first molar tooth.
2. What might be done to improve the position of the forceps in the hand in Fig. 4.33?

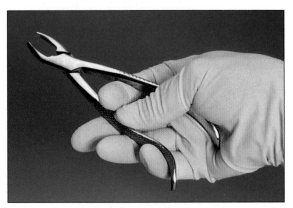

Fig. 4.33 See question 2.

3. What positions are appropriate for extraction of a lower right molar by a right-handed person?
   (a) Position of the operator relative to the patient?
   (b) Angulation of the back of the chair?
   (c) Height of the tooth relative to the operator?
4. In what direction should a maxillary first premolar be displaced?
5. What clinical features may suggest that an extraction could be more difficult?
6. How can dry socket be:
   (a) Diagnosed?
   (b) Prevented?
   (c) Treated?

Answers on page 263.

5 Removal of unerupted teeth

G. R. Ogden

- Although any tooth may become impacted or displaced, those most commonly affected are the lower third molars, maxillary canines, maxillary second premolars and supernumerary teeth.
- An impacted tooth, which may be unerupted or partially erupted, is one that fails to achieve a normal, functional position. This may be due to lack of space, obstruction by another tooth or bone or an abnormal path of eruption.
- Impacted teeth vary greatly in their likelihood of causing problems and in difficulty of removal.
- It is necessary to consider clinical and radiological factors when deciding whether (and, if so, how) to remove an impacted tooth.
- Postoperative management is more complex than for routine extractions.

ASSUMED KNOWLEDGE

It is assumed that at this stage you will have knowledge/competencies in the following areas:

- clinical and radiological anatomy of the jaws, ages of tooth eruption and relationship of teeth to adjacent anatomical structures
- pharmacology of local anaesthetic agents, antimicrobials and analgesics
- indications for local anaesthesia, sedation and general anaesthesia
- pathological processes of infection, inflammation, bone resorption and wound healing.

If you think that you are not competent in these areas, revise them before reading this chapter or cross-check with relevant texts as you read.

INTENDED LEARNING OUTCOMES

At the end of this chapter you should be able to:

1. Assess the reason why a wisdom tooth might require removal and those situations in which removal is not indicated
2. Determine the degree of difficulty and risk associated with removal of such a tooth, and the appropriate type of anaesthesia
3. Determine which patients to refer to a specialist
4. Determine which cases you can treat yourself, based upon assessment of tooth, patient and practice factors
5. Select appropriate surgical methods and techniques
6. Anticipate, minimize and recognize perioperative and postoperative complications of surgery for impacted teeth.

INTRODUCTION

Teeth fail to erupt into functional positions for a variety of reasons:

- the tooth follicle may have been displaced, i.e. the tooth occupies an ectopic position
- it may impact into an adjacent tooth, often due to overcrowding (Fig. 5.1)
- the tooth may, of course, be missing
- less frequent extraction of lower first or second molars in children (due to the use of fluoride and reduced caries) is associated with an increased incidence of impacted third molars, suggesting that crowding is a major factor.

Other reasons include retention or premature loss of deciduous teeth, tumours, cyst formation and certain developmental conditions such as cleft palate or cleidocranial dysostosis.

PREOPERATIVE ASSESSMENT OF THE IMPACTED LOWER THIRD MOLAR

History

Most patients attending hospital with impacted teeth are referred because of pain and infection, associated with partially erupted teeth (Fig. 5.2); however, many impacted or displaced teeth are unerupted and asymptomatic and therefore an incidental finding following radiographic examination. Occasionally,

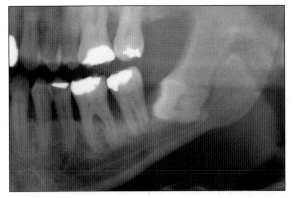

Fig. 5.1 Panoramic radiograph showing impacted lower left wisdom tooth.
Note that the inferior dental nerve canal casts a dark band over the roots of this tooth.

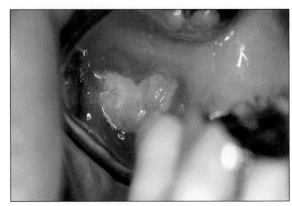

Fig. 5.2 Pericoronitis affecting a partially erupted wisdom tooth. Note the soft-tissue erythema.

unerupted wisdom teeth, in the absence of any obvious infection, can give rise to discomfort (often described by patients as 'pressure' at the back of the mouth). It is important to exclude other possible causes such as temporomandibular joint pain and pulpitis/periapical abscess from another tooth.

Intraoral anatomical factors that may influence surgical access include size of the tongue and degree of mandibular opening. The position of the impacted wisdom tooth should be noted (unerupted, partially erupted or erupted but non-functional), together with any signs of infection (e.g. caries, pericoronitis). Probing the distal aspect of the second molar will confirm whether the buried tooth is in communication with the mouth.

Pericoronitis

Pericoronitis may be defined as an infection involving the soft tissues surrounding the crown of a partially erupted tooth. It is usually caused by streptococci and anaerobic bacteria, and may be classified clinically as *acute* (the features of acute inflammation developing over hours to days, possibly with systemic involvement) or *chronic* (some redness and/or discharge of pus with few acute symptoms, lasting over weeks or months). It may be associated with poor oral hygiene, stress and upper respiratory tract infection.

Signs and symptoms of pericoronitis include swelling, soreness, erythema of the overlying soft-tissue operculum, trismus, facial swelling, raised temperature, regional lymphadenopathy and general malaise. The disorder may be precipitated by trauma from an over-erupted upper wisdom tooth or entrapment of food debris and bacterial infection of the operculum.

Pericoronitis may be treated by removal of the upper wisdom tooth (if this is traumatizing the operculum overlying the lower wisdom tooth), irrigation under the operculum with chlorhexidine, the careful application of a medicament such as trichloroacetic acid beneath the operculum, hot salt-water mouthwashes and analgesics (e.g. ibuprofen). If there is systemic involvement, then antibiotics are indicated (e.g. amoxicillin or metronidazole). Severe infections may require admission to hospital as they can spread through the fascial planes and compromise the airway (see Ch. 7).

Clinical examination assesses the wisdom tooth and excludes other causes of symptoms:

- degree of eruption of the wisdom tooth, and any associated infection
- caries or restorations in the third molar and distal aspect of the adjacent tooth
- periodontal status
- any other disease, including temporomandibular joint problems.

Radiological assessment

The radiographic examination of choice is a panoramic radiograph such as an OPT (Fig. 5.3), although periapical or oblique lateral views of the mandible may be taken as an alternative. When referring a case for treatment all recent relevant radiographs should be included to avoid further exposure to ionizing radiation.

Management of pericoronitis

- Local irrigation, hot salt-water mouthwash/chlorhexidine mouthwash
- Antibiotics if signs of spreading infection
- Analgesics (e.g. ibuprofen)
- Extract upper 8 if traumatizing lower operculum
- Remove lower 8 when infection settled

The following radiological assessment of the lower third molar should be made:

- orientation (Fig. 5.4a), with particular reference to the distinction between vertical and distoangular
- depth of the third molar below the occlusal plane (Fig. 5.4b)—the deeper the tooth the more difficult the surgery
- crown size
- follicular width
- root morphology (Fig. 5.5)—number, length, shape; fused or separate, apex curved or bulbous; loss of periodontal width—ankylosis?
- relationship to the inferior dental nerve canal (see Fig. 5.1)
- condition of crown of third molar and adjacent tooth—e.g. caries (Figs. 5.5, 5.6)
- the ratio of the distance between the distal aspect of the lower second molar and ascending ramus compared with the mesiodistal diameter of the third molar (Fig. 5.4c) (a ratio greater than 1:1 is associated with easier access)
- depth of bone between the tooth and the lower border of the mandible.

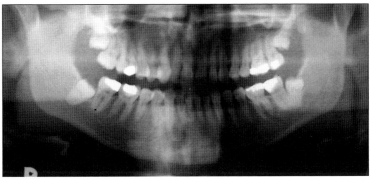

Fig. 5.3 A mesioangular impacted lower third molar on the right and distoangular impaction on the left. (Note the unerupted third molars in the maxilla.)

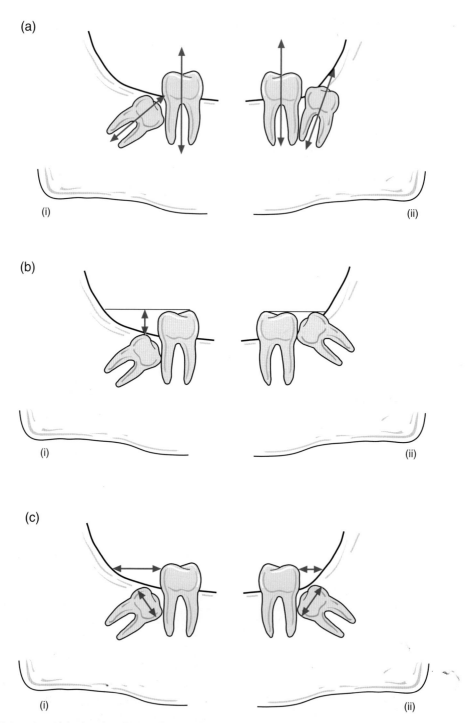

Fig. 5.4 (a) Orientation of third molar: (i) towards second molar; (ii) away from second molar. (b) Increased depth of crown of right third molar (i) from occlusal plane compared to left third molar (ii). (c) Distance between anterior ramus and distal aspect of second molar compared with width of third molar crown: increased surgical access for right third molar (i) but reduced access for left third molar (ii).

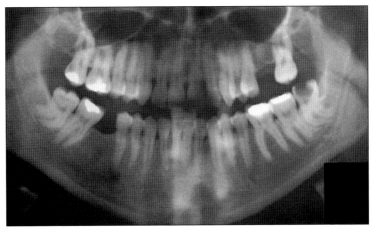

Fig. 5.5 Marked curvature of the roots of the lower third molars. Note gross caries affecting the lower left third molar.

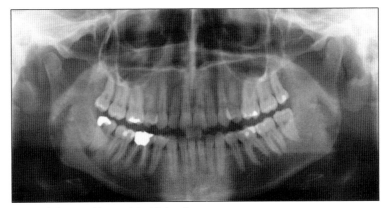

Fig. 5.6 A vertically positioned abscessed lower right third molar.

Clinical assessment

- Complaint: pain; exclude other causes such as temporomandibular disorder, pulpitis/abscess of other teeth
- Previous medical history: for example, drug therapy
- Dental history: difficult extractions, postoperative infection or bleeding, etc.
- Extraoral features: lymphadenopathy, trismus, swelling
- Intraoral features: pericoronitis/trauma from upper 8, eruption status of lower 8, caries in 8 or 7 or pocketing
- Tests: panoramic radiograph, systemic temperature if other signs of infection

Diagnosis

From the clinical and radiographic examination, a decision on whether to remove the impacted third molar needs to be made (discussed below). If there is pain/discomfort, the cause (e.g. caries) should be identified and treated. Trauma to the operculum of the lower third molar may be eliminated by either extracting or grinding down the cusps of the maxillary third molar. Pericoronitis may require irrigation with chlorhexidine, antibiotics (if systemic involvement) and analgesics. The decision whether to prophylactically remove non-diseased third molars is discussed below in greater detail, although in general their removal is not indicated because they are usually symptomless.

Patient preference should be taken into account when deciding on the form of anaesthesia: local anaesthesia, intravenous sedation, general anaesthesia.

Reasons for removal

The US National Institutes for Health (NIH) consensus on indications for removing wisdom teeth (published in 1980) (see also SIGN 2000 and NICE 2000) listed the following points as definite indications for removal:

- any symptomatic wisdom tooth, especially where there has been one or more episodes of infection such as pericoronitis, cellulitis, abscess formation or untreatable pulpal/periapical pathology (Fig. 5.6)
- where there are caries in the third molar and the tooth is unlikely to be usefully restored or caries in the adjacent second molar tooth which cannot satisfactorily be treated without the removal of the third molar (Figs. 5.5, 5.7)
- periodontal disease due to the position of the third molar and its association with the second molar tooth (Fig. 5.8)
- dentigerous cyst formation or other related oral pathology, such as ameloblastoma or keratocyst (Fig. 5.9)
- external resorption of the third molar, or of the second molar where this would appear to be caused by the third molar.

Other indications for removal include:

- orthodontic abnormalities—for example, tooth must be removed to create space in the maxillary or mandibular arch. There is, however, little evidence that the removal of third molars in the lower arch will prevent, limit or cure imbrication of the lower anterior teeth
- removal of the third molar prior to orthognathic surgery
- fracture of the mandible in the third molar region. If the tooth is not helping to splint the fracture, then it should be removed.

Contraindications to removal

Removal is not advisable:

- for patients whose unerupted or impacted third molars would be expected to erupt successfully and have a functional role in the dentition
- for those with no history or evidence of pertinent local or systemic pathology
- where the medical history makes the removal of third molars a greater risk to the overall health of the patient than the benefits would justify
- where there is an increased risk of significant complications, e.g. a high risk of permanent inferior alveolar nerve damage or fracture of the mandible (Fig. 5.10).

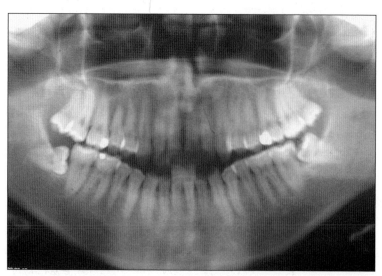

Fig. 5.7 Mesioangular impacted lower left third molar with distal caries on adjacent molar. Note horizontal impacted right third molar.

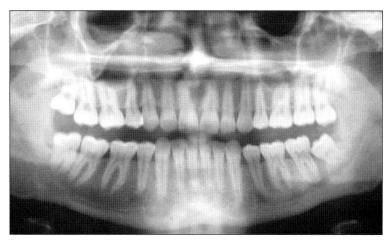

Fig. 5.8 Severe periodontal bone loss between an impacted third molar and carious second molar.

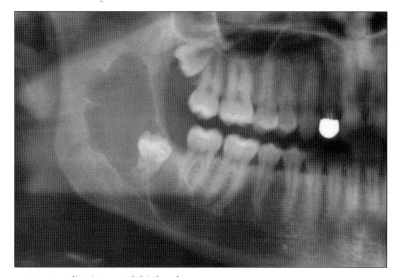

Fig. 5.9 Dentigerous cyst surrounding impacted third molar.

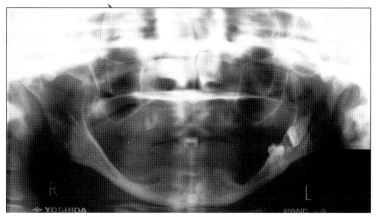

Fig. 5.10 A severely resorbed mandible. The horizontal third molar and impacted second molar occupying the full depth of the mandible show an increased risk of jaw fracture. (Note retained roots in the maxilla.)

There is no strong indication to extract asymptomatic contralateral or unerupted maxillary teeth simultaneously if they are disease-free.

Informed consent for the removal of wisdom teeth

Prior to any surgical procedure the patient should be made aware of the benefits and risks of treatment as well as the possible sequelae of other options (including no treatment).

Thus patients should be warned to expect pain, swelling, bruising, difficulty in opening the mouth and possible damage to the lingual or inferior dental nerve ('numbness in the tongue or lip'). Effects on 'quality of life' issues that may occur (interference with eating, socializing) and time off work, if applicable, should also be mentioned.

Factors influencing the decision to refer to a specialist include:

- operation likely to take longer than 30–40 minutes
- patient refuses local anaesthesia and requests a general anaesthetic
- patients who are very anxious
- procedure considered too complex for local anaesthesia
- presence of a relevant medical condition— e.g. previous radiotherapy to the jaws, haemorrhagic disease.

Type of impaction

Lower third molars may be impacted mesioangularly (Fig. 5.3, right), vertically (Fig. 5.6), distoangularly (Fig. 5.3, left), horizontally (Fig. 5.10) or ectopically placed.

One simple method of determining the type of impaction involves comparing the distance between the roots of the third and second molar (a) with the distance between the roots of the second and first molars (b) (Fig. 5.11). If (a) is greater than (b) it is a mesioangular impaction; where (a) is less than (b) it is a distoangular impaction; where (a) is equal to (b) it is a vertical impaction. If the first molar is missing, the impaction can be determined by comparing a line drawn down the long axis of both the second and third molars: if parallel, it is vertical; if lower 8 leans towards lower 7 it is mesioangular; if the

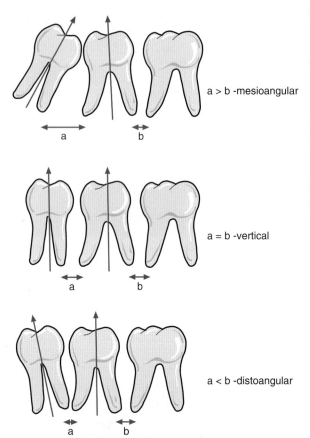

a > b -mesioangular

a = b -vertical

a < b -distoangular

Fig. 5.11 The author's method to determine the type of impaction of a third molar by reference to spacing between the roots of the molar teeth. See text for details.

lower 8 long axis diverges from that of the 7, then it is a distoangular impaction.

The difficulty associated with removing distoangularly impacted teeth should not be underestimated. Although their impaction may appear mild, the path of withdrawal towards the ramus is often associated with more bone removal and reduced surgical access. Horizontal impactions are more difficult to deal with than mesioangular impactions.

A horizontal tooth (i.e. where the line down the long axis of the tooth is roughly parallel with the occlusal plane) usually has its crown facing the second molar but occasionally lies buccolingually (Fig. 5.12). An occlusal view can be taken to identify which way the crown lies. Pell and Gregory (1933) have classified the position of the impacted lower wisdom tooth according to (1) distance between

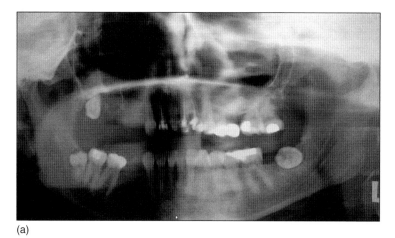

(a)

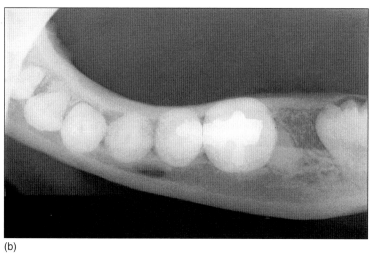

(b)

Fig. 5.12 (a) Panoramic radiograph and (b) mandibular occlusal radiographs of a buccolingually inclined lower left third molar.

distal surface of lower second molar and anterior aspect of ramus and (2) depth of the occlusal surface of the wisdom tooth in comparison to the occlusal plane of the second molar.

SURGICAL ASSESSMENT

Once the decision has been made that a patient will benefit from removal of a wisdom tooth, the difficulty of the surgery should be assessed in order to determine who should perform it, to select the mode of anaesthesia and to advise the patient concerning the likely outcome. The following method allows the operation to be planned in reverse as the flap size and shape will depend upon the bone removal, which depends upon the position of the tooth. A radiograph is essential before such assessment, and

should show the whole tooth and its association to neighbouring structures (e.g. ID canal, adjacent teeth and preferably the lower border of the mandible).

Path of withdrawal/eruption

This depends upon the root curvature, although in practice taking the direction in which the tooth would erupt is probably just as informative.

Obstacles to removal

Those obstacles identifiable on a radiograph may be external to the tooth (extrinsic) or due to the tooth itself (intrinsic).

Extrinsic factors include depth of bone, adjacent teeth and proximity of the inferior dental canal. In addition, the distance between the ascending ramus and second molar influences access. Radiographic signs of intimate involvement between the inferior dental nerve and wisdom tooth include darkening of the root, a break in the white cortical line of the canal and deviation of the canal (Fig. 5.1).

Intrinsic factors include hooked or bulbous roots, roots curving in opposite directions, caries (Fig. 5.5).

Method of overcoming obstacles

Most mildly impacted wisdom teeth can be elevated following removal of sufficient overlying bone. In more severe impactions the whole crown may require sectioning and removal before elevation of the remaining roots.

Sometimes the roots may appear to diverge only to meet again at the apices. The inter-radicular bone can prevent such a tooth being elevated, and thus may require vertical division, allowing the elevation of one root at a time.

Position of instrument to elevate tooth

This is usually on the mesial aspect of the wisdom tooth, although as the tooth moves, a better application point may be obtained buccally. It usually requires bone removal. During the operation it is sometimes necessary to drill such a point into the tooth itself—i.e. to elevate along the path of withdrawal.

Bone removal

The assessment should indicate the site and amount of bone required to be removed, to the maximum diameter of the crown or maximum bulbosity of the root.

Flap design

The size and shape of the flap depends upon the extent of the operation. It must provide access without subjecting the soft tissues to undue tension or trauma. The wound margins should ideally rest on bone to promote rapid primary healing.

SURGICAL REMOVAL OF LOWER THIRD MOLARS

Flap design

A full mucoperiosteal flap should be raised to give adequate access to the site where bone is to be removed. It should be broader at the base to ensure good blood supply and the margins should be capable of being supported on bone following surgery.

Where the tooth is not distoangularly impacted, a triangular flap is preferred. However, with distoangular teeth the proximity to the distal root of the lower second molar argues for the envelope flap.

If the tooth to be removed is partially erupted, then its gingival margin should be included in the flap. If unerupted, the incision starts from the distal aspect of the second molar.

> **Surgical assessment of third molars**
>
> - Type of impaction
> - Path of eruption
> - Obstacles to removal:
>   Intrinsic, e.g. curved roots, caries
>   Extrinsic, e.g. depth of bone, adjacent teeth, inferior dental canal
> - Position of instrument to elevate tooth
> - Bone removal
> - Flap design

Triangular flap (Fig. 5.13)

Keeping a finger on the external oblique ridge to place the soft tissues under tension and define the bony landmarks, the scalpel blade is inserted onto bone at a point immediately distal to the second molar. The incision is extended down to bone, along the external oblique ridge (upwards, outwards and backwards) for approximately 1 cm. The incision must not be carried directly backwards in the line of the posterior teeth as the mandible flares laterally and there is a risk of damage to the lingual nerve. The lingual nerve may lie on or near the alveolar crest in up to one in five cases.

The anterior relieving incision curves down from the distal aspect of the lower second molar towards the buccal sulcus. It should not be extended too far towards the sulcus as this can result in troublesome bleeding. The mucoperiosteal flap is raised (using a Howarth's or similar periosteal elevator), starting in the anterior relieving incision.

Opinion varies as to whether the lingual tissues should be protected by insertion of a retractor between periosteum and bone. Traditionally this has been done in the UK, although it is less common in Europe

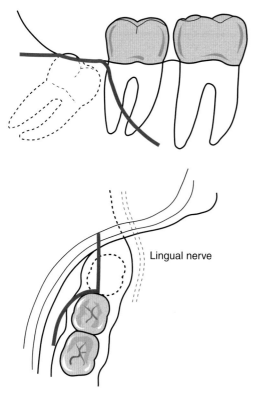

Fig. 5.13 The triangular flap used to gain access for the surgical removal of an impacted lower right third molar. (Top) Buccal aspect of incision. (Bottom) Distal relieving incision viewed from above. Note the position of the lingual nerve as the mandible flares laterally.

and the USA. Where a lingual retractor has been placed, temporary lingual nerve dysaesthesia can be expected in approximately 10% of cases. This is probably due to blunt trauma but also possibly to stretching of the nerve or compression against the mandible if trapped between bone and retractor. There is *no* evidence that the incidence of permanent nerve injury is higher without a retractor. Avoidance of a lingual nerve retractor may reduce this temporary dysaesthesia although it does not guarantee that the lingual nerve will not be damaged: for example, the nerve may be damaged whilst suturing if it is near the alveolar crest. Although inexperienced operators generally find inserting a lingual nerve retractor difficult (e.g. problems finding the correct tissue plane, or where the lingual ridge is undercut), it does improve visibility by retracting the lingual tissues. A lingually placed retractor may reduce the likelihood of permanent anaesthesia if the lingual

plate is penetrated by a bur. However, this may be at the expense of increasing the chances of a temporary paraesthesia due to blunt trauma from the retractor. It is essential to check that there is no soft tissue lying between the retractor and lingual bone. Where there has been infection of the surrounding soft tissues the flap may be more difficult to raise due to fibrous tissue.

Whether a lingual retractor is used or not, it is important to avoid penetrating the lingual cortical plate with the bur because this is often associated with permanent damage to the lingual nerve.

Envelope flap (Fig. 5.14)

Once again a distal relieving incision is made. However, with this flap the incision is taken around the gingival margin of the lower second and first molars to include the papilla between the first molar and second premolar. A Warwick-James elevator is

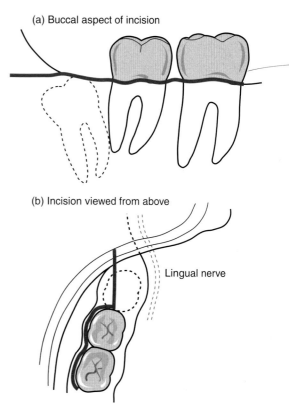

Fig. 5.14 The envelope flap used in third molar removal.
(a) Buccal aspect of incision.
(b) Incision viewed from above. The posterior incision should flare laterally to avoid damaging the lingual nerve.

used to free up the interdental papillae and the gingival margin prior to flap reflection with a periosteal elevator.

This flap is particularly indicated where it is predicted that much bone will need to be removed just distal to the lower second molar—for example, a distoangular or horizontally inclined third molar—because a triangular flap could leave mucosa overlying a site requiring bone removal. Furthermore, the relieving incision might not rest on bone following removal of the tooth, thus potentially delaying healing. Hence the value of an envelope flap, which has adequate bone support, although it is important to ensure that postoperatively the suture distal to the second molar replaces the gingival margin and papillae with sufficient tension.

Following reflection of the mucoperiosteal flap, if there is insufficient access, then the distal relieving incision may be extended. This is more easily done by inserting a buccal retractor (e.g. rake) and cutting up the external ridge (with either blade or scissors), whilst keeping the flap extended outwards under tension. If there are no obstructions, the tooth may be elevated using a Coupland's elevator placed mesially and then down the long axis of the tooth, buccally. This displaces the tooth upwards, as the instrument is driven down and rotated.

Bone removal

If the tooth cannot safely be elevated intact, then bone is usually removed using a round bur. If operating under general anaesthesia some prefer the use of chisels.

The bur should rotate in the correct direction and at maximum speed. Cutting instruments that introduce air ('air rotor') should not be used because they can result in surgical emphysema. The handpiece should not rest on the soft tissues of the cheek and lips, because burning could occur if it overheats. Adequate delivery of sterile saline through an integral part of the handpiece or from a syringe should ensure that the debris is flushed away and that the bone and bur do not overheat. The patient should be warned to expect the sound of the drill and the assistant should endeavour to keep all excess fluid sucked away. The crown of the impacted tooth should be exposed (usually to the cementoenamel junction) by removal of surrounding bone: (a) mesially (to

create a point of application but beware of adjacent root of second molar); (b) buccally (cutting a trough or gutter around the tooth to the root furcation); (c) distally (remember that, even if the lingual tissues are retracted, the lingual nerve may not be adequately protected, hence ideally the lingual plate should not be breached). If lingual tissues are not retracted, access to distolingual bone is severely restricted.

Distoangularly impacted third molars, particularly if partially erupted, may appear relatively straightforward to the inexperienced. However, more distal bone is usually required to be removed than with a mesioangular impaction, and it may be better to remove the crown and roots separately, once the tooth has been mobilized.

Tooth division

If the roots are not fused then a choice between sectioning the tooth in the vertical axis (with a bur or, if operating under GA, an osteotome; thus removal in two halves) or horizontal axis (removal of the whole crown and then elevation of the roots) should be made. The choice will to some extent depend upon the inclination of the crown, and the root apices. When using a drill it is easier to cut at an angle approximating to that which the drill takes on entering the mouth. It is easier to section the crown off a distoangular or horizontal tooth (Fig. 5.15) and to split a mesioangular tooth along its length (Fig. 5.16).

When cutting into enamel, with practice it is possible to 'feel' when the bur has reached the enamel on the lingual aspect of the tooth, which, ideally, should not be breached. The crown can be split and removed from its other half (if vertically sectioned) or from the root (if horizontally sectioned) by inserting a Coupland's elevator. The patient should be warned to expect a cracking sound due to splitting of the tooth. In older patients there may be an increased risk of mandibular fracture due to possible ankylosis, reduced mandibular thickness and less flexible bone. Where there is a large distal restoration on the second molar, the patient should be warned that it could be dislodged by elevating the tooth (Fig. 5.17).

Following removal of the crown it may be necessary to remove more bone (buccally, mesially and/or distally) to obtain a point of application for removal of the root. A point of application cut into

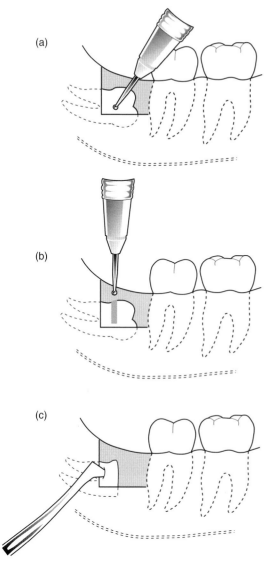

Fig. 5.15 Surgical approach to a horizontally impacted third molar.
(a) The overlying bone is removed to expose the crown;
(b) then the crown is sectioned from the roots.
(c) The roots have been divided, and are shown being removed separately with an elevator.

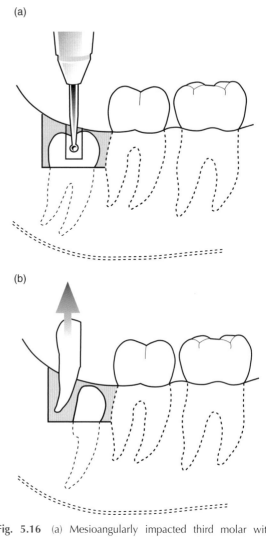

Fig. 5.16 (a) Mesioangularly impacted third molar with separate roots sectioned longitudinally with a bur. (b) The distal half is removed with an elevator before removal of the mesial half.

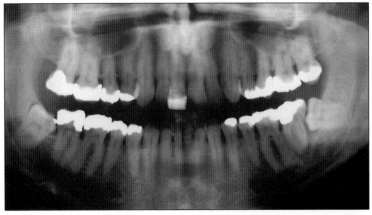

Fig. 5.17 The distal amalgam on the lower right second molar is at risk of being dislodged when elevating the mesioangularly impacted third molar.

the root may allow its removal using a Cryer's or Warwick-James elevator. Sometimes the individual pulp canals can be visualized and a cut made between them buccolingually. This should be deep enough to allow the insertion of a Coupland's elevator which, when rotated, splits the roots. Do *not* use the adjacent molar as a fulcrum. Once one root is removed the other may be elevated, by inserting either a Cryer's or Warwick-James elevator in the space cut around the root.

If the apex (or apices) fracture then they are best removed at the time. Exceptions include a vital tooth in which the fragment is small and the surgeon considers the inferior dental nerve to be at risk by its removal, or where under local anaesthesia the patient would find further surgery unduly stressful (Fig. 5.18). The patient should always be informed of this decision, which should be recorded in the notes, and told to return if symptoms arise. It is wise to take a periapical radiograph after surgery.

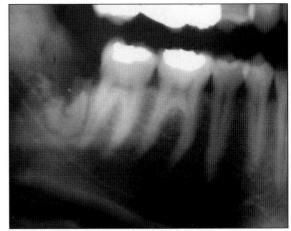

Fig. 5.18 The removal of this lower right third molar under local anaesthesia has proved impracticable.
Options include leaving the root (decoronation) or removal under IV sedation or general anaesthesia at a later date.

Wound debridement

Check that the whole of the tooth, including all roots, has been removed. The buccal and lingual margins of the socket should be smoothed using a round bur, bone file or rongeurs to remove loose, sharp bits of bone or any that has been devitalized. The wound should be irrigated with sterile saline, paying particular attention to the area underneath the soft-tissue flaps. The sequestration of small pieces of bone may cause severe discomfort out of all proportion to their size and can foster infection over a period of months postoperatively.

Mild oozing occurs from the socket immediately following removal of the tooth but brisk bleeding should be controlled before suturing the flap.

Although it is often thought that the follicle and associated fibrous tissue should be removed ('to avoid cyst formation'), there seems little evidence to suggest that its complete eradication is required, particularly if it would lead to damage to the lingual nerve. If fibrous tissue cannot be easily removed from the lingual soft tissues (e.g. with a scalpel or a pair of Fickling's forceps) then it is probably best left, although obviously infected or granulation tissue should be removed and submitted for histopathological examination.

Bone removal with chisels (the lingual split technique)

When used by specialists operating under general anaesthesia, this technique may be faster than the use of a bur. However, the extent of bone removal is less predictable than with a bur.

Briefly, a 5-mm chisel and mallet are used to create a vertical step cut at the distal aspect of the second molar. With the bevel facing downwards, a horizontal cut is made from the lowest point of the vertical step cut, backwards to just beyond the third molar. The buccal bone can then be removed, usually in one piece. It is important to ensure that the chisel is not parallel with the internal oblique ridge as this might fracture the mandible. The chisel is placed diagonally across the mandible, distal to the third molar. The angulation of the chisel will determine the depth of lingual bone split (i.e. the more vertical the chisel, the greater the depth of bone). It is not unusual for the lingual plate thus fractured to contain the lingula. The tooth can then usually be rolled out in a lingual direction. Using this technique, the lingual nerve must be protected.

Perioperative drug therapy

Various drugs may be given perioperatively just before, during or at completion of treatment to help to reduce complications.

Analgesics

Despite the availability of a reasonable spectrum of analgesics patients often experience pain. There is some evidence that preoperative analgesia leads to less pain and reduced analgesic consumption. Aspirin or ibuprofen appear effective. When taken postoperatively, soluble aspirin would appear to be better than paracetamol.

Steroids

Steroids (e.g. dexamethasone 8 mg) reduce facial swelling and discomfort if given at the time of operation, although not all surgeons routinely use them. They do not appear to delay wound healing.

Antibiotics

Although some favour the routine use of prophylactic antibiotics there is no strong evidence that it reduces the infection rate. Indiscriminate use increases the risk of unwanted side effects such as allergy/anaphylaxis or emergence of bacterial resistance. Some surgeons reserve the use of antibiotics for an operation which has taken longer than expected, if the bone appears more dense, in older patients and when using chisels.

Prophylactic antibiotics are recommended in a patient who has had radiotherapy involving the jaw bone or who is at risk of infective endocarditis. In general, short courses of high doses appear to be better than long courses of low doses. Preoperative antibiotics appear more efficacious than those given postoperatively. The latter appears not to contribute to better wound healing or less pain.

Closure

Although healing by primary intention is the ideal, in practice this is rarely achieved because the wound margin does not always rest on bone. Where a partially erupted tooth existed, a choice between complete closure or retaining the gap needs to be made. If the gap is retained then food debris may collect, causing pain, halitosis and bad taste. However, whilst primary closure may lead to faster healing there may be more pain and tethering of the cheek.

Sutures may be either resorbable (e.g. polygalactin) or non-resorbable (e.g. silk). A 3/0 suture should be used. The first suture should be placed just distal to the second molar, from buccal to lingual tissue. If a triangular flap is used, the anterior relieving incision rarely requires suturing. However, the distal relieving incision usually does.

Summary of surgical removal

- Flap design—triangular or envelope
- Bone removal and tooth division: round bur cooled and irrigated with saline
- Tooth removal
- Wound debridement
- Suture
- Drug therapy (e.g. antibiotics, analgesics, steroids)?
- Postoperative instructions
- Write up notes
- Review?

POSTOPERATIVE CARE AND COMPLICATIONS OF REMOVAL OF LOWER THIRD MOLARS

In addition to general issues of postoperative care dealt with in Chapter 4, there are certain specific points that relate to third molar surgery (Table 5.1).

The patient should be reminded of the most common complications—pain, swelling, bruising, trismus and possible alteration of sensation to the lip and tongue.

Other factors that require consideration relate to quality-of-life issues, for example, time off work, enjoyment of food, interference with oral functions, in particular ability to eat. There is a significant deterioration in oral health-related quality of life during the first postoperative week, which should be considered when obtaining informed consent.

Some surgeons do not routinely review patients after third molar surgery if they have used resorbable sutures. It is essential that the patient knows how to contact their surgeon in the event of difficulties and that they are aware that they should return if there is any sensory loss.

The lingual plate of bone can be very thin, with the possibility of displacing the apices lingually. Should this happen, a finger placed lingually can push it back into the socket; failing this a lingual flap can be raised to retrieve it. Transient dysaesthesia of the lingual nerve is highly likely.

If a root should fracture *do not* try to drill it away: remove more bone and elevate the root whole. If it is very small and near the inferior dental nerve then it is probably best left (see Ch. 4). There is a risk of mandibular fracture in the atrophied (usually edentulous) jaw or where a deeply buried tooth lies near the lower border (Fig. 5.10). In the event of a fracture, repair with miniplates is usually the treatment of choice—this is a task for a hospital specialist. Both hard (e.g. second molar roots) and soft tissues (e.g. lingual nerve) can be damaged. Be especially aware of distal restorations on the second molar when elevating at the mesial aspect of the wisdom tooth.

If any of the above occur, the patient should be informed before leaving the surgery. Ideally the problem should be corrected on the day of surgery and may require referral to a specialist. Such events should be recorded in the notes.

Bruising (ecchymosis) is common, tracking along the tissue planes and resolving usually within 2 weeks. However, pooling of blood within the soft tissue to form a haematoma may require incision and evacuation of the blood clot, which is prone to infection and slow to resolve. Infection of the soft tissues may result in secondary haemorrhage, cellulitis or abscess formation but this seldom occurs before 48 hours after surgery. Where signs of systemic involvement are present (pyrexia, lymphadenopathy) antibiotics should be prescribed and good oral hygiene advised. With persistent infection, check that no root, necrotic bone or foreign body has been retained.

Rarely, osteomyelitis (or actinomycosis) may occur (see Ch. 7).

Delayed wound healing may occur with or without pain. Institute good oral hygiene plus mouthwashes. Ensure that the wound heals (i.e. exclude tumour).

Lingual and inferior alveolar nerve damage may occur. The lingual nerve is at risk from: (1) 'bruising' or stretching, following the use of periosteal elevator; (2) a bur through the lingual plate; (3) suturing. It is surprising how infrequently patients complain of buccal nerve dysaesthesia. Loss of fungiform papillae is the only clinical sign associated with lingual nerve anaesthesia, with their return linked to nerve regeneration (Fig. 5.19). Patients with no sign of recovery of sensation should be referred to a specialist with a view to possible nerve repair. Spontaneous recovery is unlikely after 6 months.

Difficulty in opening the mouth usually resolves over 2 weeks but may require 'encouragement' through

Table 5.1 Problems associated with third molar surgery

Intraoperative	Postoperative
Haemorrhage	Pain
Fractured root apex	Swelling
Damage to adjacent tooth or soft tissue	Bruising
Fracture of the mandible	Trismus Anaesthesia of labial or lingual nerves Infection of soft tissue or bone

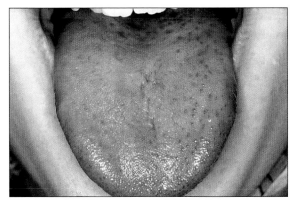

Fig. 5.19 The loss of fungiform papillae (on the right) is associated with lingual nerve damage whilst their return is linked to nerve regeneration.

the use of a trismus screw or wooden spatulas. Swelling also usually resolves within 2 weeks. It can be reduced by perioperative administration of steroids.

Removal of lower wisdom teeth may be associated with bone loss distal to the second molar, with loss of periodontal attachment.

There is little evidence to suggest that the complication rate is significantly higher in any particular group, such as older patients.

MAXILLARY THIRD MOLARS

Indications for removal

Extraction is indicated if the tooth is erupted and causing trauma to the cheek or operculum overlying the lower wisdom tooth. Unerupted third molars are often asymptomatic and unless there is associated pathology (Fig. 5.20) they should be left, regardless of whether the lower third molars are to be removed under general anaesthesia.

Surgical access (Fig. 5.21)

Access is difficult due to the posterior position and further restricted by the coronoid process, particularly when the mouth is fully open. Erupted teeth can be extracted with forceps, rather than an elevator (to reduce the possibility of a fractured tuberosity). Unerupted teeth that are to be removed require a flap in which the incision runs from the distopalatal aspect of the third molar to its mesiobuccal corner, continuing in the same direction towards the buccal sulcus. The flap may be raised using a Howarth's

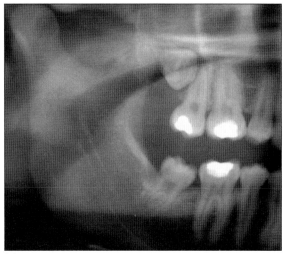

(a)

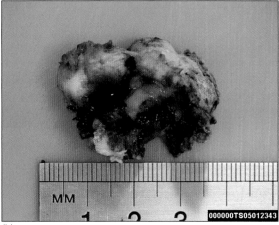

(b)

Fig. 5.20 Bad taste associated with unerupted upper third molar. Little radiographic (a) or clinical evidence for the large dentigerous cyst (b) removed with the wisdom tooth.

elevator. The tooth must be prevented from being pushed into the infratemporal fossa by inserting the Howarth's elevator behind the tuberosity (otherwise a Laster's retractor may be used). If there is overlying bone it is usually thin and can be removed with a chisel (which may be hand-held rather than being tapped with a mallet); rarely, a bur is needed. A mesial application point is established and the tooth elevated distobuccally using a Warwick-James or Cryer's elevator. A flat mesial surface is associated with more difficulty in inserting an elevator. The flap falls back in on itself and many surgeons feel it does not normally require suturing. However,

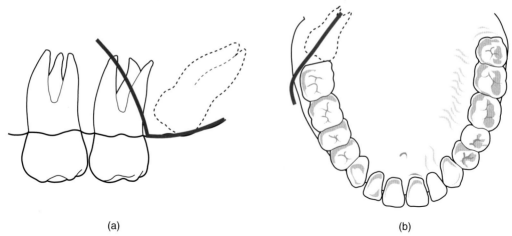

(a)   (b)

Fig. 5.21   Flap design for surgical access to an impacted maxillary third molar.
(a) Incision for buccal approach to unerupted maxillary third molar.
(b) Distal relieving incision extending from the mesiobuccal aspect of the second molar backwards in a distopalatal direction.

sometimes an extensive incision tends to bleed at its limits, and such an incision should be sutured. An envelope flap may be used, which has a distal relieving incision and extends around the gingival margins of the teeth. Access can be extremely good but it may take longer to raise and repair. A flap with both mesial and distal relieving incisions increases access still further but can be difficult to repair.

Complications

Excessive bleeding may occur, from either the buccal sulcus incision or tearing of the palatal tissue as the tooth is elevated. Pressure and suturing should suffice.

Fracture of the tuberosity (Table 5.2) is more likely if a fully erupted tooth is elevated backwards. If the fragment is small and the tooth roots are fused to the bone the tooth should be removed with the bone fragment and the mucosa sutured. Larger pieces of bone, if still attached to periosteum, may be replaced and, if the tooth is erupted and vital, it should be splinted in place and surgically removed at a later date. Check for an oroantral communication after extraction, particularly where the roots are in close proximity to the maxillary antrum.

A maxillary third molar may be displaced either backwards into the infratemporal fossa lateral to the pterygoid plates or, rarely, into the maxillary antrum. Antibiotics should be prescribed to reduce

Table 5.2 Complications associated with other impacted teeth	
Maxillary third molar	Maxillary canine
Fracture of tuberosity	Damage to adjacent teeth
Oroantral communication	Palatal haematoma
Displacement	Perforation of floor of nose
	Perforation of maxillary antrum

the risk of infection that might spread through the fascial planes. Removal of such a tooth is a task for a hospital specialist. Once located using two radiographic films at right angles to one another, a needle is inserted until it contacts the tooth. The surgeon then blunt dissects down onto the tooth to remove it.

IMPACTED MAXILLARY CANINES

Radiographic examination

The main methods of localization are (1) use of parallax or (2) two films taken at right angles to one another. Parallax movement can be assessed in both the horizontal and vertical planes by taking two periapicals with differing X-ray tube angles or an anterior and an oblique occlusal view (Fig. 5.22). If the unerupted tooth appears to move in the same direction as the X-ray tube, then it is lying palatally. A panoramic radiograph plus an anterior occlusal or lateral skull radiograph may also be used. A vertex occlusal view is best avoided, as it requires a large dose.

Surgical extraction

Canines lie buccal to the arch in approximately one in five cases. If the crown is easily palpable, then a semilunar incision, at least 0.5 cm above the gingival margin of the erupted teeth, may be used. Otherwise an incision is taken around the gingival margin of the erupted teeth. This is cut one tooth behind and one in front of where the unerupted canine is lying, with an anterior relieving incision carried up towards the buccal sulcus. The bone is usually thin and may be removed using a Coupland's elevator or bur to uncover the crown prior to elevation. Depending on the patient (e.g. maturity), this may be carried out under local anaesthesia.

Most canines are palatally impacted. Where a unilateral canine is impacted the incision may be taken around the palatal gingival margin from the first molar on the impacted side to the canine on the opposite side. Where bilaterally impacted maxillary canines are to be extracted, then the flap margin may extend from the first molar on the left side to the first molar on the right side. This is usually carried out under general anaesthesia.

The flap is raised by inserting the convex surface of a Warwick-James elevator and peeling back the gingival margin. The Howarth's can then be used to complete the raising of the palatal flap. The neurovascular bundle issuing from the incisive foramen can safely be cut with a blade (bleeding uncontrollable by pressure may require bipolar coagulation) and rarely gives rise to clinically perceptible anaesthesia.

Bone may be removed with a bur to expose the whole of the crown (from incisive edge to coronal aspect of root, taking care not to damage adjacent roots). The tooth may be removed with a Warwick-James elevator, taking care to palpate the adjacent teeth for movement. Occasionally it may be helpful to use both Warwick-James elevators together to alter the direction of displacement. The elevator must be kept against *sound* bone. If adjacent teeth begin to move, stop and section the crown from the root. Once the crown is sectioned further bone removal may be required to obtain an application point on the root.

Mould the palatal flap back (pressure from an assistant's finger whilst suturing the papillae may help reduce the likelihood of a palatal haematoma). Ensure there is no bleeding from the flap before suturing. Take deep bites of palatal tissue and place interrupted sutures through the papillae. The knots should lie buccally to avoid irritating the tongue.

Complications

There is a risk of damage to adjacent teeth and roots (Fig. 5.23; see also Table 5.2). A palatal haematoma may occur as the flap is readily displaced downwards into the mouth. If it arises there is a risk of infection.

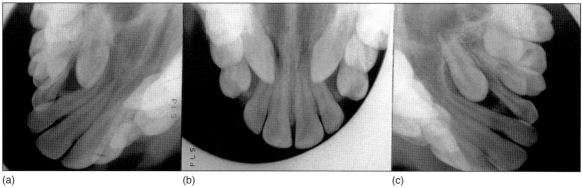

(a)   (b)   (c)

Fig. 5.22 Use of (a, c) oblique maxillary occlusal and (b) anterior maxillary occlusal views to identify palatal positioning of upper left and upper right canines by parallax. See text for detail.

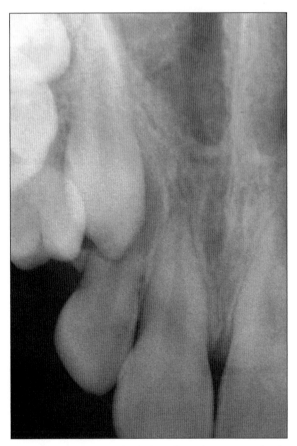

Fig. 5.23   Resorption of right lateral root by unerupted right canine.

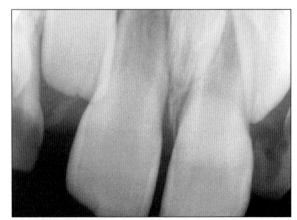

Fig. 5.24   Midline maxillary supernumerary tooth.

Perforation of the floor of nose or maxillary antrum may occur with extensive or careless bone removal. Bone loss may lead to periodontal pocketing. This is very rarely a problem clinically but may merit referral to a periodontal specialist.

OTHER BURIED TEETH

These include second premolars, supernumeraries (Fig. 5.24), supplemental teeth and, from time to time, almost any tooth. The tooth is located by palpation and radiography; occasionally parallax views may be required. Treatment options, as for buried canines, include (1) leaving it, if it is not resorbing the adjacent teeth and its removal might damage adjacent structures; (2) orthodontic alignment; (3) removal; (4) transplantation.

Surgical removal

It is difficult to raise a lingual flap in the lower arch, as it easily tears and suturing is difficult. In addition, for both upper and lower premolars lingually inclined, the apex is buccally placed and it is often that part of the tooth which is most troublesome to remove. A buccal approach involves raising a flap one tooth posterior to the impacted tooth to one tooth anterior, using a buccal relieving incision. This should gently curve away from the mental nerve region. In the lower arch the mental nerve should be identified so that it can be protected whilst bone is removed. The crown can be sectioned if necessary, the root elevated, the wound cleaned and sutured. The patient should always be warned of possible mental nerve para/anaesthesia when removing impacted lower premolars.

Supernumerary teeth are relatively common in the anterior maxillary region, lying palatal to or between the permanent teeth. Removal is indicated if they are interfering with the eruption of a permanent incisor. Otherwise mere presence does not warrant removal. Where other unerupted developing teeth are present, great care is needed to remove the correct one.

A decision to remove any buried tooth should involve a balanced judgement of the risk of damage from the tooth itself and the risk of damage from the surgery. Surgery should not proceed unless it is judged that the benefits of removal exceed the risks of surgery.

FURTHER READING

Carmichael F. A., McGowan D. A. (1992) Incidence of nerve damage following third molar removal. *British Journal of Oral and Maxillofacial Surgery* 30: 78–82.

McGrath C., Comfort M. B., Lo E.C., Luo Y. (2003) Changes in life quality following third molar surgery—the immediate postoperative period. *British Dental Journal* 194: 265–268.

McGurk M., Haskell R. (1997) How clinical research changed the habit of a lifetime. *British Dental Journal* 183: 121.

Mercier P., Precious D. (1992) Risks and benefits of removal of impacted third molars. A critical review of the literature. *International Journal of Oral and Maxillofacial Surgery* 21: 17–27.

National Institute for Clinical Excellence (NICE) (2000) *Guidance for removal of wisdom teeth. Technical Appraisal Guidance No. 1.* NICE, London.

Ogden G. R. (1989) Atrophy of fungiform papillae following lingual nerve damage—a poor prognosis? *British Dental Journal* 167: 332.

Ogden G. R., Bissias E., Ruta D. A., Ogston S. (1998) Quality of life following third molar removal: a patient versus professional perspective. *British Dental Journal* 185: 407–411.

Ong K. S., Seymour R. A., Chen F. G., Ho V. C. (2004) Preoperative ketorolac has a preemptive effect for postoperative third molar surgical pain. *International Journal of Oral and Maxillofacial Surgery* 33: 771–776.

Orr D. L. (1998) Protection of the lingual nerve. *British Journal of Oral and Maxillofacial Surgery* 36: 158.

Pell G. J., Gregory G. T. (1933) Impacted mandibular third molars: classification and modified technique for removal. *Dental Digest* 39: 330–338.

Petersen L. J., Laskin D. (1980) NIH consensus development conference on removal of third molars. *Journal of Oral Surgery* 38: 235–236.

Robinson P. P., Smith K. G. (1996a) Lingual nerve damage during lower third molar removal: a comparison of two surgical methods. *British Dental Journal* 180: 456–461.

Robinson P. P., Smith K. G. (1996b) A study on the efficacy of late lingual nerve repair. *British Journal of Oral and Maxillofacial Surgery* 34: 96–103.

Rood J. P., Nooraldeen Shehab B. A. A. (1996) The radiological prediction of inferior alveolar nerve injury during third molar surgery. *British Journal of Oral and Maxillofacial Surgery* 28: 20–25.

Ruta D. A., Bissias E., Ogston S., Ogden G. R. (2000) Assessing health outcomes after extraction of third molars: the post-operative symptom severity (PoSSe) Scale. *British Journal of Oral and Maxillofacial Surgery* 38: 480–487.

Savin J., Ogden G. R. (1997) Third molar surgery–a preliminary report on aspects affecting quality of life in the early post-operative period. *British Journal of Oral and Maxillofacial Surgery* 35: 246–253.

Scottish Intercollegiate Guideline Network (SIGN). Management of unerupted and impacted third molar teeth. Report no. 43, Royal College of Physicians, Edinburgh. [Online]. 2000. Available at: URL:http://www.sign.ac.uk

Shepherd J., Brickley M. (1994) Surgical removal of third molars. Prophylactic surgery should be abandoned. *British Medical Journal* 309: 620–621.

Thomas D. W., Hill C. M. (1997) An audit of antibiotic prescribing in third molar surgery. *British Journal of Oral and Maxillofacial Surgery* 35: 126–128. (See comment S. F. Worrall (1998) *British Journal of Oral and Maxillofacial Surgery* 36: 74.)

Von Wowern N., Nielsen H. O. (1989) The fate of impacted lower third molars after the age of 20. *International Journal of Oral Maxillofacial Surgery* 18: 277–280.

Zeitler D. L. (1995) Prophylactic antibiotics for third molar surgery: a dissenting opinion. *Journal of Oral and Maxillofacial Surgery* 53: 61–64.

ACKNOWLEDGEMENTS

Dr D Thomson and Dr E Connor, Dental Radiology, Dundee Dental Hospital for Fig. 5.1.

SELF ASSESSMENT

1. How may pericoronitis be diagnosed and how might you treat it in a lower third molar?
2. What are the indications for removal of a third molar?
3. What adverse events may arise as a consequence of not removing an impacted lower wisdom tooth?
4. What factors should be taken into account when deciding whether to refer a patient with an impacted tooth to a specialist?

5. Of what should a patient be warned before agreeing to the surgical removal of a third molar?

6. What radiographic signs are helpful in advising patients of an increased likelihood of inferior dental nerve damage following removal of a lower wisdom tooth?

7. List three radiographic measures that have been shown to correlate with difficulty of removal of a lower third molar.

8. How might the lingual nerve be damaged in removing an impacted lower wisdom tooth?

9. What are the arguments for and against routine antibiotic therapy when surgically removing teeth?

10. What postoperative complications can arise following removal of an impacted lower wisdom tooth and how would you manage each?

11. Outline the various ways in which the risk of litigation can be reduced following third molar surgery.

12. Describe your incision for a buccal flap when removing a third molar, explaining why the incisions are so sited.

Answers on page 263.

6 Surgical endodontics

I. R. Matthew

- Surgical endodontics is a term for surgical procedures undertaken on the roots of teeth and the periapical tissues.
- The aim of surgical endodontics is to prevent noxious substances from within the root canal of a tooth causing inflammation in the periodontal ligament and beyond.
- The objective of surgical endodontics is to achieve a satisfactory seal of the root canal and thus prevent noxious substances entering into the adjacent tissues.
- Surgical endodontics is indicated when conventional endodontics has failed or is impracticable.
- Surgical endodontics may also be indicated to manage other conditions, including lateral root perforation, root resorption, a fracture of the apical third of a root, curettage and biopsy of periapical pathosis.

ASSUMED KNOWLEDGE

It is assumed at this stage that you will have knowledge/competencies in the following areas:

- dental anatomy
- diagnosis and treatment of disease of the pulpal, radicular and periapical tissues
- conventional endodontics.

If you think that you are not well equipped in these areas, revise them before reading this chapter or cross-check with texts on those subjects as you read.

INTENDED LEARNING OUTCOMES

At the end of this chapter you should be able to:

1. Describe the principles of surgical endodontics
2. Select suitable cases for surgical endodontics
3. Recognize those cases for whom referral to a specialist in oral surgery is indicated
4. Explain a surgical endodontic procedure to a patient (informed consent)
5. Diagnose and manage complications of surgical endodontics
6. Evaluate the outcome of surgical endodontics.

INTRODUCTION

Success rates for contemporary endodontic therapy are in excess of 90%, depending on the skill of the clinician and the teeth involved. Surgical endodontic procedures are usually undertaken when conventional (orthograde) endodontics has failed. However, the chances of successful re-treatment of a tooth with a failed root filling are higher when non-surgical endodontics is repeated (wherever possible) rather than by undertaking a surgical approach. Surgical endodontics may therefore not be the first option when conventional root canal treatment fails.

Non-surgical endodontics attempts to eliminate the bacteria by cleaning and shaping the root canal to remove infected dentine, disinfecting the canal and sealing with a root filling. If non-surgical endodontics fails, it is usually because of the persistence of noxious substances (toxins and other by-products of bacteria) within the root canal system. If a root canal therapy fails and the tooth cannot be retreated, surgical endodontics may be indicated to eliminate the noxious substances from the root canal system. Where surgical endodontics is indicated, it is desirable that a root filling has been inserted first to improve the chances of success.

Surgical endodontics may be indicated in the management of a lateral root perforation or a horizontal fracture of the apical third of the root, root resorption or persistent periapical pathosis (e.g. inflammatory cyst or granuloma, or a periapical neoplasm).

Surgical endodontics is usually undertaken under local analgesia, with or without sedation. A patient with a pre-existing extensive inflammatory cyst might be more appropriately managed under general anaesthesia. Prerequisites for surgical endodontics are an experienced dental surgeon and trained assistant, a compliant patient who is medically fit and a range of suitable surgical instruments and root-end filling materials.

AIMS AND OBJECTIVES OF SURGICAL ENDODONTICS

The *aim* of surgical endodontics is to restore the integrity of the supporting tissues of a tooth or teeth with chronic pulpal or periapical disease, where non-surgical endodontics has failed and re-treatment cannot be undertaken or is contraindicated.

The principal *objective* of surgical endodontics is to enhance the lifespan of the tooth by removing causes of chronic periapical or periradicular inflammation. This is achieved by creating an effective seal of the root surface and thereby eradicating noxious substances present within the root canal of a tooth.

PRINCIPLES OF SURGICAL ENDODONTICS

Apicectomy

Apicectomy is the surgical removal of the apical portion of a tooth. To achieve this, access to the root apex is gained via a mucoperiosteal flap and then bone is removed around the root apex. The aim of apicectomy is to eradicate persistent infection in the periapical tissues.

The objectives of apicectomy are to:

- eliminate the 'apical delta' of minor root canals that cannot be effectively sealed by conventional endodontics (Fig. 6.1)
- excise a root apex that cannot be sealed successfully due to anatomical anomalies such as marked root curvature.

Root-end (retrograde) filling

A root-end filling is a restoration placed into the cut surface of the root after apicectomy of the root apex to occlude the root canal apically. The root-end filling requires a small cavity to be prepared in the root surface with a bur or ultrasonic instrument, and a suitable restorative material is placed in the

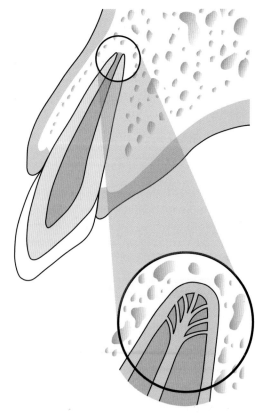

Fig. 6.1 The apical delta of root canals is a potential area for leakage despite conventional endodontics. Apicectomy aims to minimize leakage at this site.

cavity. The objective of placing a root-end filling is to achieve a satisfactory seal of the root surface.

Apicectomy may be undertaken alone but it is preferable wherever possible to place a root-end filling after apicectomy to improve the chances of gaining a satisfactory apical seal. These techniques may be performed in conjunction with the placement of an orthograde root filling at the time of surgery. This may be necessary if it has not been possible to disinfect the root canal during conventional endodontics and the patient has persistent periapical inflammation (the patient usually complains of pain and swelling that resolves only if the root filling is removed and the tooth is left on open drainage).

INDICATIONS FOR SURGICAL ENDODONTICS

Failed conventional endodontics

Typical reasons for failed endodontics include inadequately filled canals, coronal leakage, root fracture, missed canals, restoration failures, fractured instruments and post-perforations.

The signs and symptoms of chronic pulpal or periapical disease may persist after conventional endodontic treatment. The cause of endodontic failure is sometimes evident on radiographic examination. If it is feasible to retreat a tooth with a failed root filling via an orthograde (coronal) approach, then this should be attempted first. If re-treatment by non-surgical endodontics is impracticable or is unlikely to have a successful outcome, then surgical endodontics may be indicated.

Conventional endodontics is impracticable

Reasons for this may be many.

Anatomical

- A calcified root canal
- An impassable pulp stone
- Marked curvature of a root canal
- Incomplete apical development.

Pathological

- Inability to disinfect the root canal
- Inability to control persistent inflammatory changes in the periodontal tissues

- Root resorption
- Persistent pathological changes at the apex of a tooth (e.g. a dental cyst that does not resolve after conventional endodontics).

Operator-induced (iatrogenic)

- Surgically accessible perforation of the root
- Irretrievable root-filling materials. For example, noxious materials used in non-surgical endodontics (e.g. endomethasone paste) may be expressed into the apical tissues, or gutta percha extruded through the apex may cause compression of the inferior alveolar neurovascular bundle.
- Fractured reamer or file that cannot be retrieved by non-surgical endodontics.

Traumatic

- Horizontal fracture of the apical third of a root, with pulp necrosis.

CONTRAINDICATIONS FOR SURGICAL ENDODONTICS

Rarely, local anatomical or pathological conditions are a contraindication for surgical endodontics—for example, proximity of the periapical tissues to the maxillary antrum or mental foramen may necessitate removal of the tooth. Psychological conditions might compromise the success of surgical endodontics (e.g. a pronounced gag reflex). Some medical conditions may contraindicate any outpatient oral surgery procedure in general dental practice. Examples include haemorrhagic disorders, previous radiotherapy to the face and jaws, unstable angina, a compromised immunological state (e.g. due to steroids for rheumatoid arthritis, or disease of the immune system). An emerging concern is the patient taking bisphosphonates, in whom there is a risk of osteonecrosis. However, the relative risk of osteonecrosis is uncertain at present. Other medical conditions may be relative contraindications to surgical endodontics—e.g. myocardial or valvular disease. Each case should be judged on its merits. If there is any doubt about the suitability of a patient for surgical treatment, then the patient should be referred to a specialist.

Factors influencing the decision to undertake surgical endodontics

- Inappropriateness of repeating conventional (non-surgical) endodontics
- Systemic disease (e.g. cardiovascular, metabolic, endocrine or haematological disease)
- Local anatomy (e.g. the maxillary antrum, mental or inferior alveolar neurovascular bundle, or adjacent teeth)
- General state of the dentition (e.g. coexisting active caries or periodontal disease)
- Periodontal and periapical disease of the affected tooth
- Associated apical dental disease (e.g. pathological resorption of adjacent teeth)
- Surgical access
- Poor patient compliance
- The consequences of delaying treatment
- The potentially adverse influence of coexisting periodontal disease such as horizontal or vertical bone loss on the prognosis of surgical endodontics (Fig. 6.3)

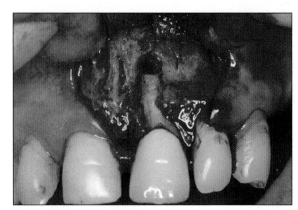

Fig. 6.3 A flap has been raised here, exposing a lack of labial bone, which reduces the chances of success for surgical endodontics.

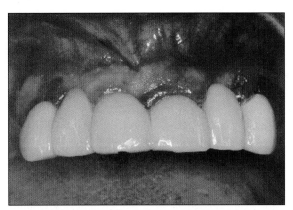

Fig. 6.2 A shallow sulcus like this, especially if teeth are proclined, makes access for surgical endodontics very difficult.

Local contraindications

- Access to the periapical tissues may be limited, in which case extraction of the tooth may be indicated.
- Anatomical structures may compromise flap design, e.g. a short sulcus depth (Fig. 6.2), or prominent fraenal and muscle attachments.
- Anatomical structures in close proximity which might be compromised during surgery (e.g. the inferior alveolar or mental neurovascular bundles, or the maxillary antrum).

TREATMENT PLANNING FOR SURGICAL ENDODONTICS

Careful preoperative planning is the key to success.

History

The patient may complain of pain, swelling, halitosis or an unpleasant taste (which may be indicative of discharge of pus) and tenderness or mobility of the affected tooth during mastication.

Clinical examination

In the presence of an acute apical abscess, there may be erythema or swelling of the soft tissues at the apex of the affected tooth. The periapical soft tissues may be tender to palpate, and the tooth is likely to be tender to percussion. A sinus may be present on the buccal aspect of the affected tooth, although this is not always the case. Occasionally pus from a maxillary incisor may discharge through a pathological sinus into the floor of the nose. Pus from a maxillary premolar or molar may discharge into the maxillary antrum, or rarely, on to the face (see Ch. 7).

A periodontal examination should be undertaken. Healing of the periapical tissues may be compromised if there is coexisting periodontal disease, which may manifest as either horizontal or vertical bone loss around the tooth.

Radiographic examination

Radiographs demonstrate both anatomical and pathological features at the apex of the tooth (Fig. 6.4). A radiograph may demonstrate an incompletely sealed root canal, or bone loss around the apex of the tooth involved. If there is chronic apical disease, a lesion with the physical characteristics of a cyst may be identified at the apex of the tooth. Rarely, the cause of a failed root filling cannot be established through clinical or radiographic examination but it may become apparent when surgical endodontics is undertaken. For example, a root fracture not detectable clinically or radiographically may be identified on surgical exploration.

The operator should also consider the position of the apex of the tooth in a mesiodistal direction. If the apex of the tooth to be treated is inclined towards an adjacent tooth root, there is a risk of damaging the adjacent root structure.

Case selection

For optimal results in general practice, surgical endodontics should be confined to the maxillary anterior sextant. Teeth more posteriorly placed pose clinical problems that diminish the chances of success, such as narrow or curved roots in mandibular incisors, or restricted access to the palatal root of maxillary

premolars and molars. It may be difficult to seal a lateral root perforation because of restricted access. As experience is gained through graduate training, it becomes possible to undertake more demanding surgery.

Referral of patients for surgical endodontics

Patients are referred for specialist care if the primary care clinician has inadequate experience to undertake the surgery, if there is any doubt about the patient's medical history or if there are anatomical or pathological features that may complicate surgery. For example, there may be marked root curvature, or the apex of the root may be close to an anatomical structure such as the mental neurovascular bundle.

Extensive bone removal may at times be required to gain access to a retruded root apex, for example a proclined mandibular incisor. Errors in identifying the correct root apex might result in surgery being undertaken in an adjacent tooth root. Identification of the apex of the root can be difficult if a periapical bone defect is small.

Pathological conditions, such as a large (more than 1 cm in diameter) radiolucent lesion (e.g. cyst or granuloma) involving the apices of several teeth, may be difficult to treat under local analgesia; pain control may be inadequate due to the extent of the lesion. General anaesthesia is then considered.

Advice to the patient before surgery

Reported success rates for surgical endodontics vary between 0 and 90%, depending on the criteria for success and the presence of a conventional root filling. Incomplete sealing of root canals may contribute to failure, but the prognosis for successful retreatment is good if an unsealed root canal is identified. However, the success of surgical endodontics without a root filling present is less predictable.

The prognosis should be discussed with the patient preoperatively. However, no guarantee of a successful outcome should be given, because circumstances may change due to factors identified at the time of surgery, such as a root fracture.

Complications

Patients should be informed of pain, swelling and bruising of the face arising after surgery. Damage

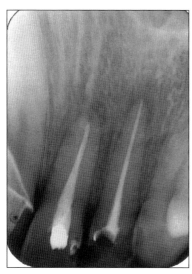

Fig. 6.4 Preoperative radiograph of upper left central and lateral incisors before surgical endodontics.

to adjacent teeth may occur through carelessness or difficulty in locating the apex of the tooth to be treated. This latter complication should be anticipated preoperatively. Contraction of the mucoperiosteal flap may occur through scarring as it heals, leading to unsightly recession around the gingival margin (Fig. 6.5). A judicious approach to flap design, reflection, retraction and careful suturing of the flap after surgery should avoid this problem.

Trauma to the infraorbital, inferior alveolar or mental neurovascular bundles during surgery may result in temporary or permanent nerve damage. This may manifest as paraesthesia (a 'pins and needles' sensation), anaesthesia (absence of sensation) of the soft tissues served by the neurovascular bundle or hyperaesthesia (pathological increase in sensitivity of the skin). The problem is most likely to occur with the mandibular premolar or molar teeth. Damage to a neurovascular bundle can have profound medicolegal consequences; loss of sensation may markedly affect quality of life. The risk of trauma to the nerve may therefore outweigh the benefits of surgical endodontics, and the patient should be aware of this.

If the maxillary antrum is breached (this may occur when operating on a maxillary second premolar or first molar) and the antral lining is inadequately anaesthetized, there may be discomfort when coolant spray enters the antrum during removal of bone. Additional local anaesthetic solution applied to the infraorbital, middle and posterior superior alveolar nerves should relieve the pain.

Root-filling material may enter into the maxillary antrum. This can precipitate a chronic infection (sinusitis) or create a chronic oroantral fistula.

A patient's signed, written consent should be obtained for all surgical endodontic procedures (with written evidence of an outline of potential complications discussed).

Perioperative medication

The drugs prescribed will vary according to the individual preferences and specific needs of the patient, some of whom may have coexisting medical disease. Anxiolytics (e.g. benzodiazepines) may be prescribed to reduce patient anxiety. An antimicrobial mouth rinse, e.g. aqueous chlorhexidine gluconate 0.2%, is recommended for routine use before surgery.

Instrumentation

A tray of sterile surgical instruments is required (see Appendix A). Loupes or an operating microscope will magnify the surgical field during surgery, and has been shown to increase the chances of success of surgical endodontics. Adequate lighting is essential; a fibreoptic light source attached to a headband or loupes is ideal. A miniature contra-angled handpiece with a small (size 1 or 2) rose head bur is used to cut a retrograde (retrograde means directed backwards) cavity in the apical portion of the tooth. A straight surgical handpiece is unsuitable if access is restricted. A standard air-rotor should never be used to cut bone and dentine, because there is a risk of surgical emphysema, tissue space infection and even death. An air-driven, backward-venting surgical turbine is acceptable. Ultrasonic dentine-cutting devices that have a fine tip to abrade the dentine and form a retrograde cavity exist.

SURGICAL PROCEDURE

Local anaesthesia

Conventional techniques (infiltration and regional block analgesia with aspiration) are applicable. There are a few points of particular relevance to surgical endodontics. Topical anaesthetic gel is recommended, especially in the anterior maxilla where the injection

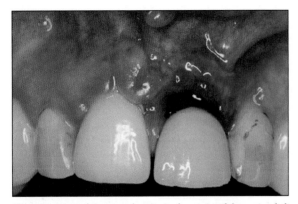

Fig. 6.5 Loss of tissue at the gingival margin of the upper left central incisor following surgical endodontics.

may otherwise be painful. A local anaesthetic solution with vasoconstrictor (e.g. 1:80000 epinephrine) provides a relatively bloodless field during surgery. The vasoconstrictor acts most efficiently by infiltration at the site of surgery, but sufficient time to achieve vasoconstriction (at least 5 minutes) should elapse before surgery commences.

Satisfactory analgesia is required of both the buccal and palatal (or lingual) soft and hard tissues. The tissues should also be anaesthetized lateral to the surgical field, where the relieving incisions are to be made. Pain cannot sometimes be controlled where granulation tissue is present around the apex of the tooth: a swab soaked in local anaesthetic solution with vasoconstrictor is then applied directly onto the granulation tissue before curettage.

Factors to consider in flap design

- Depth of the buccal sulcus may comprise access to the periapical tissues if it is shallow.
- Position and size of the labial fraenum and muscle attachments will influence the position of relieving incisions.
- Location of important structures (e.g. the mental nerve bundle) should be considered in order to avoid iatrogenic damage.
- Size of any periapical lesion present may require a broader-based flap.
- Number of teeth to be treated should be taken into consideration.

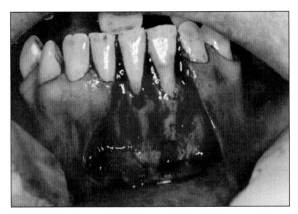

Fig. 6.6 A three-sided flap raised for apicectomy of lower incisors. The flap is reflected well beyond the apices to gain sufficient access.

The viability of a mucoperiosteal flap depends on the blood supply from the base of the flap in the buccal sulcus. The flap is designed with a broad base to ensure an adequate blood supply. Relieving incisions are made deep enough into the sulcus to provide access to the periapical tissues (Fig. 6.6), and the incisions cut through oral mucosa and periosteum down to bone. The margins of the flap will rest on sound bone after surgery is completed; otherwise an unsightly dehiscence might develop (i.e. breakdown of the soft tissue, exposing underlying bone or root).

Flap design

There are three principal flap designs for surgical endodontics (Fig. 6.7):

- 'two-sided'
- 'three-sided' (trapezoidal)
- semilunar.

See also Chapter 4, pages 37–38.

'Two-sided' flap

A relieving incision is made in the oral mucosa of the buccal sulcus, and the incision is extended around the gingival margin of the tooth to be treated (Fig. 6.7a). Preservation of the gingival attachment is preferred wherever possible. An advantage of this type of incision is the ease of repositioning of the flap after surgery. In most circumstances access to the apical tissues is satisfactory. If access is not sufficient, the gingival margin incision can be extended distally as far as is required, but failing that, a second relieving incision may be used; the flap is now a three-sided design.

'Three-sided' (trapezoidal) flap

The three-sided flap (Figs 6.6, 6.7b) provides excellent access for most surgical endodontic procedures. There should be no undue tension on the flap while it is being retracted.

A relieving incision should be avoided over thin oral mucosa where the surface of a root is prominent (such as the canine eminence), because the reduced blood supply may result in delayed healing or wound dehiscence. A disadvantage of a three-sided flap is the risk of postoperative recession at the gingival

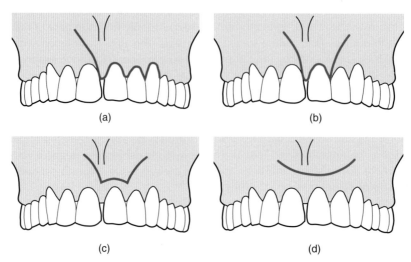

Fig. 6.7 (a) A two-sided flap, with a broad base and a gingival margin incision that can be extended around the gingival margin. (b) A three-sided flap, with divergent relieving incisions. (c) The Luebke-Ochsenbein flap, which aims to combine the benefit of avoiding the gingival margin, with the access provided by a three-sided flap. (d) The semilunar flap.

margin. This is distressing for some patients, and may require a new crown or veneer to improve aesthetics. The flap can be more difficult than the two-sided design to reposition accurately.

A modification of the three-sided flap leaves a 3- to 4-mm rim of gingival tissue in situ. This design (the so-called Luebke-Ochsenbein flap design) usually provides satisfactory access to the apical tissues (Fig. 6.7c). Although this flap is prone to wound dehiscence, it usually gives a good aesthetic result.

Semilunar flap

The semilunar design avoids the gingival margin, and there is less risk of recession of the gingival tissues after surgery (Fig. 6.7d). However, there are three main disadvantages of the semilunar flap design:

- surgical access to the apical tissues may be restricted
- it is often difficult to ensure the incision line ends up resting on bone
- the flap sometimes results in wound dehiscence.

Flap reflection

The periosteum should be raised with care because tears can result in more postoperative pain and swelling. Flap reflection may be difficult if a sinus

is present, or if fibrous scar tissue is present after previous surgery. The sinus or scar tissue is dissected from the flap with a scalpel or blunt-tipped dissecting scissors, and the resultant defect is sutured at the end of the procedure. A conventional flap retractor (e.g. the Bowdler-Henry rake retractor) is satisfactory, but specific apicectomy retractors exist.

Bone removal

If there has been loss of buccal bone through pathological resorption, it is relatively simple to determine the site of bone removal. Otherwise, it may be possible to identify the apex of the tooth if a sharp probe is pushed through the buccal cortical plate to identify the pathological cavity around the tooth apex. A medium size (5 or 6) round bur is then used to create a window in the buccal bone and expose the apical tissues, including any granuloma (Fig. 6.8).

If there has been no pathological resorption of buccal bone, the position of the tooth apex is determined using the average crown–root length for the tooth to be treated. Alternatively, the preoperative radiograph is used to work out the approximate crown–root length, taking into consideration the magnification factor of the X-ray apparatus used.

It can be difficult to identify the apex during bone removal, especially if there is persistent oozing of

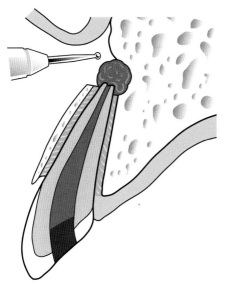

Fig. 6.8 Bone removal with a round bur, to expose the granuloma, after reflection of the flap.

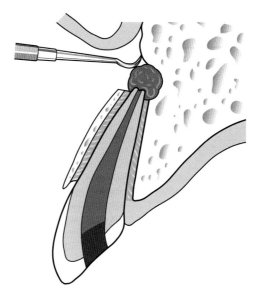

Fig. 6.9 A Mitchell's trimmer or similar curette is used to separate the granuloma from bone.

Apicectomy

The apical portion (3 mm or more) of root is excised to obliterate the apical lateral root canals (Fig. 6.10). The length of the root, the amount of bone support and the extent of root filling are considered when planning the position of the apicectomy. A flat fissure bur (size 4 or 5) in a straight handpiece is suitable for the apicectomy cut.

blood from adjacent bone. Haemostatic material (e.g. oxidized regenerated cellulose) or a gauze swab soaked in local anaesthetic solution, packed gently into the bony cavity, may help to control bleeding if left in place for 30–60 seconds. The apex of the root may then be identified more easily. Once haemorrhage is under control, blood will ooze gently from the cut surface of the bone but not from the surface of the root, thus aiding its identification.

Factors to consider when removing buccal bone

- Curvature of the root apex
- Mesial or distal inclination of the root
- Foreshortening of the apex due to natural anatomical variation or following root resorption
- The position of a root fracture in relation to the tooth apex

---

Curettage of the apical tissues

Curettage is undertaken to remove foreign bodies such as excess root-filling material within the tissues. Any periapical soft tissue is removed with a curved excavator or a Mitchell's trimmer, and is sent for histopathological examination to confirm that it is granulation tissue (Fig. 6.9).

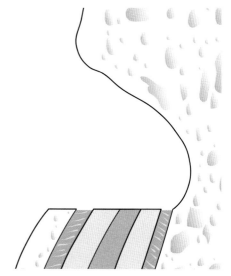

Fig. 6.10 The apex is cut off at a bevel of about 45°, leaving a wide-open cavity in the bone for access.

A bevel is made so that the entire root surface can be seen (Fig. 6.11). The angle of the bevel depends upon the tooth to be apicected. For example, an upper lateral incisor tends to be more retroclined than an upper central incisor, so a more oblique angle of bevel is required for a lateral incisor. The angle of the bur cut relative to the long axis of the tooth is generally 45° for maxillary teeth and greater than 45° for mandibular teeth.

The surface of the apicected root is examined to exclude a root fracture before the retrograde cavity is cut. Methylene blue dye aids identification of a root fracture. The dye will stain the fractured surface of the root clearly.

Root-filling material present in the canal will be visible once the apicectomy cut has been made. It can be difficult to confirm that the root filling has adequately sealed the remaining portion of the root. Even with loupes it is not possible to identify microscopic leakage. It is therefore prudent to place a root-end filling after apicectomy.

Retrograde cavity preparation

A retrograde cavity approximately 2–3 mm deep is prepared in the cut surface of the apex of the root (Fig. 6.12) to accommodate the root-end filling. A miniature rose head bur or ultrasonic cutting tip is used to cut retentive axial cavity walls to contain the root-end filling.

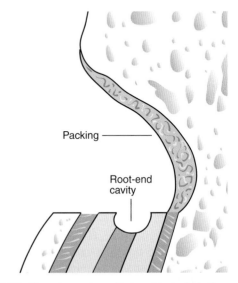

Fig. 6.12 The retrograde cavity is cut to include the margin of the canal at the apex, but avoiding the margin of the root itself.

Packing

Root-end cavity

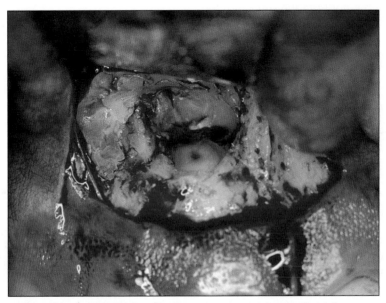

Fig. 6.11 The apex has been resected and the back of the bone cavity has been packed with bone wax (this must be removed after placement of the root-end filling).

Temporary obturation of the bone cavity

The exposed bone cavity is temporarily obturated in order to avoid spillage of retrograde root-filling material and to reduce moisture contamination from bleeding (Fig. 6.12). It is especially important to obturate the bone cavity when the lining of the maxillary antrum has been breached, to prevent ingress of foreign material into the antrum. Ribbon gauze (¹/₄ in.) is packed into the bone cavity, leaving the retrograde cavity preparation exposed. However, ribbon gauze is easily displaced; bone wax is as an acceptable alternative. All traces of bone wax should be removed before wound closure because it can delay healing and cause infection and chronic pain due to a foreign body giant cell reaction. Cotton wool is unsuitable to obturate the bone cavity; cotton fibres may remain in the wound and incite a chronic inflammatory (foreign body) reaction.

Root-end filling

A root-end filling is inserted into the retrograde cavity preparation to seal the root surface (Figs 6.13, 6.14). Many dental materials have been used, including dental amalgam, gutta percha, gold foil, polycarboxylate cement, Intermediate Restorative Material (IRM®), Super EBA® (ethoxybenzoic acid) cement, composite resin, glass ionomer cement, Cavit®, Restodent® and

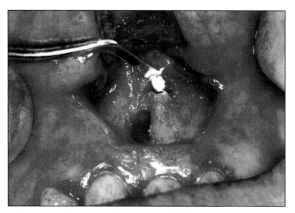

Fig. 6.14   Placement of a retrograde filling using IRM.

other zinc oxide/eugenol mixtures. Though expensive, mineral trioxide aggregate has shown great promise as an 'ideal' root-end filling material.

Debridement

After the root-end filling is inserted, the tissues are irrigated with sterile saline. An excavator can be used to remove debris, but a Briault probe is preferred to remove fine particles of filling material because it minimizes inadvertent packing of these into bone surface. Debris can also be displaced with a fine jet of sterile saline.

Some clinicians take a radiograph at this stage. This provides an opportunity to correct an inadequate apical seal before wound closure. Residual other radio-opaque debris within the apical tissues will also appear on the radiograph and can be removed before wound closure.

Wound closure

The interdental papillae are first repositioned to their correct anatomical location. Simple interrupted sutures may be placed to secure the edges of the mucoperiosteal flap. Any dehiscence caused by excision of a sinus or fistula tract can also be sutured. Resorbable sutures are suitable.

Once the mucoperiosteal flap has been repositioned and sutured back into place, gentle pressure is applied to the flap for a few minutes with a moist gauze swab to obtain haemostasis. If a postoperative radiograph was not taken before wound closure, this is usually done now.

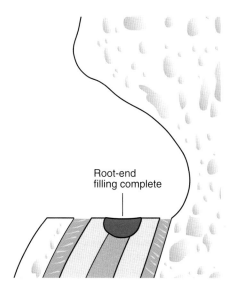

Root-end
filling complete

Fig. 6.13   The root-end filling has been placed; all debris and the packing have been removed.

Summary of surgical procedure

- Control of pain and anxiety
- Mucoperiosteal flap (two-sided, three-sided, semilunar or a variant)
- Bone removal with burs
- Curettage of any apical soft tissue
- Apicectomy (at least 3 mm to remove the apical delta) and bevelling at 45° or greater
- Retrograde cavity preparation
- Control of bleeding and of spillage of filling material
- Root-end filling with a suitable dental material
- Removal of all debris
- Wound closure

POSTOPERATIVE CARE

Postoperative instructions are given after surgery is completed. If the apicected tooth is to be crowned, it is preferable to wait at least 6 months after surgical endodontics to ensure a satisfactory outcome. A patient who wishes to have a crown made sooner should be advised of the guarded prognosis and possible failure of the surgical endodontic procedure.

Postoperative infection

Antibiotics given to prevent postoperative wound infection after surgical endodontics is controversial. If antibiotics are to be prescribed, it is suggested that they should be given preoperatively to provide adequate tissue concentrations at the time of surgery. If infection occurs postoperatively, an appropriate antibiotic is prescribed, the dosage and route being selected according to the severity of the infection.

ASSESSING THE OUTCOME OF SURGICAL ENDODONTICS

Follow-up

The success of surgical endodontics is determined from the patient's history and subsequent clinical and radiographic examinations. The patient returns for review 7–10 days after surgery, after 4 weeks (when all swelling and tenderness due to the surgery should have subsided) and after 6 months (which allows a reasonable period for signs of recurrent infection to appear).

Criteria for success after surgical endodontics

There will be complete resolution of symptoms if surgery is successful. Pain will subside, and there will be no further swelling or discharge of pus. Periodontal pocket depths should be within acceptable limits, according to the patient's general periodontal status. The soft tissues will have healed well without unsightly wound breakdown or gingival recession. The tooth will be in satisfactory function, without evidence of mobility. Any sinus or fistula will have resolved completely.

Ideally, there should be complete regeneration of periapical bone and an intact lamina dura after surgical endodontics (Fig. 6.15). However, a persistent apical radiolucency after surgery does not necessarily indicate an unsuccessful outcome. The capacity for bone regeneration diminishes with age, and sometimes surgical endodontics is successful even though a bone defect persists at the apex of the affected tooth. This is the main reason why the criteria for success should not be based solely on radiographic appearance.

Summary of criteria for success after surgical endodontics

- Uncomplicated healing of the surgical site
- Absence of persistent pain or discomfort
- Absence of soft tissue or bony infection (no sinus or discharge of pus)
- Satisfactory function of the apicected tooth
- Absence of tooth mobility
- Radiographic evidence of complete bone repair

Repeat radiographs

If the patient has no symptoms, it is reasonable to repeat radiographs no more than annually for 2–3 years.

COMPLICATIONS AND DIFFICULTIES OF SURGICAL ENDODONTICS

Discharge of pus

Pus will exude from a sinus associated with the tooth that has been apicected, sometimes preceded

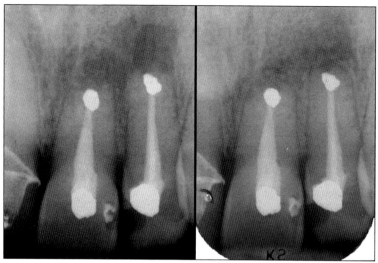

Fig. 6.15 Radiographs taken at 1 week and 6 months after apicectomy and retrograde root filling of the upper left central and lateral incisors. The bone has not returned completely to normal density at 6 months, but a lamina dura has reformed around the apices.

by an acute abscess at the site of the apicectomy. Radiographic examination of the tissues is undertaken to identify the cause of the recurrent infection, with a gutta percha point passed through the sinus to identify its origin.

Recurrent apical infection may arise through failure to curette adequately the apical tissues before wound closure, or failure to remove the apex of the tooth after apicectomy. It may also be due to an inadequately sealed root canal. In some cases the cause is not clear. If pus continues to discharge, the prognosis is poor. A repeat apicectomy might be indicated to explore and debride the apical tissues.

Perforation of the lining of the maxillary antrum

This may occur during surgical endodontics on the root of a maxillary canine, premolar or molar that is related closely to the maxillary antrum. The patient may experience pain if coolant spray from the handpiece contacts an inadequately anaesthetized maxillary antral lining. This is usually resolved by additional local anaesthetic nerve blocks.

If the lining of the maxillary antrum is breached during surgery, the apicected root tip or retrograde filling material might be displaced into the antrum. The perforation must be temporarily occluded during surgery to avoid this.

Haemorrhage

Haemorrhage may occur at any time during the surgery, e.g. during flap incision, bone removal or during excision of granulation tissue or a cyst in the apical tissues. Haemorrhage is less likely to be problematic if local anaesthetic solution with vasoconstrictor is administered (ideally epinephrine unless contraindicated). Haemorrhage during surgery is occasionally troublesome enough to delay the procedure, requiring the use of local measures as outlined in Chapter 4.

Pain during curettage of granulation tissue

The options are to:

- inject local anaesthetic solution directly into the soft-tissue mass (this is not ideal, because most of the solution is spilled)
- pack the cavity with ribbon gauze soaked in local anaesthetic solution for 1–2 minutes.

Surgical emphysema

Surgical emphysema is a rare complication of surgical endodontics; it is characterized by a marked and sudden swelling of the soft tissues. Crepitus may be elicited on palpation. Surgical emphysema occurs through entrapment of air within the soft tissues, and may be caused:

- by the use of a forward-vented air-driven handpiece (such as an air rotor for restorative procedures) instead of a slow-speed electric motor. A conventional high-speed handpiece should *never* be used during oral surgery
- if an oroantral communication has been created. Air may enter the tissues via the maxillary antrum if the patient blows his/her nose or sneezes.

Surgical emphysema may be distressing for the patient, and reassurance is required. There is a risk of infection spreading through the tissue planes, and antibiotics are prescribed to prevent this from happening.

Damage to adjacent teeth

It is occasionally difficult to identify the apex of the tooth to be apicected, particularly if there is extensive haemorrhage from the cut surface of the alveolar bone. Damage to an adjacent tooth root is possible. However, this may be avoided by judicious sectioning of the root surface after it has been identified, ensuring that the bone cut does not extend too far laterally.

Failure to apicect the tooth completely

This may occur if haemorrhage restricts the surgeon's view of the apical tissues. Control of haemorrhage is important at all times, and is usually achieved by following the techniques described earlier. A fibreoptic light source used in conjunction with loupes usually ensures satisfactory illumination and magnification of the surgical field.

Inadequate placement of the retrograde filling

A root-end filling may inadvertently be deposited in adjacent alveolar bone, particularly if the apical tissues are obscured by haemorrhage at the time of placement of the retrograde filling. This complication typically arises through inexperience, and further surgery may be required to provide a satisfactory

apical seal. For this reason, it is appropriate to take a postoperative radiograph immediately prior to wound closure.

Recession of the gingival margin

Recession of the gingivae may arise because of inadequate repositioning of the mucoperiosteal flap, a compromised circulation to the flap during surgery through excessive retraction or poor design, or contraction. The recession may leave an unsightly cosmetic result, which may require correction by crown lengthening and provision of a porcelain veneer or crown. The patient should be made aware of the possibility of gingival recession as part of informed consent.

Summary of complications and difficulties

- Recurrent apical infection
- Perforation of the sinus lining
- Haemorrhage
- Pain during curettage
- Surgical emphysema
- Damage to adjacent teeth
- Failure completely to apicect the tooth
- Unsatisfactory placement of the root-end filling
- Recession at the gingival margin

REPEAT APICECTOMY

Several surgical endodontic attempts may occasionally be undertaken to treat recurrent infection or persistent tenderness of the apical tissues. A successful outcome after repeat apicectomy cannot be assured, and it is rarely achieved unless the reason for failure of the initial surgical endodontic procedure can be diagnosed and corrected. Repeat apicectomy should therefore be reserved for patients in whom the outcome of a second surgical procedure carries a good prognosis. Furthermore, it is unusual for an apicectomy to be successful after more than two attempts, and the patient's expectations of success should not be raised after a second surgical endodontic procedure has failed.

ADVANCED PROCEDURES

Closure of lateral perforation

An iatrogenic defect in the surface of the root due to instrumentation can result in local infection and inflammation, similar to a failure of apical sealing. Provided that access is adequate, such perforations may be sealed by techniques similar to retrograde root filling (Fig. 6.16). If the perforation is directly on the mesial or distal aspect of the root, and particularly if the perforation is large or the roots are close together, access is often so poor that a satisfactory result cannot be achieved. However, such defects can sometimes be managed by conventional endodontics.

Hemisection and root amputation

These procedures may be indicated if an adequately root-filled molar has a periodontal furcation involvement, a vertical root fracture, or a single root which is not otherwise amenable to endodontics. The lesion is managed by removing the involved root (and the overlying crown), and then sealing and preserving the remaining root and crown (Figs 6.17, 6.18). A full periodontal assessment is necessary before planning these procedures.

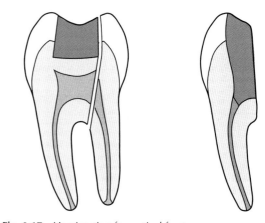

Fig. 6.17   Hemisection for vertical fracture.

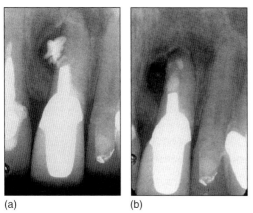

(a)   (b)

Fig. 6.16   (a) A perforation has occurred at the side of the root during preparation for a post and material has been extruded into the periodontal ligament. (b) Following sealing of the perforation and the apex with IRM® there has been bony repair.

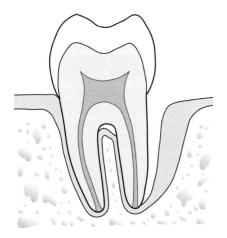 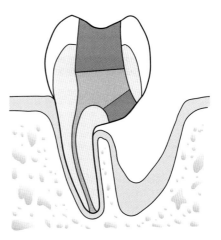

Fig. 6.18   Root resection followed by sealing of a tooth.

Intentional replantation

The tooth is extracted; surgical endodontics is performed on the apical root structure and the tooth is replaced in its socket. This procedure is indicated if the root apices are close to an important anatomical structure, such as a mandibular molar with roots close to the inferior alveolar canal. However, the tooth should be anatomically suitable for extraction without fracture of a root or excessive dilation of alveolar bone.

FURTHER READING

Beckett H. (1996) Impact of a restorative dentistry service on the prescription of apical surgery in a district general hospital. *Annals of the Royal College of Surgeons of England* 78: 369–371.

Bell G. W. (1998) A study of the suitability of referrals for periradicular surgery. *British Dental Journal* 184: 183–186.

Briggs P. F., Scott B. J. (1997) Evidence-based dentistry: endodontic failure—how should it be managed? *British Dental Journal* 183: 159–164.

El-Swiah J. M., Walker R. T. (1996) Reasons for apicectomies. A retrospective study. *Endodontics and Dental Traumatology* 12: 185–191.

Harty F. J., Pitt Ford R. T. (eds) (1997) *Harty's endodontics in clinical practice*, 4th ed. Wright, Oxford, UK.

Jou Y. T., Pertl C. (1997) Is there a best retrograde filling material? *Dental Clinics of North America* 41: 555–561.

Koseoglu B. G., Tanrikulu S., Subay R. K., Sencer S. (2006) Anesthesia following overfilling of a root canal sealer into the mandibular canal: a case report. *Oral Surgery, Oral Medicine, Oral Pathology, Oral Radiology, and Endodontics* 101: 803–806.

Kost W. J., Stakiw J. E. (1991) Root amputation and hemisection. *Journal of the Canadian Dental Association* 57: 42–45.

Longman L. P., Martin M. V. (1991) The use of antibiotics in the prevention of post-operative infection: a reappraisal. *British Dental Journal* 170: 257–262.

Maltezos C., Glickman G. N., Ezzo P., He J. (2006) Comparison of the sealing of Resilon, Pro Root MTA, and Super-EBA as root-end filling materials: a bacterial leakage study. *Journal of Endodontics* 32: 324–327.

Penarrocha M., Garcia B., Marti E., Balaguer J. (2006) Pain and inflammation after periapical surgery in 60 patients. *Journal of Oral and Maxillofacial Surgery* 64: 429–433.

Torabinejad M., Pitt Ford T. R. (1996) Root end filling materials: a review. *Endodontics and Dental Traumatology* 12: 161–178.

Tsesis I., Rosen E., Schwartz-Arad D., Fuss Z. (2006) Retrospective evaluation of surgical endodontic treatment: traditional versus modern technique. *Journal of Endodontics* 32: 412–416.

Watzek G., Bernhart T., Ulm C. (1997) Complications of sinus perforations and their management in endodontics. *Dental Clinics of North America* 41: 563–583.

USEFUL WEB SITES

American Association of Endodontists: http://www.aae.org

Interactive Endodontics: http://www.endodontics.com

INTERACTIVE COMPUTER-AIDED LEARNING PROGRAMS

Aspects of Minor Oral Surgery (AMOS) may be downloaded via http://www.dentistry.bham.ac.uk/ecourse/cal/p-amos-aspectsofminororalsurgery.asp

SELF-ASSESSMENT

1. What specific problems may be encountered in apicectomy of:
   (a) a mandibular central incisor,
   (b) a mandibular second premolar, and
   (c) a maxillary first premolar?
2. What are the advantages and disadvantages of using a two-sided flap for apicectomy?
3. Why might the bone cavity be packed before placing a root-end filling? Suggest some materials that may be used.

4. What evidence, found 1 month postoperatively, might indicate failure of apical surgery?
5. At what times after surgical endodontics should radiographs be taken, and why? What radiographic features suggest success?

Answers on page 264.

7 Spreading infection

J. Pedlar

- Infection around the mouth is responsible for much of the diagnostic and treatment demand made upon dentists.
- Most infection, in the form of caries and periodontal disease, *does not* cause serious infective problems beyond the periodontium.
- This chapter is about the cases in which infection is found beyond the periodontium, in the soft tissues of the mouth, face or neck, or bones of the jaws.
- These infections can be a serious hazard to health and, rarely, to life.

ASSUMED KNOWLEDGE

It is assumed that at this stage you will have knowledge/ competencies in the following areas:

- anatomy of the face and jaws and the planes and spaces of the neck
- immunology and pathology of inflammation
- microbiology of the orofacial region
- pharmacology of antimicrobials, antipyretics
- clinical features and management principles for local 'dental' infections.

If you think that you are not competent in these areas, revise them before reading this chapter or cross-check with relevant texts as you read.

INTENDED LEARNING OUTCOMES

At the end of this chapter you should be able to:

1. Recognize clinical features typical of infection of dental origin in terms of anatomical distribution; time scale; relationship of pain, swelling, trismus, etc.; a cause: dental pain, treatment, site of origin
2. Distinguish clinical patterns of spreading infection, abscess formation and bone infection and plan appropriate investigations
3. Distinguish the clinical pattern of infection of dental origin from those seen in infection of the salivary glands, of skin origin, or neoplastic disease
4. Distinguish patterns of presentation of infection that are unusual and elect to investigate them further
5. Predict the likely behaviour of an infection
6. Select cases requiring surgical treatment (including drainage) and describe how this would be performed
7. Select cases requiring antimicrobial chemotherapy and suggest a regimen
8. Select cases requiring inpatient treatment and suggest what that treatment would be.

CLINICAL FEATURES OF INFECTION

Local features

Many signs of infection (Fig. 7.1) are those of inflammation (pain, swelling, redness, heat), but not all inflammation is in response to infection: all these signs can be seen in rheumatoid arthritis. In infection you may also find suppuration (pus formation), an obvious cause and a greater systemic response.

The pain tends to be throbbing or aching or tenderness. Its severity depends upon the pressure of fluid within the tissue and changes with time.

Where swelling is largely due to oedema it is relatively soft. It tends to move within the tissues and accumulates at sites least constrained by fascia, as for instance, lips and eyelids (Fig. 7.2).

Some swelling is due to the cellular infiltrate of inflammation. This is more firm and is described as 'indurated' (hard). This induration is not due to fibrosis, but nevertheless may take days or weeks to resolve in infections in which it is a prominent part.

For swelling due to oedema or to cellular infiltrate it is difficult to define the precise margin of a swollen area: there is a gradual change at the edge towards normality.

Many infections form pus; this adds to the swelling. A collection of pus is called an abscess. When close to the surface it may cause a yellowish discolouration of the overlying mucosa but, when deeper, all that will be seen is the redness of inflammation. Swelling due to pus has a very different feel to it from that due to inflammatory exudates. It is described as 'fluctuant', but that encompasses several different sensations detected by the examining fingers (Fig. 7.3). Classically, fluctuance is determined by placing two fingers at the sides of a swelling and detecting fluid movement caused by a third finger on the centre. That is not easy inside the mouth, where it may be possible to detect fluid movement only by running one finger along the swelling. For deeply placed abscesses in the neck, the feeling is more like tense springiness.

The redness (and local heat) of inflammation is due to increased blood flow. There is no local increase above body core temperature and thus for intraoral locations there may be no local 'heat'.

Bacterial infections of dental origin have a characteristic natural history. The time scale is typically hours to days, from the first symptoms to the first request for medical or dental assistance. If infection is initially periapical there may be considerable pain, while exudate and pus are under pressure within bone, followed by a reduction in pain and rapidly increasing facial or neck swelling as the infection escapes bone and pressure reduces. At this stage the external swelling is largely due to oedema, and therefore soft. Over a period of 1–5 days pus may form centrally within this swelling: this *localization* is associated with developing pain, local tenderness and fluctuance. Oedema and pus may spread inwards towards the pharynx as readily as outwards towards the face.

When infection shows no significant localization of pus and has a greater tendency to spread it is called *cellulitis*. Where the predominant feature is pus formation it is called an *abscess*. However, almost all infections show elements of both and any infection

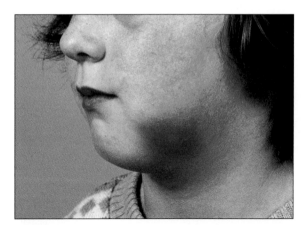

Fig. 7.1 An acute facial infection of dental origin.

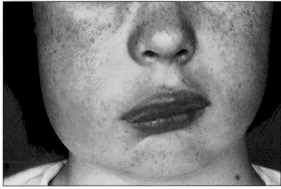

Fig. 7.2 A spreading infection or 'cellulitis' with marked oedema, particularly seen in the lips.

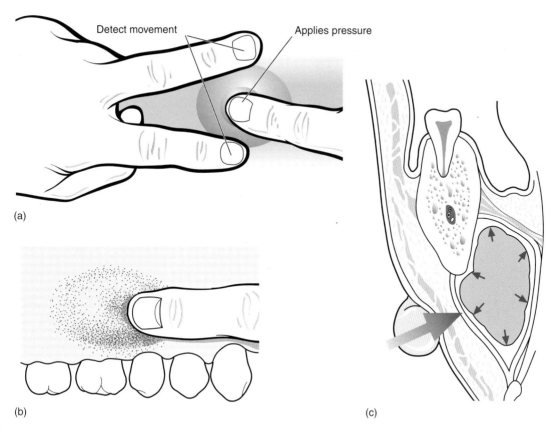

Fig. 7.3 Eliciting 'fluctuance'.
(a) Classical use of three fingers, the outer of which detect fluid movement as the central one applies pressure.
(b) Inside the mouth one finger may be run across the surface to detect fluid movement.
(c) For a deeply placed neck abscess, fluctuance is felt more as 'springiness'.

starting as a cellulitis tends to localize over a period of days.

Spread of infection

Pus tends to move under influences such as pressure, gravity, local heat or muscle layers towards surfaces. When it reaches a surface (internal or external) it bursts out or *discharges*, but often with large abscesses it takes days to drain and spontaneous drainage is unreliable. Pus is an effective defence against spreading infection.

Most suppurative dental infections discharge into the mouth via a *sinus*, sometimes without obvious acute infection (Fig. 7.4), and usually onto the labiobuccal aspect of the alveolus. Apical infection from maxillary lateral incisors is more likely to drain palatally and from any tooth may point lingually, palatally or even onto the skin (Fig. .5). The commonest site of discharge onto skin is the point of the chin, arising from infection at the apex of a mandibular incisor. However, it is when, rarely, the infection tracks beyond the alveolus but does *not* readily escape onto a surface that the infections described in this chapter develop. The interlinked planes and spaces to which dental infections may spread have few absolute boundaries but can be summarized by considering the example of the third molar.

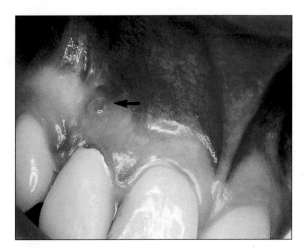

Fig. 7.4 An intraoral sinus (arrow).

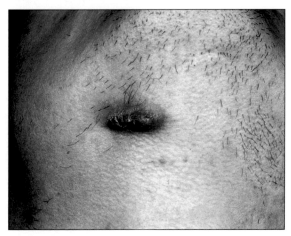

Fig. 7.5 An extraoral sinus (beneath the mandible on the right side, related to apical infection on a lower molar).

The crown of the part-erupted mandibular third molar, particularly if distoangular, may be below the attachment of buccinator/superior constrictor, allowing infection to escape laterally to the buccal space (Fig. 7.6), posteriorly to the masticator space or posteromedially to the lateral pharyngeal space. The masticator space is the potential space surrounding the ascending ramus and the elevator muscles of the mandible. Infection (whether or not pus has formed) makes these muscles resistant to lengthening, resulting in limited mouth opening, called *trismus*. Trismus in odontogenic infection indicates involvement of masticatory muscles.

Apical infection from the lower wisdom tooth may escape laterally to the buccal space, producing swelling of the cheek above the lower border of

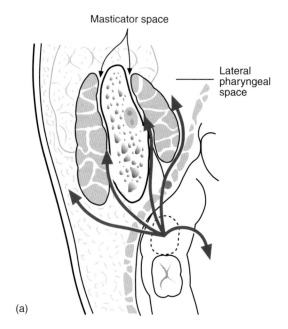

(a)

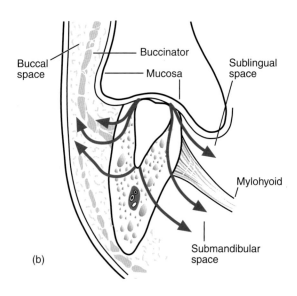

(b)

Fig. 7.6 Routes of spread of infection from a lower third molar.

(a) When seen in horizontal section, infection may track laterally into the buccal space, posteriorly, either side of the mandible into the masticator space, further medially into the lateral pharyngeal space or lingually into the sublingual space.

(b) When seen in coronal section, routes to the buccal, submandibular and sublingual spaces are visible.

Spaces into which infections typically track from the teeth

Mandibular third molar (apical or pericoronal infection)

- Sublingual
- Submandibular
- Buccal
- Masticator
- Lateral pharyngeal (open inferiorly to mediastinum)
- Retropharyngeal (open inferiorly to mediastinum)

Maxillary third molar

- Lateral pharyngeal
- Retropharyngeal
- Masticator
- Buccal

Maxillary canine and premolar

- Buccal/canine

Summary of local features

- Pain, swelling, redness, heat of inflammation
- Suppuration (formation of pus)
- Swelling caused by oedema, cellular infiltrate and pus
- Trismus if masticatory muscles involved
- Dysphagia if sublingual, submandibular, lateral pharyngeal or masticator spaces involved

---

the mandible. As the apex is below the attachment of mylohyoid, infection tracking medially enters the submandibular space, producing swelling in the neck, but sometimes upward bulging of the floor of the mouth too.

Infections involving the lateral pharyngeal or retropharyngeal spaces are of particular concern, because of the risk of respiratory obstruction and because they may track downwards directly into the mediastinum, resulting in life-threatening mediastinal infections.

Occasionally infection arising from a maxillary canine or premolar may spread upwards and backwards to involve the orbit. If there develops a thrombophlebitis of the ophthalmic veins or the deep facial vein, such infections may spread to the cavernous sinus.

Recognizing these clinical features should enable you to describe an infection in terms of its spread (i.e. the spaces involved) and its tendency to localization or further spread, then with the duration thus far and the level of systemic upset, make an estimate of the severity of the infection. For all infections of dental origin, there should also be an identifiable cause: a part-erupted third molar; a non-vital tooth with its apex beyond muscle attachments; a site of injection; a fracture; a foreign body.

Systemic features

A raised body core temperature is common in infections of all types. The normal temperature varies widely according to the metabolic rate and the time of day. The upper limit of the normal range is 37.0°C but this may actually be a raised temperature for some individuals, and a 'normal' temperature may be higher than this such as at the time of ovulation in women. Therefore take temperature only as a guide and watch for changes over time. Temperature may be measured sublingually, provided that the mouth will open satisfactorily and it is not too painful. Endaural (within the ear) measurement can also be accurate and convenient if the equipment is available. Alternatively, take the axillary temperature, allowing for it being about 1°C below core temperature.

A substantial abscess may cause temperature 'spikes' (Fig. 7.7) on a daily basis. A single temperature reading taken at a trough between such spikes will be misleading. The pulse and respiratory rates rise with or slightly ahead of the temperature.

The malaise (feeling unwell) that is standard with infections such as influenza is often not a prominent feature of bacterial odontogenic infection. If the infection is severe, a greyish pallor of the face may be evident, but again this is relatively unusual and less than that with viral infections.

Regional lymph nodes are usually enlarged and tender, although if there is much neck swelling individual groups of nodes may not be distinguishable on palpation. Almost all cervicofacial infections drain to the jugulodigastric node in the upper part of the deep cervical chain, but mandibular infections tend to go first to the submandibular nodes (or anteriorly, to the submental nodes). Facial skin infections may drain to the facial node.

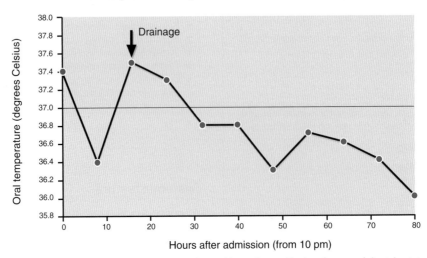

Oral temperature for a patient with a submandibular abscess

Fig. 7.7 A spiking temperature (oral measurement) in a patient with a submandibular abscess of dental origin.

Summary of systemic features

- Temperature above 37.0°C
- Normal daytime body temperature range approximately 36.0–37.0°C
- Raised pulse and respiration rates
- Regional lymphadenitis (submandibular, jugulodigastric depending on site)
- Possible malaise and pallor, but less than would be expected of viral infections

PATTERNS OF PRESENTATION

Alveolar abscess

This infection is largely confined to the mouth, with swelling centred around the alveolus near the cause. Usually within 2 days of appearance of first symptoms pus forms and becomes evident as a fluctuant swelling on the labiobuccal aspect of the alveolus. The degree of systemic disturbance is often slight.

Cellulitis

The overlying skin is swollen and oedematous (*pitting* occurs in some cases), with particular swelling of lips and eyelids. There is usually no true fluctuance (unlike the abscess, although most infections do form some localized fluid collection) and the devel-opment tends to be more open-ended, with a progressive spread to involve adjacent spaces, cross the midline and eventually down the neck. Often the systemic upset is more severe than with an abscess.

Cervicofacial space abscess

There is less oedema, and the infection seems more deeply placed than that of a cellulitis because there is less skin inflammation, but the clinical signs and the symptoms depend upon the spaces involved. Both masticator and lateral pharyngeal space infections are associated with severe trismus. In either case the abscess cavities may be inaccessible to the examining finger, preventing identification of fluctuance. Lateral pharyngeal abscesses and sublingual space infection may cause severe pain on swallowing. Sublingual space infection also causes raising of the floor of mouth and the tongue.

DISTINGUISHING INFECTIVE FROM NEOPLASTIC DISORDERS

There is usually no difficulty in distinguishing infective from other disorders. However, confusion can arise in the slower, lower-grade infection and the superficial infected tumour. Secondary malignancies are less common in the mouth than primaries, and by arising within bone may cause confusion.

Generally, infection develops over a few days, but responds to removal of the cause and/or drainage of pus. Malignancies develop over weeks to months and do not respond to treatments suited to infections. Induration is common in long-standing infection, and may persist for days to weeks after treatment, but should show signs of improvement with treatment. By the time tumours are evidently infected, they are usually obviously ulcerated, which would be rare for an infection of dental origin.

Lymph node involvement may also reveal differences between tumours and infection. Usually, dental infections cause lymphadenopathy in the upper part of the cervical chain and submandibular nodes. Infected lymph nodes are likely to be enlarged, firm or rubbery in consistency, tender, usually mobile, while neoplastic lymph nodes are often enlarged, hard in consistency, non-tender, fixed, especially in advanced disease. A lesion associated with enlarged nodes lower in the neck, or showing spread upwards or backwards in the face or neck, should arouse suspicion.

The rule must be: if infection is responding poorly to what should be satisfactory treatment, neoplasia should be considered.

INVESTIGATION

Microbiology

The identity and antibiotic sensitivity of the causative microorganisms is commonly determined from pus samples. To sample with a swab (Fig. 7.8), soak it in pus from the main abscess cavity and not from the skin or mucosal incision, to avoid contamination by surface organisms. In samples left open to the air, oxygen kills the anaerobes and drying kills most other bacteria; therefore swabs must be sent for culture within 1 hour, in an appropriate transport medium, to the microbiology laboratory. Aspirates of pus taken with a syringe and needle are more readily protected from the air and may be more reliable, but still require rapid attention. For a spreading infection, without pus, the organisms can often be grown from a blood sample. This procedure is best performed in hospital. On occasion organisms might be sought in tissue washings or biopsies.

For most minor infections of dental origin, culture of microorganisms adds little because, by the time sensitivity results are known (2–3 days), the local treatment and antibiotics have substantially resolved the infection. This is not a safe approach with extensive infections, which have a low, but real, incidence of serious outcomes.

Response to infection

Reduced resistance should be considered in those with severe infection. The normal response to acute bacterial infection includes a considerable increase in circulating blood white cells, particularly the neutrophil polymorphs. (An increase in lymphocytes is associated with viral infections.) A full blood count will also demonstrate anaemia (if present), or a reduced white cell count. A blood film will identify abnormalities of red or white cell morphology. If the infective nature of the condition is doubted, C-reactive protein (CRP) may be a helpful guide to the severity of inflammation. Urinalysis or a fasting blood sugar estimation may detect previously undiagnosed diabetes, but remember that severe infection itself tends to raise the blood sugar level. Also consider the recent use of corticosteroids, alcohol or drug abuse or HIV infection.

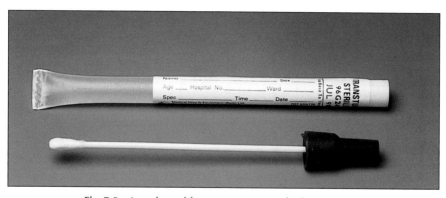

Fig. 7.8 A swab used for transport to microbiology.

SURGICAL TREATMENT OF INFECTION

Early removal of the 'cause', such as by tooth extraction, is important in management of dental infections. If the severity or spread of infection makes local anaesthesia, access for extraction or induction of general anaesthesia impracticable or dangerous, this treatment may be delayed.

Drainage of pus is an essential part of the treatment of suppurative infections. Sometimes it may be appropriate to encourage spontaneous drainage, particularly in small, localized, superficial abscesses, but usually active surgical intervention is required.

Drainage of intraoral abscesses (Fig. 7.9) may be performed using local anaesthetic injected close to the site of incision (for large, deeply placed abscesses, general anaesthesia may be required). Topical ethyl chloride anaesthetizes only to a very shallow depth. The blade of the scalpel is inserted parallel to the gingival margin, directly into the abscess to the full depth in its long axis, then used to cut outwards towards the surface. This should be followed immediately by a flow of pus. Gently opening the cavity allows the pus to drain. If a pus sample is to be

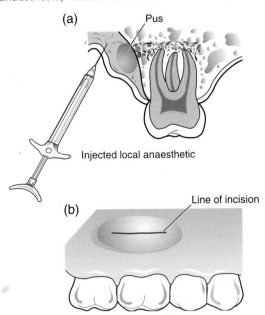

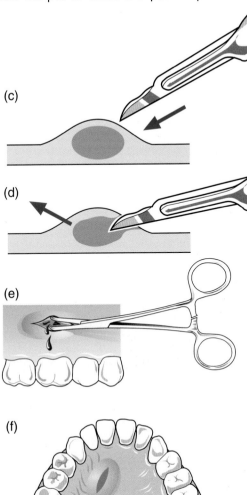

Fig. 7.9 Drainage of an intraoral abscess.
(a) Local anaesthetic is injected lateral to the abscess.
(b) The incision is made parallel to the gingival margin, at the lower end of the abscess cavity.
(c) The scalpel is pushed into the abscess lengthwise and positively, then
(d) cuts outwards, reducing pressure on the abscess.
(e) The abscess cavity is opened with curved artery forceps, scissors or sinus forceps.
(f) In the palate, it can be helpful to remove an elliptical window of mucosa to prevent the wound resealing.

collected, it may be taken at any time up till now. The base of the abscess cavity is usually bare bone. If no discharge of pus occurs, it is likely either that there is no pus in the lesion (yet) or that the incision is not deep enough.

For small abscesses a drain is not usually necessary.

Anaesthesia

The author prefers to use local anaesthetic injected close to the abscess or, if this is not practicable, general anaesthesia. Some prefer to relieve pain with a topical spray of ethyl chloride (to lower the mucosal temperature below 4°C); however, this provides little pain relief. Topical local anaesthetics work to a depth of several millimetres and can be satisfactory for very superficial abscesses.

Drains

Larger and deeper abscesses tend to seal off shortly after drainage, leaving pus inside or still forming: something must be done to hold the cavity open. In the mouth a corrugated rubber or tubular plastic drain (Fig. 7.10)—or, in desperation, the finger of a sterile rubber glove—may be used. These must be sutured in for at least 24 hours. For palatal abscesses, it is more convenient and successful to excise an ellipse of mucosa from the centre of the abscess so that when the mucosa is pushed flat by the tongue the wound cannot seal.

Larger abscesses

Cervicofacial space abscesses require a more vigorous approach to drainage, and even the buccal space abscesses, which can theoretically be incised intraorally, are better approached from outside the mouth. Usually this will be under general anaesthesia on an inpatient basis.

The incision should be placed in a neck crease to leave the least evident scar (Fig. 7.11). To approach a submandibular abscess, make the incision at least two fingers' breadth below the angle of the mandible to avoid the marginal mandibular branch of the facial nerve. The nerve may also be displaced downwards by the swelling of tissue above, and in inflamed tissue its identification is near impossible.

As pus tends to track downwards under gravity, it is usual to make the incision at the lowest (most dependent) part of the expected cavity. For buccal space abscesses the incision may also be placed in the neck to hide it in a skin crease.

Once the skin incision is made, the abscess is approached by blunt dissection using scissors or a curved haemostat. This involves pushing the end of the instrument into the wound with the tips together, then forcibly opening the instrument to develop a plane of dissection. This is repeated until the abscess cavity is reached. Blunt dissection minimizes the risk of injury to nerves and vessels. A sample of pus should be taken by aspiration at this time, reducing the likelihood of skin contamination.

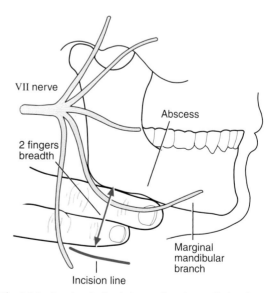

Fig. 7.11 Landmarks for drainage of a submandibular abscess. The marginal mandibular branch of the facial nerve dips below the lower border of the mandible. The incision line should be at least two fingers' breadth below the lower border.

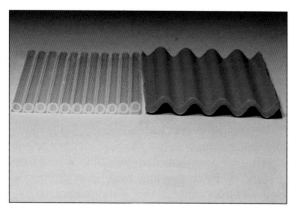

Fig. 7.10 Corrugated rubber and tubular plastic drains.

When the cavity is entered, the access should be enlarged to enable the little finger to be inserted to explore the cavity and gently disrupt any fibrous septae between locules of pus. Some operators irrigate the cavity with saline at this stage to reduce residual contamination.

A drain should be cut that will extend from the deepest part of the cavity beyond the skin edge. This is sutured in place with a material which can be found easily for removal (such as black silk), but *the wound is not closed*. A non-adherent dressing is placed over the wound and an absorbent dressing placed over that. Some surgeons prefer to seal a stoma bag over the wound to collect the pus. The drain is usually removed after 24–72 hours, depending upon the size of the abscess and its tendency to continue draining. Some surgeons will shorten the drain daily, to allow the deeper part of the wound to fill with inflammatory tissue first. The wound often continues to discharge for a week or more after the drain is removed and the dressings need to be changed daily (or sooner if soaked) until the wound dries.

Summary of surgical treatment

- Remove the cause (tooth or root) early
- Small abscesses are incised using injected local anaesthetic
- Ensure continued drainage; if necessary place a drain
- For neck abscesses beware the VII nerve
- Use blunt dissection to find the abscess cavity

MEDICAL AND SUPPORTIVE TREATMENT

Antibacterial chemotherapy is central to the treatment of bacterial infection. However, antibiotics may be over-prescribed and there are certainly circumstances when antibiotics are unnecessary.

Antibacterial drugs should be used when:
- the infection is of bacterial origin
- there is significant regional lymph node or systemic reaction (raised temperature)
- spread is significant
- appropriate local treatment has not been successful
- resistance to infection is reduced
- there is a risk of infection at distant sites (e.g. the endocardium).

Antibacterials should not be used to control pus (indeed they will not), but on occasion will prevent spread of infection while awaiting localization. If antibiotics are used to control an abscess, the abscess may go 'quiet', but it will become painful and obviously infected again within days of ceasing the antibiotics. Such a persistently swollen, tender, indurated mass is sometimes called an 'antibioma', but should not be confused with a tumour, from either its name or its appearance.

Choice of antibiotics

The initial choice of antimicrobial drug is empirical. Most infections of dental origin are caused by a mixture of organisms and both aerobes and anaerobes can often be cultured. In mixed infections, eliminating one organism can be effective in treating the infection, because of synergism between the organisms.

Factors that determine the choice of antimicrobial drug include:

- efficacy against a range of organisms isolated from dental infections
- safety and adverse reactions
- compliance
- cost.

A common first choice is *metronidazole* (note: this is active only against anaerobes). For mild infection it may be given orally at a dose of 200–400 mg three times a day for 5–7 days. Metronidazole should be taken with or after meals as it is irritant to the stomach. It produces an unpleasant reaction with alcohol and patients should therefore be advised to avoid alcohol while they are taking the drug. Compliance is likely to be poor in patients who drink a lot of alcohol.

The broad-spectrum penicillin *amoxicillin* covers a range of organisms wider than that of the basic penicillin, penicillin V, but is still well tolerated orally (and with less tendency to cause diarrhoea than oral ampicillin). It is given at a dose of 500 mg three times daily.

The cephalosporins, such as *cefradine* (250–500 mg four times daily), also have a wider range of activity against oral organisms than penicillin V, and there is some evidence that they may be more effective clinically than either amoxicillin or metronidazole. However, the differences appear to be small and, although cephradine is not an expensive drug it does cost more than penicillin V and metronidazole.

Where it is necessary to ensure a high and consistent blood level of an antibiotic, it is usual now to administer the drug intravenously. This implies hospital admission.

Because the initial choice is empirical, there is a tendency to use two antibiotics in combination when an infection is severe and there is a risk of serious outcome. Again there are arguments for and against a variety of combinations of drugs. The author's choice for intravenous use is metronidazole 500 mg 12-hourly and ampicillin 500 mg 6-hourly.

Alternative drugs are needed in cases of adverse reaction or if the organisms isolated are not sensitive to the first-choice drugs. Consideration may be given to macrolide antibiotics such as erythromycin (for oral use) or clarithromycin (parenteral), tetracyclines, lincosamides and occasionally the aminoglycosides. Reference may be made to texts on microbiology and therapeutics, and consultant microbiologists will advise in cases of difficulty.

Failure to control an infection with antibiotics may be due to:

- a substantial residual collection of pus
- use of inappropriate antibiotic
- inadequate dose of drug (either by prescription or by failure of compliance)
- course too short
- persistence of a 'cause'.

Supportive care

The role of supportive care is more difficult to prove. There is little evidence that bed rest affects the outcome of dental infections. However, it is unlikely that taking vigorous exercise is beneficial.

Fluid intake, on the other hand, is of great importance. A patient with a painful mouth and face, especially if it is painful to swallow, often eats nothing and drinks too little, resulting in dehydration over a period of days. Fluid requirements are increased if the temperature is raised, so rehydration is essential. The average adult requires about 2.5 L of fluid per day, but if pyrexial that may rise to 3 or 3.5 L. If adequate fluid cannot be taken by mouth, it must be given intravenously, which implies hospital admission.

Patients with dental infections rarely become dangerously pyrexial (temperature exceeding 40°C), but if they do it is necessary to reduce the temperature with aspirin or paracetamol, or by sponging with tepid water and circulating air over the body.

CASES REQUIRING INPATIENT MANAGEMENT

Localized dental infections in fit individuals are usually managed in dental practice. There are certain cases, however, in which outpatient management is impracticable or unnecessarily risky.

Good reasons for hospital admission include:

- considerable systemic reaction in terms of fever or malaise
- failure readily to control an infection, or rapid or extensive spread
- significant dysphagia or any dyspnoea
- signs of dehydration or reluctance to drink
- suspected reduced resistance to infection
- need for general anaesthesia for drainage.

Usually on admission the following will be done:

- venous access established
- fluid loss replaced intravenously (often with normal saline)
- haematological investigation, and occasionally blood culture
- antibiotics given intravenously
- investigation whether drainage is required and arrange as necessary
- consideration made of how and when any 'cause' can be eliminated.

Each case is treated individually and reviewed to ensure earliest recognition of problems. The patient is discharged when the infection is under control, any drainage has been performed and risk of relapse is small.

SPREADING CELLULITIS IN THE FLOOR OF THE MOUTH (LUDWIG'S ANGINA)

A cellulitis starting in the floor of the mouth (Fig. 7.12), often arising from a mandibular molar and not readily localizing, has the potential to threaten life by obstructing the airway.

Clinical signs include:
- oedema of both sides of the floor of the mouth
- tongue lifted up

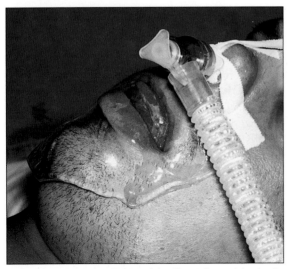

Fig. 7.12 A severe cellulitis of the floor of mouth and sub-mandibular space (Ludwig's angina).
The tongue protrudes from the mouth and there is extensive oedema below the chin. The patient has been intubated to protect the airway. An inert jelly covers the mouth to prevent drying.

- involvement of both submandibular spaces
- oedema spreading down the neck over a period of hours
- firmness, redness and tenderness in the neck with loss of definition of anatomical structures, particularly if it reaches the sternal notch
- progressive trismus
- high temperature (not always)
- marked pain or difficulty on swallowing
- difficulty with speech or breathing.

This condition requires urgent action:

- Admission to hospital
- High-dose intravenous antibiotics, usually ampicillin and metronidazole initially
- Intravenous fluid replacement
- Assessment of whether drainage is required
- Consideration of airway management (this might be endotracheal intubation or tracheostomy) if there is a significant risk of obstruction

Corticosteroids have been advocated to reduce swelling in these cases, but they reduce resistance to infection and the available evidence on their efficacy is not conclusive.

OSTEOMYELITIS

Osteomyelitis is defined as the spreading infection of bone marrow. Although the clinical features of osteomyelitis are different from those of soft-tissue infections, the disorder may start in the same way and it is valuable to distinguish this infection early. The cancellous bone of the jaw (usually the mandible) seems well protected from apical infection, which usually moves rapidly out into soft tissue. However, sometimes this protection fails, allowing intraosseous spread.

This may simultaneously cause thrombosis of veins in the marrow and stripping of periosteum by pus (Fig. 7.13). The blood supply to the mandible is substantially from the inferior alveolar artery in young people, but becomes progressively dependent on the periosteum and muscle attachments with age. Spreading infection with thrombosis and periosteal stripping thereby causes loss of blood supply to the infected area, resulting in bone necrosis.

Osteomyelitis sometimes occurs as an acute infection; it is more likely to do so in the maxilla in children. In that case the infection is particularly severe and probably of different pathogenesis from

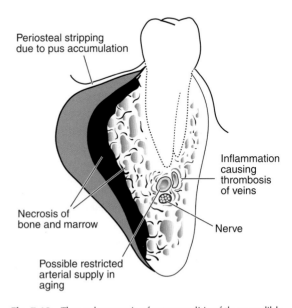

Periosteal stripping due to pus accumulation

Inflammation causing thrombosis of veins

Necrosis of bone and marrow

Nerve

Possible restricted arterial supply in aging

Fig. 7.13 The pathogenesis of osteomyelitis of the mandible. Inflammation causes thrombosis of vessels in the marrow; periosteal stripping by pus (or surgery) causes loss of periosteal blood supply, with consequent necrosis of bone. This encourages continuance of infection as well as bone resorption.

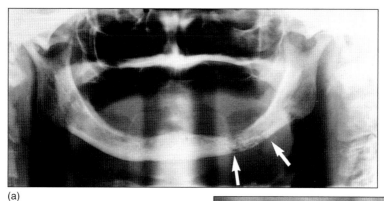

(a)

the chronic mandibular disease. Occasionally osteo-myelitis may involve the periosteal surface of the bone exclusively, or appear solely as a sclerotic reaction of the marrow.

Clinical features

The clinical features are thus those of infection in general, plus tenderness of more teeth than would be expected, possibly mobility of teeth, loss of function of the inferior alveolar nerve and *numbness of the lower lip*. Because of periosteal inflammation and stripping there is a firm or woody expansion of the affected bone area, with no clearly defined junction between the swelling and normal bone. The overlying skin may be mobile, provided there is little acute infection. If the infection is not rapidly resolved, bone resorption becomes evident on radiographs (Fig. 7.14a), necrotic bone may separate as a *sequestrum*, and new bone may form on the inner aspect of the stripped periosteum and may become visible on tangential radiographs (Fig. 7.14b). Eventually the weakened mandible may fracture.

Time scale is important in the diagnosis of osteomyelitis. It often takes weeks from the first symptoms till a clear diagnosis is made, even though the condition is obviously infective early on.

Predisposing factors

Factors predisposing to osteomyelitis include those which make any infection more likely (e.g. use of corti-costeroids or alcohol dependency) and anything which tends to open up the marrow space widely (fracture or surgical removal of a tooth), or increased density of bone, such as in Paget's disease or osteopetrosis.

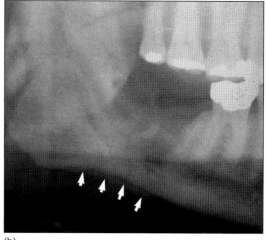

(b)

Fig. 7.14 (a) Typical radiological appearance of osteomyelitis. Patchy bone resorption is highlighted by arrows. (b) A thin layer of subperiosteal bone (arrows) has formed at the lower border of the mandible in a patient with osteomyelitis.

Clinical features of osteomyelitis of the mandible
• Signs of infection • Reduced sensibility in the lower lip • Tenderness and mobility of adjacent teeth • Patchy, irregular bone loss • Sequestration • Periosteal thickening • Subperiosteal new bone • Pathological fracture

Treatment

The investigation and management of osteomyelitis are best performed within a hospital setting.

Treatment relies upon antibiotics, maintained for 6–8 weeks. The initial choice of antibiotic is usually empirical. *Penicillin V* is safe and well tolerated, with a reasonable spectrum of activity against oral microorganisms and appears to be effective in this condition. The *tetracyclines* are bound in bone by chelation of calcium, but are inactive in that form; they have, however, been very successfully used in osteomyelitis. The *lincosamides* achieve high bone concentrations, but there is a small risk of pseudomembranous colitis on long-term use. The *cephalosporins* and *penicillins* also have their advocates. The initial choice may not be that critical, but the causative organism should be identified and antibiotic treatment modified accordingly.

Any controllable predisposing factor (such as anaemia) should be dealt with early in the management of osteomyelitis.

Surgery is necessary if a substantial sequestrum forms. Occasionally, in resistant cases, it is necessary to remove the lateral cortical plate of bone to allow access for granulation tissue to the remaining bone. Pathological fractures require immobilization and often bone grafting once the infection is settled.

Treatment of chronic osteomyelitis of the mandible

- Antibiotics (penicillin) for 6–8 weeks
- Removal of sequestrae as they form
- Control of predisposing factors

ACTINOMYCOSIS

Actinomycosis is a specific infection caused by *Actinomyces* species, often arising from a dental source. It differs from many infections of dental origin in being *much slower in onset* and *more chronic in its course*. Microbiological diagnosis can be difficult and the clinical signs vary, making this a diagnosis about which one may be uncertain.

If the infection has followed a specific event such as a fracture of the mandible, the time scale is usually a few weeks. There is often low-grade swelling, tenderness and induration (hardening) of the skin of the face or neck. Sometimes this is localized to an area as small as 3 cm, but it can be much more extensive. Often, then, over a short period pain increases, a fluctuant abscess forms superficially and the abscess discharges, only to build up again over days to weeks. The classical actinomycosis (Fig. 7.15) with multiple discharging sinuses and pus containing yellow 'sulphur granules' is relatively rare but is easily identified when seen.

Treatment is with oral penicillin for a period of about 3 months, with surgical drainage of pus as appropriate. If there is a dental cause, it should be treated early.

Actinomycosis: summary

- Infection developing over several weeks often arising from a 'dental' cause
- Induration leading rapidly to discharge over 1–2 days at the end of that time
- Oral penicillin for 3 months
- Drainage of pus as appropriate
- Removal of the 'cause'

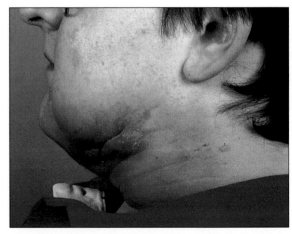

Fig. 7.15 Actinomycosis, with multiple submandibular sinuses, in a patient who did not seek treatment for a fractured mandible 3 months previously.

NECROTIZING INFECTIONS

Severe necrotizing infections are rare now in Europe, but are still common in parts of the world where poor nutrition is widespread. The mildest form seen is acute necrotizing ulcerative gingivitis, which is well covered in periodontal texts.

Cancrum oris or 'noma' is extremely destructive of facial soft tissue, especially around the mouth, and is recognized largely by that feature.

Treatment is with antibiotics (metronidazole and penicillin) in the first instance to control the infection, surgical removal of non-vital tissue (debridement) and closure of the mucosa to the skin surfaces of the wound. Reconstruction is delayed until the general health is stabilized.

Rarely, necrotizing infections caused by a mixed growth of *Staphylococcus aureus* and a β-haemolytic *Streptococcus* may start from minor skin abrasions. This has been called 'synergistic gangrene'. Like cancrum oris, it is usually an indication of a severe underlying reduction in infection resistance. The prognosis is extremely grave.

MRSA

Infections of the head and neck, particularly hospital-acquired wound infections, may be caused by methicillin-resistant *S. aureus* (MRSA). This organism is remarkably resistant to a range of antibiotics and is prevalent in hospitals because of the widespread use of antibiotics. Infections of this type are a particular risk to the elderly or debilitated patient in hospital. Efforts must be maintained to minimize spread of such infection by strict hygiene measures, by identifying and isolating those with the infection and by careful wound care to encourage rapid healing where infection has occurred.

FURTHER READING

Adekeye E. O., Cornah J. (1985) Osteomyelitis of the jaws: a review of 141 cases. *British Journal of Oral and Maxillofacial Surgery* 23: 24–35.

Calhoun K. H., Shapiro R. D., Stiernberg C. M., Calhoun J. H., Mader J. T. (1988) Osteomyelitis of the mandible. *Archives of Otolaryngology* 114: 1157–1162.

Fazakerley M. W., McGowan P., Hardy P., Martin M. V. (1993) A comparative study of cephradine, amoxycillin and phenoxymethyl penicillin in the treatment of acute dentoalveolar infection. *British Dental Journal* 174: 359–363.

Har-El G., Aroesty J. H., Shaha A., Lucente F. E. (1994) Changing trends in deep neck abscess. *Oral Surgery* 77: 446–450.

Lewis M. A. O., MacFarlane T. W., McGowan D. A. (1990) A microbiological and clinical review of the acute dentoalveolar abscess. *British Journal of Oral and Maxillofacial Surgery* 28: 359–366.

Lindner H. H. (1986) The anatomy of the fasciae of the face and neck with particular reference to the spread and treatment of intraoral infections (Ludwig's) that have progressed into adjacent fascial spaces. *Annals of Surgery* 204: 705–714.

Wannfors K., Gazelius B. (1991) Blood flow in jaw bones affected by chronic osteomyelitis. *British Journal of Oral and Maxillofacial Surgery* 29: 147–153.

Young P., Smith S. P., Caesar H. (1995) Airway management in Ludwig's angina. *British Journal of Hospital Medicine* 54: 239.

SELF-ASSESSMENT

1. The patient shown in Fig. 7.16 gave a 24-hour history of increasing facial pain and swelling, following discomfort from a carious left maxillary canine.
   (a) What clinical type of infection does this mostly represent?
   (b) Why is the lower eyelid more swollen than the cheek?
   (c) Which anatomical space does the infection occupy?
   (d) What investigations are indicated?
   (e) Why is this unlikely to represent tumour?
   (f) What are likely to be the main elements of treatment?

2. Figure 7.17 shows a man who gave a 2-week history of increasing pain, right facial swelling and trismus associated with soreness around a lower third molar. His interincisal opening was measured at 8 mm.

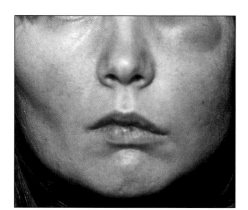

Fig. 7.16 See question 1.

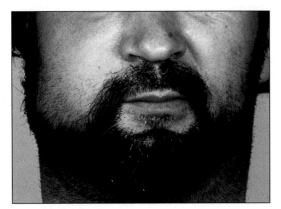

Fig. 7.17 See question 2.

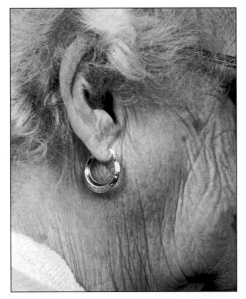

Fig. 7.18 See question 3.

(a) What anatomical spaces may be involved, in view of the trismus?

(b) What questions should be asked to clarify the spread of infection?

(c) What imaging techniques might clarify the spread of infection?

3. The patient shown in Fig. 7.18 gave a 6-day history of increasing pain and swelling of the side of the face.

(a) Why does this not seem likely to be of dental origin?

(b) What anatomical structure is likely to be infected?

(c) What question might you ask to confirm that anatomical observation?

4. A patient attends with a 3-day history of pain and swelling of the face centred buccally to a carious upper premolar. Examination reveals tender, firm or tense swelling of the cheek and a 3-cm swelling intraorally, which is tender, fluctuant and red, buccal to the apex of the tooth. The tooth is carious and non-vital and has an apical radiolucency.

(a) What is the diagnosis?

(b) What surgical treatment would you perform on the day?

(c) How would you prevent pain during that procedure?

(d) What would you expect to find at the base of the wound created?

5. (a) What antibiotic regimen would you choose for control of a cellulitis of dental origin, with minimal systemic disturbance (temperature 37.5°C, pulse 80 beats/minute), confined to the buccal space in an adult allergic to penicillin, but otherwise fit and well?

(b) How long should you leave the patient before review?

6. A 60-year-old woman attended with a 2- to 3-week history of left facial pain and swelling following an ulcer at the margin of an ill-fitting lower complete denture. The swelling was centred around the buccal aspect of the premolar region. There had been some tingling of the lower lip. She had a long history of asthma. The retained root of the lower left second molar was removed surgically as treatment for this infection. A radiograph taken 1 month later showed moth-eaten radiolucencies.

(a) What disease process(es) do you think is (are) responsible for the clinical and radiographic features?

(b) What further questions might you ask?

7. A patient describes pain and swelling in the side of the neck and face, following a blow to the jaw. The symptoms subsided over several days, then slowly and progressively worsened over the next 8 weeks, with discharge from the neck for 4 weeks.

(a) What aspects of this story are unusual for a dental infection?
(b) What sort of infection might this be?
(c) What additional questions would you ask?
(d) What investigations would you do?

(e) In the light of your preferred diagnosis, what treatment would you recommend?

Answers on page 264.

8 Oral lesions: differential diagnosis and biopsy techniques

C. G. Cowan
J. Marley

- A wide variety of lesions arise from the soft tissues, e.g. mucosa and submucosal structures, or hard tissues, e.g. bone or odontogenic tissue in the orofacial region.
- Patients often first present to the general dental practitioner and it is essential that the clinician can recognize the abnormal and begin developing a differential diagnosis.
- This requires understanding of the possible pathological diagnoses and the ability to make appropriate deductions from:
  - Clinical history and symptoms
  - Clinical signs, e.g. site, consistency, colour and anatomical relationships.
- Definitive diagnosis often requires special investigations, such as radiology or biopsy.
- Management will depend on the clinical significance of the diagnosis, the presence or absence of related symptoms, the site and size of the lesion, and, in many cases, will require referral to a specialist.

ASSUMED KNOWLEDGE

It is assumed that at this stage you will have knowledge/competencies in the following areas:

- anatomy of the face and jaws
- surgical sieve (see Ch. 2)
- WHO classification of odontogenic tumours and cysts
- pathological and radiological appearance of a range of oral lesions.

If you feel you are not competent in these areas, revise them before reading this chapter or cross-check with relevant texts as you read.

INTENDED LEARNING OUTCOMES

At the end of this chapter you should be able to:

1. Develop a differential diagnosis based on the history and symptoms, anatomical site, consistency, colour and other anatomical relationships
2. Plan investigations to confirm your diagnosis, including radiology and biopsy or make an appropriate referral
3. Describe the techniques of biopsy and similar investigations
4. Understand the principles of treatment and be able to equate these to your clinical competency or alternatively refer onwards
5. Either alone or in conjunction with a specialist, advise patients concerning the nature and effects of their disease, its treatment and, as necessary, a follow-up regimen.

OVERVIEW

Many oral lesions are first noticed by the patient or clinician as changes in the colour, texture or disruption of the mucosal surface, or as a swelling or asymmetry of the orofacial structures. When involving or arising from the underlying bone, these lesions may produce a variety of radiological changes, including radiolucencies with or without opacities, evidence of expansion and bone loss in the form of erosion or resorption.

Securing the diagnosis is fundamental to safe and successful management of the patient and will depend on a clear and concise history, careful clinical examination and the use of additional special investigations including radiography, biopsy and other laboratory and diagnostic techniques. Within this spectrum, biopsy is a commonly performed test and is detailed later in this chapter. Should the lesion appear malignant, biopsy should not be performed in general practice, but the patient should be referred immediately for a specialist opinion (see Ch. 10). This approach avoids the need for the general practitioner to break unexpected/distressing news with the consequent requirement to explore the management options with a now anxious patient.

All referrals require clear and concise details, but where malignancy is suspected, direct contact should be made with the specialist by telephone or fax.

SOFT-TISSUE LESIONS

Diagnosis

Soft-tissue oral lesions are common, often symptomless, slow-growing lumps and are first noticed by the clinician at a routine examination so the clinical history might not contribute greatly to making the diagnosis. Pain is unusual and would indicate infection in a lesion such as a cyst (secondary infection, see Ch. 9). On rare occasions it may indicate aggressive behaviour, e.g. malignant tumour of minor salivary gland (Ch. 14).

Clinical examination, however, based on inspection *and* palpation referenced to site, colour and consistency provide the main pointers to diagnosis.

Site

The posterior palate, lateral third of hard palate and upper lip are particularly high-risk sites for minor salivary gland tumours. The lower lip is a common site for mucoceles, whilst the buccal mucosa is a common site for fibroepithelial polyps particularly when associated with missing teeth.

Colour

Colour will distinguish between fibroepithelial polyps (pink) (Fig. 8.1) and the white rough cauliflower presentation of viral papillomas (warts) (Fig. 8.2). Mucous cysts tend to be translucent with a bluish colour (see Figs 14.7, 14.8) and haemangiomas and 'venous lakes' (Fig. 8.3) dark blue. Pyogenic granulomas (Fig. 8.4) and giant-cell epulides (Fig. 8.5) normally present as maroon/red.

Anatomical relationships and consistency

Lesions may also be distinguished by their depth within the oral tissues and their relationship to adjacent structures. This will differentiate superficial lesions such as fibroepithelial polyps, viral papillomas and epulides (gingival swellings) from submucosal lesions. Palpation is essential to define the lesion's consistency and distinguish between discrete and diffuse swellings, or whether the lesion is mobile

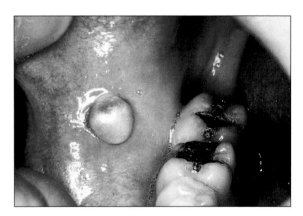

Fig. 8.1   Fibroepithelial polyp, right buccal mucosa.

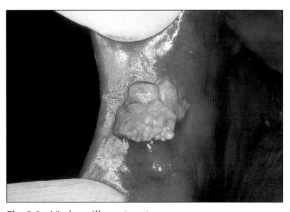

Fig. 8.2   Viral papilloma (wart).

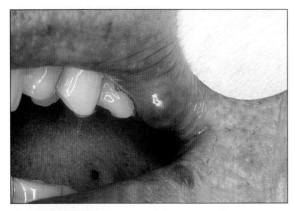

Fig. 8.3 Degenerative 'venous lake' in upper lip.

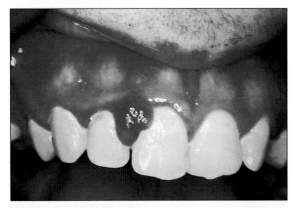

Fig. 8.4 Pyogenic granuloma.

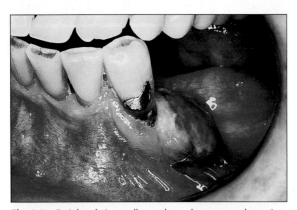

Fig. 8.5 Peripheral giant-cell granuloma, lower premolar region.

or attached to deeper structures. Solid submucosal lesions can be reactive (e.g. lymph nodes) or neoplastic arising from any of the submucosal structures (e.g. adenomata of minor salivary glands and neurilemmomas). All submucosal swellings that are solid have the potential to be neoplastic and must be investigated.

Modifying influences

The intraoral environment having given rise to lesions may in turn alter their morphology, depending on site. For example, fibroepithelial polyps can vary in presentation from 'leaf fibromas' in the palate to denture-induced hyperplasia at the periphery of a denture (see Figs 11.5, 11.6). Immature or developing polyps, particularly when arising from the gingivae, are described as pyogenic granulomas and the pregnancy epulis is a variant. They present as red, acutely inflamed lesions that are soft and bleed readily. Similar in presentation is the peripheral giant-cell granuloma although this may be more purple.

Single and multiple lesions

Almost all the lesions described so far present as single and discrete swellings. The presence of multiple lesions is of significance and indicates systemic disorders. Examples include the mucosal tags and polyps in oral Crohn's disease/orofacial granulomatosis and multiple viral papillomas of HIV infection.

White/red and pigmented lesions

White and red patches are discussed in detail in Chapter 10 (see Figs 10.1, 10.2), but it should be noted that a wide array of white patches that have no significant malignant potential can occur. The difficulty is that interpretation of this risk almost always requires a histological diagnosis. Biopsy is therefore mandatory for all unexplained lesions and the decision not to biopsy requires clinical experience in the management of these types of lesions.

A variety of pigmented lesions may present within the oral cavity; they may be blue, brown or black in colour, flat (macule), raised or granular (papule) and single or multiple. Common single macular lesions include *amalgam tattoos* and *benign naevi*. Multiple macular lesions include *racial deposits* and lesions secondary to chronic inflammatory damage to the epithelium such as *lichen planus* and *tobacco-induced melanosis*. However, in common with white/red lesions, biopsy may be indicated to confirm the diagnosis. It is essential that, as with leukoplakia, any recent history of ulceration, haemorrhage or change in the type (becomes papular) or size of a lesion is to be regarded as serious when urgent referral is mandatory.

Indication for biopsy

Where the diagnosis is clinically evident as in the case of fibroepithelial polyps, viral papillomas or mucous cysts, biopsy is not required for diagnosis although where treatment involves excision, the specimen should always be submitted for histological confirmation. If there is doubt or the lesion is arising deep to the mucosa then histological diagnosis is essential.

Summary: Soft-tissue lesions

- Site, colour and consistency are key diagnostic pointers:
  Pink, soft and superficial—innocent
  Firm/solid and submucosal—potentially neoplastic
  Dark blue/red—vascular (fluid) giant-cell lesion (solid)
  Translucent/bluish—cyst (salivary)
- Fibroepithelial polyps are treated by excision biopsy
- Peripheral giant-cell granulomas require curettage of underlying bone and may recur
- Beware change, ulceration or haemorrhage in brown, blue or blackish mucosal patches: they may represent malignant melanoma

---

TREATMENT OF SOFT-TISSUE LESIONS

General points

The primary management objective is to establish the diagnosis. This may require nothing other than clinical examination as for a squamous papilloma or mucous cyst, but often and particularly for solid/firm submucosal lesions does require biopsy. Subsequent treatment will depend not only on the clinical significance of the diagnosis but on the presence of related symptoms and the site and size of the lesion.

Lesions causing problems, or which can be anticipated to do so, will require surgery or referral. Small, innocent lesions can be left, assuming they are not causing symptoms, increasing in size or of concern to the patient in terms of function or appearance.

In general, the size and site of the lesion do not change the technique but do require careful assessment of the patient and the level of experience of the operator. Larger lesions (greater than 2 cm),

particularly submucosal ones, are more difficult to manage surgically. This is due to the access required and the risks to adjacent blood vessels and nerves. In addition they will be more difficult to repair and consequently they should not be attempted unless the operator is skilled in soft-tissue surgery and in dealing with the intraoperative and postoperative complications.

Fibroepithelial polyps, squamous papillomas and epulides

Surgical excision is the most common treatment for small lesions (fibroepithelial polyps, squamous papillomas and epulides) and is often completed as part of the biopsy (see below). It must, however, be combined with appropriate management of precipitating or causative factors. These include the elimination of chronic trauma for polyps or the removal of localized deposits of calculus for pyogenic granulomas. Peripheral giant-cell lesions will require a similar approach including curettage of the underlying bone. Epulides related to pregnancy are, unless they are large and causing distress, best left alone and removed if they persist postpartum, usually with an appropriate adjunctive periodontal therapy. Scaling and improved oral hygiene during pregnancy may reduce further growth and lessen the likelihood of surgery.

Surgical management of denture-induced hyperplasia must be combined with appropriate modification to the prosthesis such as temporary relining (Ch. 11). This is essential to retain sulcus form and prevent recurrence and is similarly so for 'leaf-fibroma' in the palate. Denture-induced hyperplasia can be extensive and, when affecting the lower jaw, is often related to other significant anatomical structures. This is particularly so in the anterior region where the main trunk of the mental nerve can be superficial due to resorption of the alveolus. The lingual nerve can also be at risk when the lingual side is operated on. In these circumstances it is important to carefully identify the edge of the hyperplastic tissue, to keep the excision superficial and to use blunt dissection to free the tissue from underlying structures (see section on biopsy).

Mucous cysts

Mucous cysts divide between the common extravasation cyst and the rarer retention cyst and present as tense bluish swellings often in the lower lip (see Fig. 14.7). These conditions are discussed in Chapter 14.

Vascular lesions

Vascular lesions are best considered as two groups: the rare haemangiomas, which can be extensive and multiple, and the common smaller degenerative malformations (varicosities) often seen on the lip in older patients (Fig. 8.3). For the former it is essential that the type, site and extent are fully evaluated, which normally requires referral to a specialist centre. For extensive and deep lesions or where there is any possibility that the haemangioma extends into bone, extractions or other surgery must be avoided until the type and extent of the vascular abnormality have been established. Conversely, discrete small lesions are easily dealt with either by excision with appropriate management of the vascular source or by cryotherapy. Indications for surgery are cosmetic or lesions that are repeatedly traumatized and bleed.

Submucosal solid lesions

All submucosal solid lesions require investigation as the probability of them being neoplastic is high. Treatment selection is very much a balance between incisional biopsy to determine the histological diagnosis first and removal of the lesion in its entirety to avoid compromise of the site in terms of further surgery by potential seeding of tumour cells (e.g. pleomorphic salivary adenoma). This is often decided by the site and size of the lesion along with the results of specialist imaging such as CT or MRI scanning. For small lesions the careful combination of sharp and blunt dissection as described below should only be undertaken by clinicians skilled in soft-tissue surgery. As stated below, the excision of lesions arising under mucoperiosteum such as the palate requires the defect to be closed either by dressing the site and allowing repair by secondary intention or by primary repair with a mucosal flap or graft. Surgery in the soft palate area can be difficult, particularly if the lesion is deep where there is a possibility of perforation through to the nasal side.

DIAGNOSIS AND TREATMENT OF HARD-TISSUE LESIONS

Overview

Hard-tissue lesions can arise from odontogenic tissue or from bone. They present a range of diagnoses from developmental lesions such as palatal or mandibular *tori* or *odontomas* (see Figs 8.6, 11.13, 11.14) and bony *exostoses*, to the rarer benign and locally invasive lesions such as *ossifying fibroma*, *ameloblastoma* and *cementoblastoma*.

This is a complex group of lesions and conditions. Readers are referred to relevant pathology and radiology texts for more detailed descriptions of the various types and their histological and radiological findings. From the clinical standpoint they can be considered according to presentation: the common single discrete lesions (odontomes, odontogenic tumours and osteomata); the rare, large and diffuse lesions (fibrous dysplasia and Paget's disease); and rare conditions with multiple lesions (Gardner's syndrome and cemento-ossifying lesions).

Often they first come to attention as a bone-hard swelling beneath the overlying mucosa, but in many cases presentation is an incidental finding on routine radiography. As the symptoms and signs have so much overlap, diagnosis is largely dependent on radiological findings and, more importantly, histology. As described below, site can be an important sign in establishing the diagnosis: not only are the lesions within this group difficult to separate, they are often clinically and radiographically similar to cysts (see Ch. 9). As with soft-tissue lesions, there will be malignant counterparts, e.g. osteosarcoma and secondary tumours, that can present in similar fashion (see below).

Odontogenic lesions

These arise as abnormalities of tooth-forming structures and form a group ranging from odontomes (which are *hamartomas*, i.e. developmental lumps, with progression limited to the normal growth period) to benign and locally invasive tumours. They can present as discrete single lesions and are often extensive. Radiographically they can be radiolucent with the characteristics of cysts (Ch. 9) or be radio-opaque or of mixed radiodensity.

Odontomes

These hamartomas (see pathology texts for subclassification) do not continue to grow. They commonly present as a chance radiographic finding, related to delayed eruption of teeth (Fig. 8.6), or as a palpable mass in the alveolar region. Occasionally they cause pain if infected. Radiographs show them to be well-circumscribed, radio-opaque lesions often with a radiolucent margin akin to the periodontal ligament of a tooth.

Clinically they can be considered as malformed supernumerary teeth and treatment should reflect this, with removal recommended if they interfere with tooth eruption or orthodontic tooth movement, or are infected. In the absence of such problems, particularly if there are risks to adjacent structures or the patient has significant co-morbidity, they may be left alone.

Benign and locally invasive odontogenic tumours

Most odontogenic tumours are essentially benign and, depending on the cellular bias, can be composed entirely of soft tissue presenting as cysts or produce, to varying degrees, radio-opaque, odontogenic hard tissue. They have similar presenting symptoms and signs to odontomata but as they are tumours they will continue to grow and present a significant challenge in terms of management. This stems from their similar presenting symptoms and signs weighed against a spectrum of clinical behaviour. The potential for local recurrence is high and in some cases such as ameloblastomas, there is a very small but significant potential for metastatic spread. Very few are suited to simple enucleation. Conservative excision (removal with aggressive curettage of the bony margins) or formal resection with a margin of sound bone are the treatment options and must be referenced to the risks of local recurrence or spread and the size and anatomical relationships of the lesion. With the extensive overlap in presenting symptoms and clinical and radiographic signs between cysts and tumours it is essential that the histological diagnosis be established prior to definitive surgery. This is particularly so with large lesions and would take the form of an exploratory procedure with an incisional biopsy.

Ameloblastomas

These are the most common of the odontogenic tumours with many, including malignant, variants (see pathology texts for subclassification). They almost always present as a radiolucency (Fig. 8.7), often at the angle of the mandible and can, in some instances, be confused with the odontogenic keratocyst or dentigerous cyst. When they are small they can be unilocular but large lesions usually take on a multilocular appearance with a less well-defined border. Resorption of cortical bone and roots of adjacent teeth are common findings. Interestingly, despite the moderately aggressive growth pattern of these tumours, they rarely cause damage to the

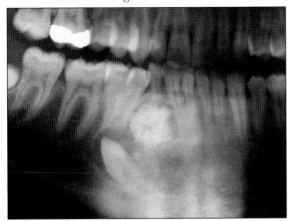

Fig. 8.6 Odontome lying above an unerupted canine and cyst.

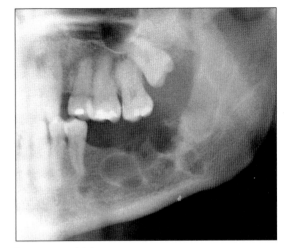

Fig. 8.7 Ameloblastoma.

neurovascular bundle, in the mandible. They tend to displace it as they enlarge, so that numbness of mental nerve distribution is a rare clinical feature compared with osteogenic malignancy or intraosseous secondary malignancies.

The most appropriate treatment is to resect the tumour with a margin of surrounding bone. For the ameloblastic fibroma conservative excision and for the unicystic ameloblastoma, enucleation alone may provide adequate treatment, but as with all this group, radiographic follow-up should be maintained for an indefinite period.

Odontogenic myxoma

This rare tumour can present with radiographic signs similar to ameloblastoma: sometimes it may display a 'soap bubble' appearance. It is benign but tends to extensively infiltrate the surrounding bone. Excision with extensive curettage may prevent recurrence but resection with a margin of bone may be required.

Adenomatoid odontogenic tumour and odontogenic fibroma

These uncommon tumours can be associated with unerupted teeth and may have tiny calcified areas. They are benign with a low potential for recurrence. Careful enucleation is usually curative.

Calcifying epithelial odontogenic tumour

This is a rare tumour usually presenting as a radiolucent area in the molar region of the mandible, but as its name suggests will have a radio-opaque element. In common with many other odontogenic tumours it has a malignant counterpart. It is locally invasive and resection with a margin of bone is recommended.

Cementifying lesions

Cementoblastomas are rare tumours and densely radio-opaque (not always homogeneous), and show a radiolucent rim in continuity with the periodontal space. They are attached to roots of vital teeth that may be resorbed and almost always occur in the first molar, or premolar region of the mandible. In contrast to most other odontogenic tumours they may present with pain.

They are benign and if the offending tooth is extracted and the lesion completely resected there should be no recurrence.

Cemento-osseous dysplasias form another group and as their name suggests are mixed and not neoplastic. They occur both as single and multiple lesions with a rare familial variant. It is important to note that they relate to apices of vital teeth and in early stages are radiolucent, mineralizing gradually as they mature. It is important therefore not to confuse them with dental cysts and apical granulomas.

Treatment of cemento-osseous dysplasia can be difficult and to be curative needs to be more extensive than would normally be associated with a reactive lesion. Indeed infection following attempts at surgical extraction may supervene, which can result in sequestration. Regular review is normally all that is required.

Osseous lesions

In common with the odontogenic lesions there is a wide variety of bony lesions ranging from discrete simple exostoses including tori (hamartomas) to rare benign growths, such as ossifying fibroma, to malignancies.

With the exception of tori, they are all considerably less common than odontogenic lesions but can present with the same signs including swellings of the jaw or displaced teeth. Radiographic findings are also similar with lesions presenting as radiolucencies, opacities or mixed appearance. Some, such as ossifying fibroma, have reasonably well-defined and corticated margins; others such as the giant-cell lesions are well defined but not corticated. Resorption of roots of adjacent teeth is associated with aggressive growth behaviour, but can occur with benign lesions and with giant cell lesions. Radiological features will be a major factor in making the diagnosis, but for most histological confirmation is necessary.

Also of note are discrete areas of dense bone within the cancellous architecture that are almost always a chance radiological finding. These are sometimes called enostoses or solitary bone islands and are most common in the mandible, though not related to the roots of teeth and do not exhibit a radiolucent rim. They are sometimes considered as the bone's response to low-grade infection but perhaps better seen as a variant of normal and therefore should be left alone. The larger and more diffuse conditions of Paget's disease, fibrous dysplasia and cherubism are rare and require specialist investigation and management (see below).

There are other intrabony lesions such as acute and chronic osteomyelitis, primary (osteogenic sarcoma) and secondary malignancies (myeloma, lymphoma and metastatic deposits from breast, bronchus, kidney, prostate or thyroid) and Langerhans cell histiocytosis, which can all present within the described spectrum of clinical and radiographic signs. It is important to be able to recognize the symptoms and signs that would warrant their inclusion in a differential diagnosis (see below).

The overlap of clinical and radiological signs makes diagnosis of this varied, complex and potentially dangerous group of lesions difficult. It is dependent on histology and sometimes other special investigations such as bone chemistry and specialist imaging such as CT and bone scans. In view of this and the often difficult decisions on treatment, and need for long-term follow-up, it is important to refer patients with these types of lesion.

Tori and exostoses

Tori and exostoses are common and non-neoplastic. They can occur singly or as multiple lesions in the midline of the palate or on the lingual aspects of the lower premolar region. In many situations they do not require any active treatment unless they are repeatedly traumatized or cause interference with the fit of dentures (see Ch. 11).

Osteomata and other benign tumours

Osteomata are benign tumours and as such will be progressive, usually as peripheral growths and should be excised. If multiple they may be a feature of Gardner's syndrome. They can present centrally with a radiographic appearance similar to that of solitary bone islands or even cementifying lesions. A rare variant is the osteoblastoma, a lesion of variable radiodensity that, like the cementoblastoma, can be painful and is also best excised. Larger lesions such as the ossifying fibroma can be treated with local excision and curettage but require long-term follow-up as recurrence is relatively common.

Giant-cell lesions

This group of lesions extend from what are considered non-neoplastic lesions such as the peripheral giant-cell granuloma (see above) and its central counterpart, to systemic lesions associated with hyperparathyroidism to rare tumours both benign and malignant.

The central giant-cell granuloma is a radiolucent soft-tissue mass arising within bone and notably has a well-defined margin that is not corticated. This derives from its osteoclastic origin, which in turn can result in resorption of adjacent teeth. It is indistinguishable histologically from the central bony masses of hyperparathyroidism. For that reason, if a histopathology report suggests a giant-cell lesion then plasma calcium, phosphate and parathormone levels should be checked to exclude hyperparathyroidism. Otherwise these are treated by local excision and curettage and this is usually successful. The true giant-cell tumour of bone is rare in the jaws; it requires a wide resection and reconstruction.

Cherubism

Cherubism is an inherited (autosomal dominant) disorder characterized by the development of bilateral symmetrical facial swellings. The swellings are composed mainly of fibrous tissue and giant cells. Cherubism is characteristically more common in males and presents in early childhood. Radiological findings are similar to those of multilocular cysts. Treatment is conservative as the lesions usually resolve as the bony tissues mature.

Fibrous dysplasia

Fibrous dysplasia, as its name suggests, is a non-neoplastic condition where bone is replaced by fibro-osseous tissue. It is of unknown aetiology but recent studies indicate a link with activating mutations affecting the alpha subunit of the g-protein GNAS1. The association is strongest with McCune-Albright syndrome but also is detected with polyostotic and monostotic fibrous dysplasia.

Fibrous dysplasia usually presents in young adults as a unilateral painless progressive swelling often affecting the maxilla. It can become disfiguring and may displace teeth and on occasion cause malocclusion. Both clinically and radiographically the margins are poorly defined and maxillary lesions can invade and obliterate the air sinus. Radiographic findings are slightly granular, medium radiodensity with loss of trabecular pattern ('ground glass' or 'orange peel' appearance) that blends into the surrounding bone. Although growth can be rapid, it is usual to defer treatment until bodily growth has ceased. At this stage the bone may be surgically reshaped for aesthetic purposes. Surgical interference during growth tends to be ineffective with recurrence almost inevitable. Uncommonly it may involve multiple sites (polyostotic). This is more common in females and can be associated with skin pigmentation and sexual precocity (McCune-Albright syndrome). There is a small risk of malignant (sarcomatous) change particularly in the polyostotic variant.

Paget's disease

Paget's disease of bone is a non-neoplastic disorder that may have a viral aetiology. It occurs in old age and whereas it may start in a single bone (monostotic), it almost always develops to involve multiple sites (polyostotic). Although most common in the lumbar spine, skull involvement is common, usually calvarium, with maxilla less common and mandible rare. Initially there is bone resorption and at this stage lesions are highly vascular. Later the bone becomes extremely dense. The level of activity of the disease may be measured with the plasma alkaline phosphatase level.

There are significant implications of Paget's disease for the dentist. In the early phase protracted bleeding may complicate extractions but later the increased bone density and the commonly associated hypercementosis can lead to difficult extractions. Deformity of bone may be evident extraorally and may interfere with the fit of dental prostheses. Bone pain can be a major problem and in extreme cases the high blood flow through active lesions can lead to 'high-output' cardiac failure. Surgical reduction is an option if there is significant oral deformity or functional impairment. The treatment of Paget's can include the use of bisphosphonate drugs, which have a high propensity to induce bony necrosis that is difficult if not impossible to treat (see Ch. 4).

Haemangioma

Intrabony haemangiomas are very rare and may present as solitary radiolucent lesions, which can in some cases be multilocular. They should always be considered in the differential diagnosis of large radiolucent areas in the jaws. They mimic cysts, giant-cell lesions and odontogenic tumours such as ameloblastomas. Aspiration should be carried out before definitive surgery to exclude haemangioma as surgery could, in high-flow lesions, lead to catastrophic haemorrhage. If a haemangioma is suspected (for instance, if there were a soft-tissue haemangioma close to the site of a radiolucency of bone), specialized imaging such as CT and angiography should be considered to define the extent of the lesion and the blood supply. Treatment, if appropriate, may extend from interventional radiology techniques such as embolization to formal surgical excision.

Intrabony and other malignancies

The most common malignant diseases in the mouth are oral squamous cell carcinoma (see Ch. 10) and salivary gland tumours (see Ch. 14).

As with any other part of the skeleton, the facial bones can be the origin of primary malignant disease such as sarcomas arising from bone or cartilage, or the site of a metastatic deposit or systemic malignant disease such as myeloma or lymphoma. In addition there is a group of diseases characterized by proliferation of antigen-presenting cells (Langerhans cell histiocytosis), which although not defined as malignant, in many ways behave as malignant disease. Readers are advised to refer to relevant pathological texts.

Because early diagnosis gives the best chance of curative treatment, it is essential that clinicians recognize the symptoms and signs that would depict malignancies of this type. Invasion with destruction of adjacent tissues is the hallmark of malignancy and is usually coupled with rapidly developing swelling. The classical clinical presentation is swelling of relatively short duration, loose and/or displaced teeth and dysaesthesia of the mental or other branches of the trigeminal nerve. Radiological signs also reflect this with irregular, 'moth-eaten' margins typical of sarcoma and secondary deposits or the circumscribed, but 'punched out' lesions suggesting multiple myeloma, all without cortication of the margin. The radiodensity will vary from totally radiolucent tumours such as myeloma, through mixed radiodensity seen with some osteosarcomas and chondrosarcomas, to the radio-opaque lesion typical of a secondary deposit from the prostate. It is important to remember that 'moth-eaten' margins with mixed radiodensity are also typical of osteomyelitis, osteoradionecrosis and bisphosphonate-induced bone necrosis. Nasopharyngeal tumours can present with painless hard enlarged cervical lymph nodes, unilateral deafness, mandibular/lingual nerve dysaesthesia and chronic progressive trismus (Trotter's syndrome). Prompt diagnosis is paramount and all of the above require urgent referral.

Even though these diseases are very rare, clinicians must maintain an index of suspicion and either arrange urgent referral or, if in doubt, contact specialists directly and discuss the clinical findings. Diagnosis of this group of diseases is complex and usually requires specialist biopsy and imaging techniques and therefore they should not be biopsied in general practice.

Summary: hard-tissue lesions

- Odontomes should be removed if infected or preventing orthodontic tooth movement
- Exostoses and tori require removal only if they are traumatized, or interfere with function or construction of dentures
- Intrabony lesions are diagnosed on radiological appearance and biopsy: true neoplasia will require excision
- Haemangiomas very occasionally occur in bone presenting as radiolucencies and should be considered in the differential diagnosis
- Intrabony malignancies, primary and secondary, are rare but can mimic other pathology

---

BIOPSY

Biopsy is defined as the complete or partial removal of a lesion for laboratory examination to aid definitive diagnosis. Whereas biopsy usually establishes the definitive diagnosis, there are occasions when the result is not clear and in these circumstances the available histological data must be measured against clinical findings.

Biopsy techniques

Excisional biopsy

This is the ideal approach for small superficial lesions less than 1 cm in diameter, where the **clinical appearance suggests that it is benign**. Most if not all of these procedures can be performed using local anaesthesia (LA). Where regional blocks are not performed, the local anaesthetic should be injected at a distance from the lesion to avoid distortion of the tissue at the operating site.

Excisional biopsy of superficial lesions

Superficial lesions such as fibroepithelial polyps and squamous papillomas that are pedunculated (arising from a narrow stalk) can be excised by simple division of the base of the pedicle where it arises from the mucosa. For papillomas that have a viral aetiology some surgeons like to use electrosurgery. For larger and sessile lesions (broad-based) excision should be based on an elliptical incision (Fig. 8.8a). This is made around the base of the lesion (No. 15 blade) and should include a 1- to 2-mm margin of normal tissue. Choice of such an incision is aimed at

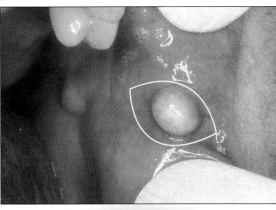

(a)

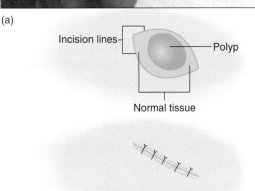

(b)

Fig. 8.8 (a) Excisional biopsy of a polyp, leaving an elliptical wound. (b) Closure of the wound, as a straight line without 'dog-ears'.

creating a wound that will appose (Fig. 8.8b) without redundant tissue (dog ears) and close without tension, because the ellipse needs to be at least twice as long as it is broad. A suture may be placed at the edge of the ellipse to hold the tissue. This will avoid crushing the specimen with tissue forceps. It can be used to retract the specimen during dissection with scissors or scalpel. When dissecting the specimen free it is important to avoid damaging underlying structures such as blood vessels and nerves by using 'blunt dissection' (described below).

Excisional biopsy of submucosal lesions

To excise submucosal lesions the covering mucosa needs to be divided to develop access and establish the plane of dissection. This is therefore more complicated than excision of superficial lesions. The orientation of the incision will be along the longest dimension of the lesion but must also take into account anatomical relationships such as the opening of the parotid duct or the mental nerve. For large or superficial lesions such as mucous cysts that have thinned the mucosa this technique can be modified to an elliptical incision to include a portion of the covering mucosa. This will reduce the risk of rupture, or perforation of the lesion at the superficial aspect, but will mean sacrificing the overlying mucosa.

To avoid distortion the outline of the incision can be marked using a surgical pen before the introduction of LA. The initial incision should divide the mucosa but not penetrate the specimen, so the depth will vary depending on the site and depth of the lesion. Superficial lesions covered by thin mucosa, as found in the floor of the mouth or lower lip, will require very careful work to avoid related anatomical structures. Following the incision, a combination of sharp and blunt dissection is required to define the plane of dissection and then deliver the lesion. In the main, blunt dissection is advised as it will define the tissue plane around the lesion and avoid damage to adjacent structures such as blood vessels and nerves.

In this technique blunt-ended scissors are introduced into the tissues at the margin of the lesion with the points together. The points are then separated, forcing the tissues apart along their natural planes and the instrument is withdrawn with the blades open so there is no cutting action. The process is best started away from the 'thin' covering mucosa or superficial part of the lesion as it is easier to get the plane identified and started. Dissection is then repeated from various angles to 'develop' the plane all around the lesion. As required, sharp dissection either with a scalpel or by cutting with scissors may also be used to finally deliver the specimen. During this stage of the process great care must be taken to prevent damage to adjacent and underlying structures, and to avoid perforating the lesion.

Incisional biopsy

This technique is indicated in cases where the diagnosis is in doubt (i.e. possible malignancy or potential for recurrence) and complete excision, in one stage under LA, is impractical in terms of size, complexity and/or the patient's ability to cope with the surgery.

Incisional biopsy of superficial lesions

In the hospital context, if there is a suspicion of malignancy, the biopsy must be taken from a representative part of the lesion and include a suitable edge of normal tissue. This allows the sample to be held at the normal tissue margin and thereby avoids introducing surgical artifact. It also gives some idea of the pattern of invasion at the interface. An elliptical incision is suitable, with a sharp dissection technique using a scalpel and scissors.

If the biopsy is of a mucosal lesion such as leukoplakia, it is important to take a deep enough specimen to get into connective tissue (approx. 6 mm) (Fig. 8.9) and to take a broad enough piece, so that after processing there will still be sufficient for a number of complete sections to be cut from it in the laboratory (at least 4 mm). Where the field of mucosal abnormality is extensive, it may be necessary to carry out multiple incisional biopsies. If this technique is carried out, it is important to draw a diagram of the lesion to make orientation clear for the pathologist.

Incisional biopsy of submucosal lesions

For large, solid submucosal swellings, particularly in the palate where the risk of minor salivary gland malignancy is high, incisional biopsy is often the procedure of choice but this decision carries significant implications for further management and therefore should be left to specialists.

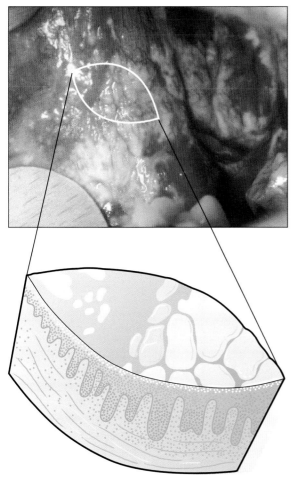

Fig. 8.9 Incisional biopsy should include a portion of normal tissue and should be large enough in all dimensions to ensure that the pathologist can see the margin of the pathological area and have sufficient tissue to take multiple sections.

Soft-tissue repair

Haemostasis is the essential first step and a period of pressure followed by suturing will achieve this in most cases. If necessary, electrocoagulation can be used but with care in areas such as the lips where nerves are superficial. Careful wound closure is important and choice of suture depends on the thickness of the mucosa. In most cases interrupted sutures using a 3/0 resorbable material on a 22-mm half-circle cutting needle is indicated but for thin mucosa such as the inside of the lip or floor of the mouth a 4/0 suture is advised.

The tension of the sutures is important and they need to be tight enough to appose the wound edges firmly but not so tight as to impair the blood supply (wound blanching). Deep sutures are only required if there is a second layer, such as tongue muscle, to repair. When repairing lip incisions avoid placing the suture through the deeper tissue as this could damage adjacent structures such as other minor salivary glands and nerves. Similarly avoid multiple or tight sutures in the floor of the mouth close to the opening of the sublingual and submandibular glands to avoid strictures.

Repairing biopsy wounds involving mucoperiosteum such as hard palate mucosa is problematic in that the wound edges cannot be approximated. They require a pack of haemostatic gauze, or other dressing such as a Whitehead's varnish (Compound Iodoform Paint) pack or a periodontal wound dressing placed over the defect, possibly supported by a healing plate. In some cases it may be preferable to cover the defect either by an advancement or transposition flap of adjacent mucosa.

Other biopsy techniques

Punch biopsy

A circular blade can be used to remove a cylindrical core of tissue as a form of incisional biopsy: this *punch biopsy* technique is more commonly used on skin.

Trephines

In this technique a core of tissue is trephined from the lesion. It may be used for soft-tissue swellings or bone. This provides sufficient material, retaining tissue architecture, for histological diagnosis and is useful for lesions where access may be difficult.

Cytology

This technique is based on microscopic sampling of tissue either by fine needle aspiration (FNA) or by using an abrasive technique such as brush or swab (exfoliative cytology). Both aim to remove cells representative of the lesion, which are then transferred to microscope slides and prepared for histo-cytological assay. These are investigations that require special equipment and skill in both taking the sample and preparing the slides and, as such, are best referred to operators with the appropriate experience. All such methods lack the advantage of maintaining tissue architecture, but offer a relatively quick and minimally invasive approach to biopsy.

Aspiration biopsy

Fine-needle aspiration cytology is a useful method for sampling soft-tissue masses in the head and neck, such as lymph nodes and salivary glands. A 10- or 20-mL syringe with a 21-gauge needle is installed into a specially designed holder which facilitates the safe and controlled introduction of the needle, and allows aspiration at variable pressures. The needle is inserted into the centre of the deep tissue mass and the plunger pulled back, drawing a small 'core' tissue sample into the needle. The needle tip is re-sited within the lesion and the procedure repeated several times. The sample is then delivered directly onto a microscope slide, spread and fixed. This is a valuable method but technique sensitive. Accurate sampling is clearly essential and on occasions where the lesion is deep it can be combined with ultrasound investigation to ensure the needle is positioned within the lesion (ultrasound-guided FNA).

Smears

Cytological smears can be used to sample the surface of epithelial lesions, especially where the lesion is not heavily keratinized, in which case it is possible to harvest cells deeper within the epithelium. The technique could be used as an adjunct to biopsy for monitoring widespread lesions, which may undergo malignant transformation. A diagnosis of malignancy based on cytology alone would be considered insufficient by most pathologists and formal histological sampling would be required before proceeding to cancer treatment.

Care of the specimen

The key to a successful biopsy is the presentation of either the entire lesion or a representative sample of tissue uncontaminated and of good quality. The sample must not be allowed to dry out and should be placed immediately in a tissue fixative (usually 10% neutral buffered formalin). These are pre-requisites for the pathologist to have tissue adequately pre-pared for histological interpretation. However, if special immunohistochemical techniques such as immunofluorescence are required, the tissue sample requires special processing and needs to be referred

---

Methods of biopsy

- **Excisional:** complete removal with surrounding normal tissue (width and depth)—for small and *presumed benign lesions*
- **Incisional:** removal of a portion of normal and abnormal tissue—for larger lesions to establish the diagnosis and subsequent treatment options including potentially malignant lesions
- **Punch:** core of abnormal tissue—rarely performed in the mouth
- **Trephine:** Removes core of tissue suitable for deep-seated lesions
- **Aspiration:** fine-needle aspiration cytology, for deep soft-tissue lesions, such as potentially malignant neck lymph nodes; technique sensitive
- **Cytology:** abrasive removal of superficial cells (±) deeper cells

---

to a hospital department. Some pathologists prefer to receive all specimens fresh, on saline-soaked gauze, provided the specimen reaches the laboratory within one hour of being taken.

In the UK there are strict regulations governing transport of the specimen to the laboratory if sent by post: all the appropriate regulations should be adhered to.

Completing a pathology request form

- Patient details: name, gender, race, age, address, medical and social history
- Clinical details
    History: symptoms, previous biopsy and treatment
    Examination: signs, size, shape, position, texture, colour
- Investigations: microbiology, haematology, radiology
- Biopsy type
- Previous biopsy number/s
- Orientation: use a diagram
- Clinical diagnosis

Also ensure that the specimen pot is clearly marked with the patient's name and other identification information (such as hospital number or date of birth)

Biopsy in general dental practice

For the practitioner to proceed with surgery he/she must have the appropriate skills to be able to complete the procedure and to deal with intraoperative and postoperative complications.

Generally excisional biopsy of superficial benign lesions is suitable for general dental practice with the more complicated submucosal excisional biopsies dependent on the training and experience of the individual. Solid submucosal lesions have a high probability of being a tumour and are best referred.

Incisional procedures by definition are aimed at establishing diagnosis. This will then raise issues with continuing care, the interpretation of potential for malignant change and the advisability of further treatment including major surgery. These points and the possibility of a diagnosis of malignancy would suggest that patients requiring this type of biopsy would be best referred.

As with all proposed treatment the patient needs to be able to give informed consent and with surgery this should be written consent. It requires clear explanation of the nature and significance of the problem, possible treatment options and the risks and benefits of surgery in contrast to no active treatment. Should the option be to refer the patient then the letter must be clear and concise and if there are concerns about a possible malignancy the specialist should be contacted by phone.

Refer patients for biopsy if:

- You lack appropriate skills/training, equipment and transport medium
- You feel that due to position and size of lesion you are unsure that you will be able to harvest a representative sample and/or repair the biopsy site
- The lesion is blistering or bullous (these require special handling of samples and/or transport medium) or if you suspect the lesion to be vascular
- You suspect the lesion to be malignant
- You are concerned about co-morbidity and/or the patients' ability to cope with the procedure

---

FURTHER READING

Barnes L. (ed.) (2005) *Pathology and genetics of head and neck tumours.* IARC Press, Lyon, France.

Cawson R. A., Binnie W. H., Barrett A. W., Wright J. M. (2001) *Oral disease clinical and pathological correlations*, 3rd edn. Mosby, St Louis, MO, Chs. 6, 7, 8 & 10.

Kramer I. R. H., Pindborg J. J., Shear M. (1992) *Histological typing of odontogenic tumours.* Springer Verlag, Heidelberg, Germany.

Peterson L. J., Ellis E., Hupp J. R., Tucker M. R. (eds.) (1997) *Contemporary oral and maxillofacial surgery*, 3rd edn. Mosby, St Louis, MO, Ch. 23, pp. 512–532.

Waites E. (2002) *Essentials of dental radiography and radiology*, 3rd edn. Harcourt Health Sciences, Edinburgh.

SELF-ASSESSMENT

1. A patient presents with a firm, pink, soft-tissue swelling, 4 mm in diameter, on the buccal-attached gingiva in the lower premolar region, which has been present for 6 months and causes difficulty with hygiene in the area.
   (a) What is the most likely diagnosis?
   (b) How would you treat it?
2. A 28-year-old male patient presents with a white, roughened, raised lump 5×5 mm^2 on the lateral border of his tongue that has been present, unchanged, for 8 months.
   (a) How would you confirm your diagnosis?
   (b) Describe how you would perform this investigation.
   (c) What would you do with the specimen?
   (d) What information would you wish to receive from the pathologist?
3. A patient presents concerned about a raised lump at the junction of the anterior two-thirds and posterior third of the tongue dorsum.
   (a) What information would you wish to elicit from the history of the present complaint?
   (b) What information would you wish to elicit when examining the lesion?
   (c) Suggest a possible diagnosis.

4. A 70-year-old patient presents with a rounded, bony hard, pink swelling of 2×2 cm^2 in the midline of the palate which is asymptomatic and has been present for many years.
   (a) What is the probable diagnosis?
   (b) Why is it unlikely to be a salivary neoplasm?
   (c) How would you treat it?

5. List the key aims in designing the incisions for biopsy of a suspected malignancy.

6. What investigations should be arranged for a suspected haemangioma of the jaw?

Answers on page 265.

9 | Cysts

J. Marley
C. G. Cowan

- A variety of cysts occur in the orofacial region and often present first to the general dental practitioner.
- Cysts are usually classified as odontogenic or non-odontogenic in origin and may present within the hard and soft tissues of the head and neck region.
- Other lesions; benign and malignant, can present with similar clinical and radiological findings (see Ch. 8). Histology is required to establish the diagnosis.
- There are two methods of treatment: *enucleation*, a one-stage procedure to remove the entire cyst, and *marsupialization*, a method of decompressing the cyst by converting it into a pouch.
- Small cysts are best treated with primary enucleation.
- Marsupialization is often the most appropriate treatment for extensive lesions, particularly for the elderly and/or patients with significant co-morbidity or if the cyst is infected or in close proximity to important anatomical structures.

ASSUMED KNOWLEDGE

It is assumed that at this stage you will have knowledge/competencies in the following areas:

- anatomy of the face and jaws

- WHO classification of odontogenic tumours and cysts
- pathological and radiological appearance of cysts and other benign oral lesions
- practice of surgical endodontics (apicectomy) (see Ch. 6).

If you feel you are not competent in these areas, revise them before reading this chapter or cross-check with relevant texts as you read.

INTENDED LEARNING OUTCOMES

At the end of this chapter you should be able to:

1. Recognize cysts according to clinical symptoms and signs, anatomical site and radiographic appearance
2. Develop a differential diagnosis based on the clinical features, anatomical site and radiographic findings
3. Understand the principles of surgical management relating to both enucleation and marsupialization
4. Propose treatment options according to probable diagnosis, anatomical relationships and size of lesion
5. Understand the level of operator experience required for surgery and recognize cases that will require referral

6. Either alone or in conjunction with a specialist, advise patients concerning the nature and effects of their disease, its treatment and any follow-up regimen.

OVERVIEW

Cysts of the face and jaws are common and present a wide variation in type. The vast majority of cysts are intrabony and odontogenic in origin and these will form the basis of this chapter with minor reference to the rarer soft-tissue cysts, e.g. dermoid and branchial cysts.

By definition true cysts are developmental or reactive lesions with the vast majority growing by fluid accumulation. This gives them their benign characteristics with the typical resorption of bone and displacement of adjacent structures such as the neurovascular bundle as a result of the pressure effect, properties that are common to benign tumours as well. There are, however, some cysts that grow by cell proliferation, e.g. the odontogenic keratocyst, and they tend to behave in a more aggressive manner with recurrence common. This cyst has been re-classified as a locally invasive tumour (Philipsen 2005), although it should be noted that unlike most tumours, this condition can be successfully treated by partial removal (see below concerning marsupialization). In addition there are tumours, locally invasive and true malignancies, that can appear cystic on presentation, e.g. ameloblastoma, adenoid cystic carcinoma and some sarcomas. Malignant change in cysts has been reported but is a very rare occurrence.

Despite these variations, presenting symptoms and signs tend to be similar. The principles of management are dictated by predicted behaviour, which in turn is dependent on histological type.

This chapter will be confined to clinical diagnosis and principles of treatment of the commonly occurring cysts of the mouth and jaws.

DEFINITION

A cyst is a pathological cavity usually lined by epithelium with fluid or semifluid contents, not created by the accumulation of pus.

DIAGNOSIS

Presenting symptoms and signs

Intrabony cysts may remain symptomless for many years and only come to light as an incidental finding on routine dental inspection or radiographic investigation (Fig. 9.1) or can present in a variety of ways described below.

Association with teeth

Radicular (dental) cysts are the most common of all cysts and are associated with a non-vital root of a tooth. Ectopic teeth can often be associated with cysts either as the primary cause as with the dentigerous cyst (Fig. 9.2) or when displaced by a cyst, such as an odontogenic keratocyst. It is important to appreciate that other more significant conditions, e.g. ameloblastoma, may also present in this manner (see Ch. 8).

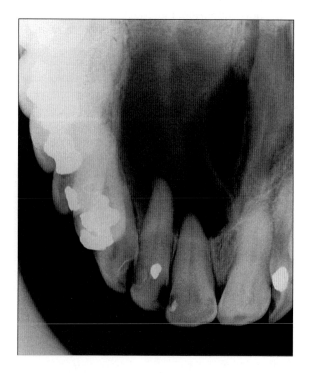

Fig. 9.1 Occlusal radiograph of a radicular (dental) cyst, displaying a well-defined radiolucency arising from a non-vital upper lateral incisor.

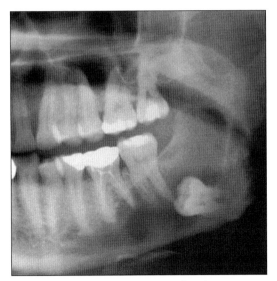

Fig. 9.2 A dentigerous cyst associated with an unerupted lower third molar.
Note the margin of the cyst at the amelocemental junction.

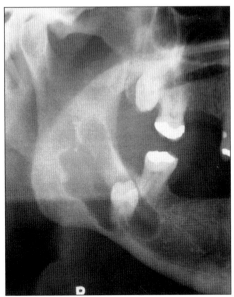

Fig. 9.3 An odontogenic keratocyst at the angle of the mandible.

Site

Many cysts show a predilection for specific areas. For example, 75% of odontogenic keratocysts present at the mandibular angle (Fig. 9.3) whilst 88% of glandular odontogenic cysts occur at the anterior mandible (Cawson et al. 2001). Some cysts are completely site-specific such as the nasopalatine duct cyst, which arises from tissues within the incisive canal, and the paradental cyst, which is associated with impacted lower third molars. Also of note is the group of cysts that present in the gingival area including the inflammatory lateral periodontal cyst (a variant of a radicular cyst), the true lateral periodontal cyst, the peripheral odontogenic keratocyst and gingival cyst of adults. These classically present coronal to the apices and in-between teeth in the premolar areas.

Site is also a major diagnostic feature for the rare soft-tissue cysts, particularly the developmental dermoid, nasolabial and thyroglossal duct cysts (see below).

Swelling

Swelling is a common presenting complaint and if extensive can cause both intraoral and extraoral asymmetry. Importantly the swelling is normally clinically discrete and well demarcated. Where there has been extensive expansion of the cyst the overlying bone will be thin or absent. In the former, the surface will feel firm but flexible, but if the overlying bone has been completely eroded it will appear as a tense bluish swelling that feels 'fluctuant' (Fig. 9.4) (see Ch. 7 for a description of fluctuance).

Patterns of growth and anatomical site

How the cyst grows and the anatomical site will dictate the extent and presentation of swelling. Cysts will expand quicker through cancellous and thin cortical bone and so tend to present sooner in the anterior region than in the posterior mandible. In contrast, the late presentation of cysts in the

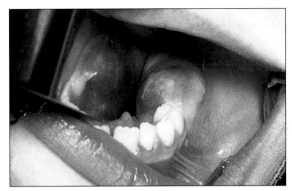

Fig. 9.4 Bluish swelling associated with an eruption cyst on a lower first molar.

posterior mandible/maxilla reflects cysts spreading along cancellous bone or into the maxillary air sinus respectively, thus making clinically obvious swelling a late feature. This can be of major significance in terms of making the initial diagnosis, primary management and follow-up, particularly for keratocysts where recurrence is common.

Cysts that develop by fluid accumulation and consequent hydrostatic pressure, e.g. inflammatory and dentigerous cysts, will develop spherically and so expand through cortical bone relatively early. In contrast, odontogenic keratocysts grow by cellular proliferation. Expansion tends be to a late feature, with the keratocyst preferentially expanding within the cancellous bone, leading to a greater antero-posterior dimension on radiographic examination.

Pain

Pain is uncommon and is usually indicative of acute infection. This can arise in any of the cyst types but is more likely in radicular cysts, which have an inflammatory aetiology. On rare occasions large mandibular cysts that become infected cause dysaesthesia in the inferior alveolar nerve distribution or acute sinusitis in the case of an infected maxillary cyst.

Lobulation

Where a radiolucency displays lobulation it is strongly suggestive of the keratocyst (Fig. 9.3), which has a pattern of cyst growth with 'invasion' of lining epithelium through the cancellous bone space leaving behind isthmi of bone.

Associated signs/symptoms

As well as eroding bone, cysts can affect the adjacent structures, teeth and neurovascular structures. Erupted teeth are occasionally loosened or displaced, sometimes enough to disrupt the occlusion or alter the shape of the alveolus and the fit of a prosthesis. Rarely cysts can resorb teeth (infection increasing the risk). In extreme cases mandibular cysts can cause so much destruction of bone that a pathological fracture occurs (Fig. 9.5).

Clinical features of jaw cysts
• Often none at all (chance finding on X-ray)   • Swelling (usually bony, smooth but later soft, bluish and fluctuant)   • Displacement of teeth   • Increased mobility of teeth   • Evidence of a cause (missing or non-vital teeth, infection)   • Rarely pathological fracture

Special investigations

Radiology is a key investigation in determining the diagnosis and the extent and anatomical relationships of the lesion. It is therefore important in treatment planning and issues relating to consent. Simple plain films such as orthopantomogram (OPT), periapical and occlusal views are normally sufficient but for extensive cysts, particularly if they may be extending into soft tissue (e.g. the lingual area or the maxillary

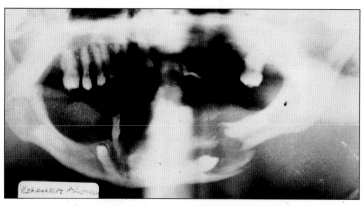

Fig. 9.5   An extensive cyst with a fracture of the mandible.

sinus and pterygoid regions), advanced imaging such as CT will be required. For further details of the radiological features of cysts, readers are referred to standard texts on dental and maxillofacial radiology. However, the general radiological features of cysts can be summarized as radiolucencies with a well-defined, corticated margin. The features of site, shape, relationship to teeth and whether there is any lobulation will all contribute to the diagnosis.

The rare soft-tissue cysts—branchial, thyroglossal and dermoid—need specialist investigation, which may include ultrasound, CT and MRI scanning.

Given the variety of cysts with their differing propensity to recur and the possibility of other cyst-mimicking pathology, a definite diagnosis is essential.

All cyst specimens should therefore be submitted for histological examination (see Ch. 8). Often this takes the form of an excisional biopsy when establishment of the histological diagnosis is coupled with complete removal of the lesion. For larger lesions it is essential to match the cyst type to the appropriate surgical treatment so it is sometimes best to perform an incisional biopsy to establish diagnosis before considering major surgery.

The diagnosis of cysts in the upper premolar and molar regions can be problematic given the relation of the maxillary antrum. On occasions aspiration biopsy can be of value in confirming presence of a cyst. This involves a small incision through the mucosa to expose the appropriate area and depending on the thickness of bone, either direct introduction of a wide-bore needle or use of a bone drill can facilitate this. Aspiration of air indicates the maxillary sinus.

Differential diagnosis of radiolucencies of the jaws

- Cysts: well defined, corticated, locular/multilocular/multilobular, displacement of adjacent structures
- Central giant-cell granuloma: well-defined boundary, not corticated
- Ameloblastoma: multilocular/unilocular, defined or diffuse edge, usually displaces adjacent structures, may resorb roots of adjacent teeth
- Ossifying fibroma: diffuse edge, mixed radiolucency/opacity
- Myxoma: soap bubble
- Multiple myeloma: multiple, punched out, rounded but not corticated

---

Fluid aspiration indicates a cyst, with mucus being suggestive of an antral mucosal cyst, straw-coloured fluid with cholesterol crystals a dental cyst and pus an infected cyst or sinus infection. No aspirate may mean the cyst contents are too viscous to be aspirated but significantly it may indicate a solid lesion and therefore a possible neoplasm.

PRINCIPLES OF TREATMENT

Depending on the experience of the operator, patients with small cysts can be treated under local anaesthesia, with or without sedation, in general dental practice. The specimen should be sent for histological analysis to confirm diagnosis and consequently whether recurrence is likely. Large lesions may require more complex investigations and treatment, best undertaken in hospital, with surgery performed under general anaesthesia.

The need to remove teeth associated with a cyst depends upon the diagnosis. Teeth are routinely retained when removing radicular cysts provided they have had good preoperative endodontics and have a good prognosis postoperatively in terms of periodontal support and suitability for restoration. However, teeth that are significantly resorbed, have been grossly displaced, lie within the cyst or significantly inhibit access to the cyst may also need to be removed.

There are two methods of treating cysts: *enucleation* and *marsupialization*.

Radiological features

- Well-defined radiolucency with a **corticated** margin
- Possibly unilocular or multilocular (or multilobular)
- Relationship with teeth
  —Radicular
  —Dentigerous relationship (dentigerous cysts and keratocysts)
  —Capable of displacing or resorbing teeth
- Relationship with adjacent structures
  —Usually displaces inferior alveolar canal
  —Extends into and displaces maxillary antrum
- Radiological signs similar to those of other lesions, cf ameloblastoma, etc. (Ch. 8)

Enucleation

Enucleation involves the complete removal of a cyst lining (Fig. 9.6). It is best used for small to medium-sized cysts and is dependent on the establishment of a blood clot in the cavity, its subsequent organization and its eventual replacement with new bone. The main limiting factor is size. Extensive defects will give rise to large clots and are prone to becoming secondarily infected with subsequent wound breakdown. The presence of pre-existing infection will also compromise primary healing. If acute the infection should be treated prior to surgery, or if chronic, by careful wound management or by marsupialization.

The cyst lining should be carefully separated from the surrounding structures in an attempt to remove the lesion intact. The success of enucleation depends on adequate access through the overlying mucoperiosteum and bone. An incision is made well clear of the margins of the cyst to ensure that the wound margin will lie on sound bone postoperatively. Access usually requires some bone removal. But if the overlying bone is thin an access point can be gained by a curette to carefully pick off a small portion of bone and allow the insinuation of a periosteal elevator under the bone edge to develop a plane of dissection. The cyst lining can then be gently pushed away and the access extended with bone nibblers. Thick bony plates are best removed by cutting an outline window with a bur. This is not extended completely through to the cyst but fractured and levered up and away from the underlying cyst using a thin periosteal elevator or a Warwick-James elevator. Again, the cyst can be separated from the bone and the access widened with surgical burs. Avoid using bone nibblers on thick plates of bone as it is possible to fracture the plate of bone.

It is important to carefully dissect away the overlying bone and expose the cyst lining without tearing it. Curettes such as a Mitchell's trimmer or Cumine Scaler are useful in teasing away the cyst lining from

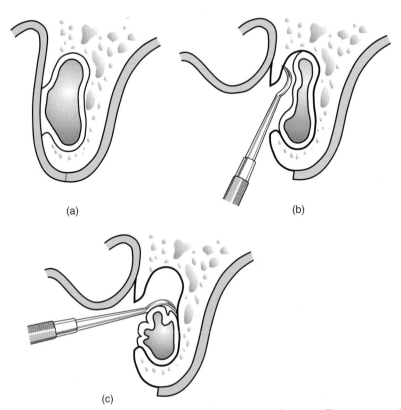

(a)

(b)

(c)

Fig. 9.6 (a–c) Cyst enucleation using a Mitchell's trimmer, with the convex surface initially in contact with the cyst and the edge against bone.

the underlying bone, but it is important to keep the edge of the instrument against bone to develop the plane of dissection around the cyst. Chronically infected cysts can be difficult as their linings may be firmly adherent to the bone, and/or the mucoperiosteal flap or adjacent palatal mucoperiosteum. In such instances it is essential to develop the plane of dissection around the margins and develop exposure using sharp and blunt dissection techniques to separate the cyst lining from the bone and soft tissues (see Ch. 8).

Healing is dependent on organization and eventual replacement of the blood clot with new bone, so wound repair and postoperative care must focus on this. The cavity must be checked to ensure all remnants of cyst lining or contents and fragments of bone are removed, particularly so if the cyst was infected. It is also important to reduce any sharp edges of the bony cavity as they can ulcerate through later and compromise healing. This can be done with bone files or carefully with a surgical bur and in principle the less bone removed the better. The edges can be checked by replacing the flap and palpating the margins; if they feel sharp through the flap they will need further attention.

Haemostasis is essential as haematomas under the flap will cause swelling and bruising that will delay healing and they are prone to infection. It is important therefore to identify any bleeding points. For general bleeding from the bony cavity a pressure pack (for 5 to 10 minutes) or bone wax for specific points will normally suffice. Soft-tissue bleeding can be controlled with diathermy but must be used with care if close to nerves. If there is persistent bleeding it is usually from the bony cavity and on occasions may need definitive packing. This can be in the form of resorbable haemostatic agents or packing such as ribbon gauze dressed with Whitehead's varnish or other antiseptic, which will need to be removed. For the former it is still appropriate to proceed with primary closure of the cavity but breakdown of the clot is now more likely and the patient should be warned about the signs of infection, pain, swelling and, depending on the site, dysaesthesia. If a non-resorbable pack is used, the treatment has, in effect, been converted to a multistage procedure. Although the cyst has not been marsupialized it will now require similar management (see below). In this case, as the cavity has no epithelial lining, initial removal of

the pack can be very painful as the pack tends to be stuck down to the raw bone and 'solid' with blood. Once the cavity granulates and develops a lining it is managed as a marsupialized cyst and dressing changes are simple and wound healing generally quite quick (see below). For large cavities an external pressure dressing (for 12 hours) taped to the skin can help to reduce risk of haematomas and swelling.

Adjunctive care

To reduce the chance of wound breakdown a course of antibiotics is usually appropriate. For small cysts this may be confined to a preoperative dose with follow-up cover for 12 hours but for extensive and/or infected lesions a 5-day course is required. Appropriate analgesia must be prescribed. Both analgesia and the choice of antibiotic will be dependent on clinical history. It is noteworthy that over-packing of the cavity can result in severe postoperative pain. This results from the already 'tight' pack expanding with the attendant inflammation. As a general rule if there is severe pain from a packed cavity, shorten but do not remove the pack and this often alleviates symptoms.

Marsupialization

Marsupialization involves the surgical excision of the superficial part of the cyst lining to convert the cavity into a pouch (Fig. 9.7). It is based on the principle that cysts will shrink to smaller more manageable size when decompressed. In some cases this process continues and the lesion resolves completely without further intervention but many require secondary surgery to remove the residual lining.

Indications

It is an ideal treatment when the cyst is large and the resultant defect from enucleation would be too large to heal by primary intention or may even require bone grafting; similarly so for infected cysts, where primary closure of the wound would not be an option. The technique also minimizes the potential for damage to adjacent structures, such as the inferior alveolar nerve during the enucleation of large cysts at the angle of the mandible, or the apices of vital teeth where the cyst extends up around

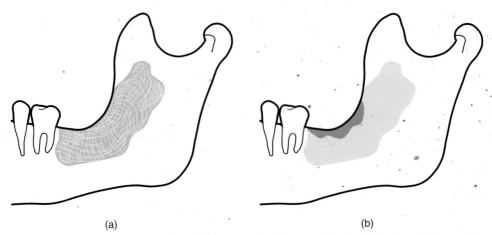

Fig. 9.7 (a) Marsupialization followed by packing of the cavity. (b) After a period of months the cavity has reduced in size; enucleation at this stage would be a much smaller operation.

them. As it can be done under local anaesthetic it is suitable for treating large lesions in elderly patients or those with major co-morbidity, thus avoiding a major procedure and a general anaesthetic. In addition, as marsupialization involves the excision of the superficial portion of the cyst lining it will establish a histological diagnosis that will determine treatment. This will also prevent more significant lesions such as ameloblastomas being enucleated rather that resected. The main drawbacks are that although the primary procedure is relatively simple there is a protracted follow-up treatment with multiple pack changes.

The first step is to create a mucoperiosteal flap that will expose the cyst or the overlying bone. The key objective is to establish an opening into the cyst that when healed will maintain a wide opening into the residual cavity (Fig. 9.8). If the opening is too small the cyst will tend to close over and therefore reform, or the opening will become a narrow inlet to the large underlying cavity. If the lumen is too narrow then the cavity cannot be adequately packed and it will also be difficult, if not impossible, to prevent infection. Also, as the wound heals there will be significant shrinkage in the size of the lumen established at operation, so adequate exposure is essential.

The cyst contents are then removed and the residual cavity packed with ribbon gauze dressed with Whitehead's varnish or bismuth iodoform paraffin paste (BIPP) and left open. In some cases dentures can

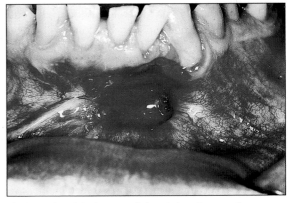

Fig. 9.8 A residual mucosal depression, 2 years after marsupialization of a 10-cm diameter cyst.

be modified, or prostheses made, to allow a temporary obturation. The wound will then heal to form an epithelial-lined pouch composed of the residual cyst lining which is then in continuity with the oral mucosa. There now follows a series of follow-up visits to change the pack and this can, depending on the size of the defect and healing potential of the patient, take anything from 3 to 12 months with pack changes every 2 to 3 weeks. The objective during this period is to pack just enough to maintain the opening but not impede healing. Patients often report the pack coming out and when the cavity is shallow enough that it can be irrigated to be kept clean, packing can be stopped. Some surgeons use a bung made of acrylic (Fig. 9.9) or periodontal

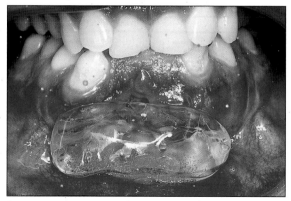

Fig. 9.9 An acrylic bung occluding the entrance to a marsupialized cyst cavity.

packing material to hold the wound entrance open, after initial pack removal, with the patient being required to wash the wound out after meals, rather than repeatedly packing the wound.

The decision about secondary surgery will depend on cyst type and speed of healing. Many surgeons will remove the marsupialized residue of cysts, such as keratocysts, which carry a significant recurrence rate, or any cyst which has not significantly closed in 12 months.

Treatment of jaw cysts

Enucleation

- A one-stage procedure to remove the entire cyst
- Suitable for small to medium-sized cysts
- Risk of damage to adjacent structures
- Removal of extensive lesions leaves large cavity prone to infection

Marsupialization

- Multistage procedure
- Less extensive surgery
- Prolonged healing period
- Protects vitality of teeth and integrity of nerves
- May require secondary surgery to remove residual lining

CYSTS AND THE MAXILLARY ANTRUM

In dealing with cysts that extend into the maxillary antrum, treatment options depend on the size of the cyst and whether it is infected. Small cysts can be enucleated and closed as a primary procedure provided the sinus has not been perforated. If, however, the cyst is large and has significantly encroached into the sinus or even replaced or obliterated the maxillary sinus then the resultant cavity will be too big to heal by primary intention. In such cases the preferred option is to marsupialize the cyst into the sinus rather than into the oral cavity, allowing the sinus to reform. The cyst cavity is therefore closed on the oral side and opened through into the antrum. This requires careful excision of the adjacent portion of the antral lining and on some occasions it will require the removal of a section of the bony periphery that delineated cyst from sinus. With large cysts, care must be taken to ensure that the orbital floor and infraorbital nerve are not compromised. The sinus will reform to include the cyst cavity. An intranasal antrostomy is often required to make sure that the antrum can drain, as a large 'closed cavity' will become infected.

FOLLOW-UP

Follow-up is required during the immediate postoperative phase for all cysts. At this stage the objective is to ensure that the wound heals (enucleation) and that the packing changes to establish the epithelialized cavity (marsupialization). In the former, should the wound break down, the cavity should be opened and packed, effectively converting the procedure to a form of marsupialization. The length of follow-up for simple cysts is debatable. Where the cyst is extensive it is best to review after 6 months to confirm progression of bone in-fill.

Long-term follow-up will be required for any cyst where there is a propensity for recurrence, such as the odontogenic keratocyst where review will extend beyond 6 months. Initially reviews should be conducted every 6 months, and then yearly with radiographic monitoring. The authors recommend a follow-up period of at least 5 years. Clearly if there is a possibility of multiple cysts (Gorlin Goltz syndrome) then follow-up will be for life and will extend to screening family members.

SPECIFIC CYST TYPES

Inflammatory cysts (radicular and residual)

These are the most common of all jaw cysts and the main issue is to combine the removal of the cyst with eradication of the cause, i.e. the products of pulp necrosis. This may mean either retaining the tooth with a combination of endodontic therapy and surgery or removal of the associated tooth at the time of the enucleation. Residual cysts are treated with enucleation alone. A decision regarding retaining teeth requires careful assessment of all factors, the state of the dentition and periodontal tissues, significance of the loss of the tooth on the dentition and the patient's attitude to treatment. The size of the cyst and the degree of infection will also influence treatment options.

Dentigerous (follicular) cysts

There are two issues specific to management of dentigerous cysts. Other lesions such as keratocysts and ameloblastomas often have ectopic teeth in dentigerous relationship, which may lead to misdiagnosis. Secondly, it may be desirable to retain the ectopic tooth and allow it to erupt into a functional position. The latter is determined by the age of the patient (and stage of root development), the tooth and dentition. The teeth commonly associated with dentigerous cysts are third molars, second premolars and canines and it would be unusual to want to retain the third molars unless the patient had oligodontia or had suffered premature loss of other teeth. In contrast, the others are often valuable and their management may be part of a treatment plan combined with orthodontics (see Ch. 12). For large cysts if the option is to marsupialize, then the tooth will have to be left *in situ* as the cyst is attached at the amelocemental junction and removal of the tooth will dislodge the main portion of the cyst lining.

Odontogenic keratocysts

These cysts present as unilocular (Fig. 9.3) or multi-loculated (or multilobulated) radiolucencies, more commonly at the angle of the mandible, often with an ectopic tooth in apparent dentigerous relationship. They are the most problematic of all cysts and this reflects their mode of growth and potential for recurrence. Odontogenic keratocysts are believed to grow by cellular proliferation rather than fluid accumulation and growth tends to preferentially extend through the cancellous bone with lateral and medial expansion occurring late. This means they often present as large cysts elongated in the antero-posterior dimension. The growth pattern also determines the recurrence rates in that there are small islands of cells outside the main cyst body. Eradication of these so-called 'daughter cysts' is difficult especially if the overlying bone has been thinned or resorbed. It is also believed that as this cyst arises from dental lamina 'rests' which are frequently found in the alveolar mucosa in the third molar region, and that many such rests persist through life, at least some apparent recurrences arise from these rests. The situation is further complicated as it can be impossible to ensure total removal if the cyst extends through bony plates into difficult areas such as the lingual side of the mandible or the maxillary air sinus.

Treatment options focus on this potential for recurrence, with some operators advocating as definitive surgery, enucleation and treatment of the cavity with Carnoy's solution (a tissue fixative), which will kill residual cells lying within bony spaces. Some will also remove any overlying mucosa with a view to removing any residual dental lamina rests. Others adopt marsupialization to shrink the cyst down and then deal with a much smaller problem of residual cyst lining that is now confined within bone. There is evidence that the histological appearance of the mucosal lining of such marsupialized cavities changes towards that of oral lining mucosa over a period of months, probably indicating that an aggressive approach to its removal is not essential. Clearly as there are significant issues in management and a real potential for recurrence, with some arguing that the keratocyst should be considered as a locally invasive tumour, it is essential to ensure the diagnosis. Careful evaluation of options is required based on preoperative investigations that may include CT to fully evaluate the extent, in particular into the lingual area of the mandible or the pterygoid and maxillary sinus regions for upper jaw cysts. It may also be advisable to perform a formal incisional biopsy of cysts likely to be keratocysts, prior to definitive surgery. This will not only confirm the diagnosis but determine the type (the rarer orthokeratotic variant has a recurrence rate much lower than that of the usual parakeratotic type).

Multiple odontogenic keratocysts

Multiple odontogenic keratocysts may be a presenting feature of basal cell naevus (Gorlin Goltz) syndrome, which is well described in other texts. This autosomal dominant trait is variable in its expressivity but salient features include:

- multiple odontogenic keratocysts
- multiple basal cell naevoid carcinomas of the skin
- rib deformities
- facial characteristics including frontal bossing, hypertelorism and mandibular prognathism
- calcification of the falx cerebri.

Where this is suspected, CT scans of the facial region will be required to identify cysts which are rarely apparent on plain views within the maxilla; referral to clinical genetics and dermatology is essential.

Nasopalatine duct cyst

These uncommon cysts derive from the ductal epithelium in the incisive canal. They are more common in males (4:1) and present either as a chance radiographic finding or as midline swelling at the incisive papilla. They can present with pain if infected and symptoms can be chronic and low grade with purulent or 'salty' discharge. On rare occasions they can cause chronic nasal symptoms. Large cysts can extend anteriorly to create swelling in the labial sulcus, enough on occasion to distend the lip. Radiographically they present with the typical features of cysts with the superimposition of the nasal spine, giving the so-called 'heart-shaped' appearance characteristic of larger cysts that have extended anteriorly. A small cyst can be confused with a large incisive foramen and the 'rule of thumb' is that the foramen is not likely to be greater than 6 mm in diameter. As with cysts arising in the gingival areas (see below) it is important to exclude other cysts, in this case radicular cysts. Precise midline positioning, positive vitality tests and intact lamina dura around the roots of the related teeth go a long way to confirming the diagnosis.

Treatment is by enucleation and given the relationship to the canal and therefore to the neurovascular bundle postoperative loss of sensation in the anterior palate is probable. Although this is unlikely to impact significantly on the patient, they must be advised of the possibility and that it may be permanent. Access is from the palatal side unless the cyst is large when both palatal and labial flaps are required. Palatal dissection is difficult and on occasions the neurovascular bundle must be divided.

Cysts arising in the alveolus of the jaw

Radiological findings can be minimal (gingival cyst of adults) or of well-defined ovoid radiolucencies (true lateral periodontal cyst, 'peripheral' or soft-tissue odontogenic keratocyst and inflammatory cyst arising from a lateral pulp canal, or periodontal pocket). Vitality tests are an essential aid to differentiation of inflammatory cysts, but all these cysts require enucleation to confirm diagnosis.

Cysts presenting in this area include the glandular odontogenic cyst and the Botryoid cyst. Surgical management is enucleation but because of their mechanism of growth, site and difficulties with access, both can recur. The bony cavities should be inspected carefully and curetted or ablated with a surgical bur (small acrylic trimming bur) to try to ensure all trace of epithelium has been removed. Recurrence is more likely when cysts are multiloculated and on occasions local resection may be needed.

Eruption cysts and the gingival cyst of childhood

The eruption cyst, which is best considered a superficial soft-tissue follicular cyst, almost always related to erupting deciduous or permanent molar teeth, is self-limiting. If, however, it is troublesome and persistent the treatment is marsupialization. The gingival cyst of childhood (Bohn's nodules or Epstein's pearls) is a developmental cyst derived from remnants of the dental lamina, which is also self-limiting.

Soft-tissue cysts

In addition to mucoceles (Ch. 14) and skin-derived dermoid and epidermoid cysts, there are a few rare developmental soft-tissue cysts comprising the nasolabial, floor of mouth dermoid, branchial and thyroglossal cysts. They all arise from remnants of embryonic epithelium and typically present as swellings that are submucosal or subdermal at the site of fusion of embryonic processes. They present complex issues in diagnosis, particularly branchial and thyroglossal cysts, with often difficult soft-tissue surgery, and should be referred to appropriate specialists. For further details readers are referred to relevant surgical texts.

Non-epithelial-lined, cyst-like lesions (aneurysmal and traumatic bone cysts)

These are rare lesions and are not true cysts but as they present radiographically in similar fashion to cysts they are therefore included in this chapter. Of these the aneurysmal bone cyst is the most significant in surgical terms as it can recur. It is highly vascular with no appreciable lumen and intraoperative haemorrhage can occur. Treatment is enucleation with curettage and follow-up.

Traumatic bone cysts in contrast are, in the majority of cases, asymptomatic chance findings, in adolescents, of poorly defined radiolucencies interdigitating with roots of associated teeth that are vital. Findings at operation are an 'empty' cavity and no further active intervention is required; the bone heals after the cavity has been opened. They are almost exclusively found in the mandible and significantly do not displace the neurovascular bundle, which can cross the cavity and therefore be at risk in terms of intraoperative haemorrhage and postoperative function.

FURTHER READING

Cawson R. A., Binnie W. H., Barrett A. W., Wright J. M. (2001) *Oral disease clinical and pathological correlations*, 3rd edn. Mosby, St Louis, MO, Ch. 5.

Donoff B. (1998) *Manual of oral and maxillofacial surgery*, 3rd edn. Mosby, St Louis, MO, Ch. 15, pp. 345–352.

Kramer I. R. H., Pindborg J. J., Shear M. (1992) *Histological typing of odontogenic tumours*. Springer Verlag, Heidelberg, Germany.

Peterson L. J., Ellis E., Hupp J. R., Tucker M. R. (eds.) (1997) *Contemporary oral and maxillofacial surgery*, 3rd edn. Mosby, St Louis, MO, Ch. 23, pp. 534–545.

Philipsen H. P. (2005) Keratocystic odontogenic tumour. In L. Barnes (ed.) *Pathology and genetics of head and neck tumours*. IARC Press, Lyon, France, pp. 306–307.

Shear M. (1992) *Cysts of the oral regions*, 3rd edn. Wright, Oxford, UK.

Shear M. (1994) Development of odontogenic cysts, an update. *Journal of Oral Pathology and Medicine* 23: 1.

Waites E. (2002) *Essentials of dental radiography and radiology*, 3rd edn. Harcourt Health Sciences, Edinburgh.

SELF-ASSESSMENT

1. A patient presents with a cyst involving the apex of the maxillary left lateral incisor.
   (a) List the possible signs and symptoms associated with this lesion.
   (b) What special investigations would you perform, and what would you expect them to demonstrate?
   (c) List the forms of treatment and the indications for these lines of treatment.
2. (a) Name two cystic lesions which may present as swellings in the palate.
   (b) What symptoms may they present with?
   (c) What investigations would you employ to confirm your diagnosis?
   (d) List the treatment for each case and any possible complications.
3. What clinical aspects of the swelling associated with jaw cysts would distinguish them from other disorders?
4. What clinical features other than swelling and infection might suggest the presence of a cyst?
5. You decide to marsupialize a cyst in the mandible that extends from third molar to third molar. What should the patient be told?

Answers on page 266.

10 Malignant disease of the oral cavity

J. D. Langdon

- Mouth cancer is relatively rare in the West, accounting for 2% of all malignant disease, whereas in Asia it is the most common malignant disease, accounting for 40% of all malignancy.
- In the West mouth cancer is becoming more common, particularly among young people.
- The overall cure rate of oral cancer has not improved dramatically during the past 40 years.
- However, the cure rate of early (small) cancers is 80%. Therefore it is important that all dental and medical practitioners can recognize suspicious lesions and refer them promptly.
- A variety of relatively common intraoral mucosal lesions carry a risk of malignant change. Other more generalized conditions predispose a person to develop mouth cancer.
- In the West, alcohol and tobacco smoking are major risk factors. Both of these habits are widespread and account for the increasing incidence of mouth cancer in young people. In Asia, tobacco chewing, often in combination with betel, is the major aetiological factor and this habit is almost universal in many communities.

ASSUMED KNOWLEDGE

It is assumed that at this stage you will have knowledge/competencies in the following areas:

- anatomy of the oral cavity, oropharynx and the lymphatics of the head and neck
- pathology of benign and malignant neoplasia including the spread of malignant disease
- mucosal diseases of the oral cavity.

If you think that you are not competent in these areas, revise them before reading this chapter or cross-check with relevant texts as you read.

INTENDED LEARNING OUTCOMES

At the end of this chapter you should be able to:

1. Describe the incidence and aetiology of oral cancer in different parts of the world
2. Differentiate mucosal lesions and conditions that have a potential for malignant change
3. Describe the role of the general dental practitioner in the prevention and screening of oral cancer
4. Recognize oral cancers presenting at different stages in various sites in the mouth
5. Describe the principles of staging of oral cancer and how this relates to the treatment and prognosis
6. Describe the advantages and disadvantages of different treatment methods

7. Plan the provision of mouth care for a patient with oral cancer
8. Determine the urgency of referral of a patient with a suspicious lesion in the mouth
9. Describe the requirements of a satisfactory biopsy and say how it should be performed.

ORAL AND OROPHARYNGEAL CANCER

In global terms, oral/oropharyngeal cancer is the sixth most common malignancy. In the Western world it accounts for only 2–4% of all malignant tumours although there is now good evidence to show that the incidence is increasing, particularly in younger people. By contrast, in Asia oral/oropharyngeal malignancy is the most common malignant tumour, which in parts of India accounts for no less than 40% of all malignancy. It is estimated that globally nearly 500 000 new cases develop annually and that in the year 2000 there were 1.5 million people alive with oral cancer at any one time.

Oral/oropharyngeal cancer is an almost entirely preventable disease, being caused by use of tobacco (with or without alcohol). In the West this is mostly cigarette smoking combined with alcohol abuse; the risk caused by both in combination is greater than the summation of the risks of each individually. In Asia and the Far East the use of Pan in its various forms and reverse smoking are the major aetiologic agents: epidemiological evidence strongly suggests that it is the presence of tobacco in the betel quid which is the major agent, although there seems also to be some relationship to the source of slaked lime and the areca nut itself. In the West, the incidence in women appears to be increasing and there is a worrying increase in the number of young patients, mostly male and particularly with tongue cancer, after a gradual fall earlier this century. This recent trend seems not to be related to tobacco and alcohol consumption and has been observed throughout Europe and North America. The general dental practitioner has a major role in prevention by advising and helping patients to cease tobacco smoking or chewing and moderating alcohol consumption.

Local control of disease at the primary site and the management of neck disease has improved; yet, despite this, cure rates and survival rates have only improved marginally in 40 years, remaining at approximately 55% survival at 5 years. Both recurrence of local disease and failure to control lymphatic metastases in the neck are early events and are a major cause of death. There is no doubt, however, that during the past 20 years great advances have been made in the management of oral cancer, and persistence of local disease and lymphatic metastasis are now less common. Why then have cure rates not improved? Field changes in the upper aerodigestive tract result in the phenomenon of multiple primary cancers. The longer a patient survives a first tumour, the greater the risk of developing a second or third primary tumour either elsewhere in the oral cavity or in the larynx, bronchus or oesophagus.

Even a patient who does not develop a second primary tumour is at risk of developing distant metastatic disease. Metastasis via the bloodstream is a relatively early event in oral cancer, although until recently rarely recognized during life. Currently 20% of all cancer-related deaths in patients with a tumour in the oral cavity/oropharynx are due to distant metastasis with no evidence of disease in the head or neck. Thus oral cancer is a 'systemic' disease from an early stage.

Resection

Surgical advances have been mainly in techniques of access surgery and in reconstruction. The widespread adoption of lip splitting and mandibulotomy has facilitated safe three-dimensional resections of tumours in the tongue and floor of the mouth in continuity with the lymphatics in the neck. A better understanding of the patterns of invasion of the mandible by adjacent tumour has allowed the development of rim resections, avoiding the sacrifice of mandibular continuity in many cases, without risking local recurrence. In recent years the development of skull base access surgery using well-established oral and facial osteotomy techniques has rendered previously inoperable tumours operable. This is particularly true for tumours extending into the pterygoid, infratemporal and lateral pharyngeal regions.

Reconstruction

Primary reconstruction is now the rule, and this is to the great benefit of patients. Earlier techniques were often unreliable and when bony reconstruction was involved it was often delayed. It was reasonably felt that before embarking on such prolonged and insecure techniques a period of time should be allowed to elapse, to demonstrate that local recurrence was unlikely before reconstruction was attempted. With current techniques based largely on muscle flaps—pectoralis major, trapezius and latissimus dorsi—and free tissue transfer based on microvascular techniques—radial forearm, lateral thigh, scapular, fibula and groin—primary reconstruction is not only reliable but produces acceptable functional and cosmetic results.

Radiotherapy

Megavoltage X-ray beams or electron beams are able to penetrate tissues and can cause cell death by producing lethal damage to DNA. Irradiated cells die as they attempt to divide and because malignant cells generally divide more rapidly than normal cells there is differential cell death. With careful planning and adjustment of dosage and frequency of treatment the tumour cells can be destroyed whilst sparing sufficient normal tissues to allow healing and repair. A typical regimen for an oral carcinoma would be a total dose of 55 Gray given by daily treatments on Monday to Friday over a 6-week period. The daily dose (fraction) is therefore only small and allows for repair of normal tissues between treatments. In most centres, surgery is the primary modality for most patients. Radiotherapy is used as a supplement when the surgical margins of the tumour are not clear or there is extensive nodal metastasis in the neck.

Although treating a cancer with radiotherapy avoids major surgery it has disadvantages:

- during treatment severe mucositis develops because the rapidly dividing mucosal cells are killed. This mucositis is very painful and oral feeding is frequently impossible
- secondary bacterial and fungal infections are common and oral hygiene is difficult to maintain
- taste becomes distorted but recovers after about 6 months
- salivary tissue is very sensitive to radiation and is permanently damaged so that a persistently dry mouth ensues if the treatment involves the radiation beam passing through the salivary glands. The latest techniques for delivering radiotherapy (intensity modulated radiotherapy—IMRT) will hopefully enable the radiotherapist to avoid exposing the major salivary glands to the radiation
- two long-term effects of radiotherapy are particularly important: capillary vessels undergo a progressive endarteritis obliterans, which results in ischaemia of the tissues with subsequent atrophy, and the bone is damaged. Irradiated osteocytes remain alive until they are stimulated to divide, at which time they die. A common stimulus to osteocyte division in the jaws is dental extractions. The bone is both ischaemic and unable to remodel, resulting in osteoradionecrosis which frequently becomes secondarily infected.

An alternative way of treating tumours with radiotherapy is to implant radioactive materials into the tumour (brachytherapy). Radioactive iridium wires are the most commonly used implants. There is a rapid fall-off of dose with distance, and the technique continuously delivers very high-dose local irradiation with very little damage to adjacent tissues. Therefore the adverse effects of conventional radiotherapy are largely avoided.

Chemotherapy

Although many single agents or combinations of drugs can result in a response rate of around 60%, there is no evidence that this results in an increase in survival time or cure rate. Some centres advocate the use of induction chemotherapy before surgery but again there is no evidence, based upon prospective studies, that this improves survival. Palliative chemotherapy using agents such as cisplatinum and 5-fluorouracil are sometimes helpful for painful or fungating tumours.

Clinical aspects

Oral cancer has a predilection for certain sites within the mouth, mostly the lateral margins and ventral tongue, floor of mouth, retromolar trigone, buccal mucosa and palate. Most—more than 85%—are mucosal squamous cell carcinomas. Malignant tumours arising in the minor salivary glands are next in frequency, with lymphomas, malignant melanomas, sarcomas and metastatic tumours making up the remainder.

PREMALIGNANT LESIONS

The association of oral carcinoma with other oral mucosal lesions has been recognized for many years. Often these lesions are in the form of white plaques ('leukoplakia') or bright red velvety plaques ('erythroplakia'), which may be present for periods of months to years before the onset of malignant change and often will be present together with the carcinoma when the diagnosis of malignancy is made. Because of this association, it has been assumed that such lesions lead directly to invasive carcinoma and hence are themselves premalignant. Some white plaques do have a potential to undergo malignant transformation and an examination of established carcinomas will show many to exist in association with white plaques. However, most oral carcinomas are not preceded by, nor associated with, leukoplakia.

Although historically oral leukoplakia has been recognized as premalignant, the risk of malignant transformation is not as great as was previously thought. Early literature suggested a 30% or higher incidence of malignant transformation of these lesions whereas more recent authors quote an incidence of 3–6%. The following oral lesions are now considered to carry a potential for malignant change:

- leukoplakia
- erythroplakia
- chronic hyperplastic candidiasis.

A further group of conditions, although not themselves premalignant, are associated with a higher than normal incidence of oral cancer:

- oral submucous fibrosis
- syphilitic glossitis
- sideropenic dysphagia.

There remains a further group of oral conditions about which there is still some doubt as to whether their association with oral cancer is causal or casual:

- oral lichen planus
- discoid lupus erythematosus
- dyskeratosis congenita.

Leukoplakia (Fig. 10.1)

Using the term leukoplakia either in a histological or clinical context is a matter of defining what is meant by the term. The World Health Organization (WHO) has defined leukoplakia as 'any white patch or plaque that cannot be characterized clinically or pathologically as any other disease'. This definition has no histological connotation.

Clinical features

Clinically leukoplakia may vary from a small, circumscribed white plaque to an extensive lesion involving wide areas of the oral mucosa. The surface may be smooth or it may be wrinkled and many lesions are traversed by cracks or fissures. The colour of the lesion may be white, yellowish or grey; some are homogeneous whilst others are nodular or speckled on an erythematous base. Many lesions are soft whereas other thicker lesions feel crusty. Induration (hardening) suggests malignant change and is an indication for immediate biopsy. It is important to recognize that it is the speckled or nodular leukoplakias which are the most likely to undergo malignant change.

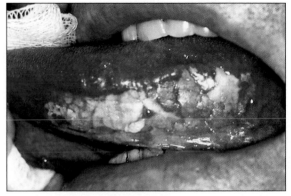

Fig. 10.1 Nodular leukoplakia of the lateral border of the tongue.

Potential for malignant change

The incidence of malignant change in oral leukoplakia increases with the age of the lesion. One study showed a 2.4% malignant transformation rate at 10 years, which increased to 4% at 20 years. It also showed that as the age of the patient increased so did the risk of malignant transformation: for patients younger than 50 years it was 1%, whereas for those between 70 and 89 years it was 7.5% during a 5-year observation period. Kramer et al. (1978) have shown that in Southern England leukoplakia of the floor of the mouth and ventral surface of the tongue, so-called 'sublingual keratosis', has a particularly high incidence of malignant change. Their study suggested that this occurrence was due to pooling of soluble carcinogens in the 'sump' of the floor of the mouth.

Aetiology

Tobacco smoking or chewing are undoubtedly important aetiological factors. In Indians who smoke or chew tobacco (often as a component of the betel quid) the incidence of leukoplakia in those of 60 years of age is 20%, whereas in those who neither smoke nor chew tobacco the incidence is 1%.

The role of alcohol in the development of oral leukoplakia is difficult to assess. Few studies have been reported, but it has been shown that in patients with leukoplakia the incidence of excessive alcohol consumption is greater than in those without leukoplakia.

Management

In any patient presenting for the first time with oral leukoplakia a careful history—particularly looking for aetiological factors—and a detailed clinical examination should precede the histological examination of biopsies of any suspicious areas. Suspicion is aroused by any areas of ulceration, induration or where the underlying tissues are bright red and hyperaemic. Vital staining with toluidine blue can be used to guide the clinician to those sites most suspicious of malignant change.

If there is a history of tobacco consumption then the patient should be persuaded to stop immediately. It has been shown that if the patient stops smoking entirely for 1 year the leukoplakia will disappear in 60% of the cases.

Whenever severe epithelial dysplasia or carcinoma-in-situ is present, surgical excision or CO_2 laser excision of the lesions is mandatory. Small lesions may be excised, the margins of the adjacent mucosa undermined and the defect closed by advancing the margins. For larger defects the area should be left to epithelialize spontaneously (alternatively the area can be skin-grafted). On the tongue the graft is quilted onto the raw area, whereas on the cheek, floor of the mouth or palate the graft can be retained in place by suturing a suitable pack overlying it.

When only mild to moderate epithelial dysplasia is present the patient should be followed up at 4-month intervals and details of the lesions recorded in the notes either photographically or diagrammatically.

Erythroplakia (Fig. 10.2)

Erythroplakia is defined as 'any lesion of the oral mucosa that presents as bright red velvety plaques which cannot be characterized clinically or pathologically as any other recognizable condition'. Such lesions are usually irregular in outline, although clearly demarcated from adjacent normal epithelium. The surface may be nodular. In some cases erythroplakia coexists with areas of leukoplakia. The incidence of malignant change in erythroplakias is 17 times higher than that in leukoplakia. In nearly every case of erythroplakia there are areas of epithelial dysplasia, carcinoma-in-situ or invasive carcinoma. Clearly all erythroplakic areas must be completely excised, either surgically or with a CO_2 laser, and the specimens submitted for careful histological examination.

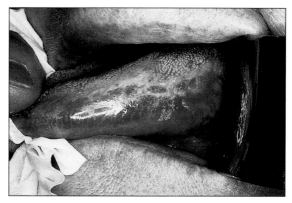

Fig. 10.2 Erythroplakia of the lateral border of the tongue. On biopsy the lesion had areas of carcinoma-in-situ.

Chronic hyperplastic candidiasis (Fig. 10.3)

In chronic hyperplastic candidiasis, dense chalky plaques of keratin are formed, the plaques being thicker and more opaque than in non-candidal leukoplakia. Such lesions are particularly common at the oral commissures, extending onto the adjacent skin of the face. In 1969 attention was drawn to the high incidence of malignant transformation in these candidal leukoplakias, suggesting that the invasive candidal infection is the cause of the leukoplakia, and not merely a superimposed infection. It has also been suggested that in such patients there may be an immunological defect which allows the *Candida albicans* to invade the epithelium and may render the patient susceptible to malignant change.

It is thought that treatment with antifungal agents to eliminate the candidal infection will reduce the risk of malignant change. However, treatment may be necessary for many months to eliminate the organisms and reinfection is a constant problem. Surgical excision is recommended for persistent lesions.

Oral submucous fibrosis (Fig. 10.4)

Oral submucous fibrosis is a progressive disease in which fibrous bands form beneath the oral mucosa.

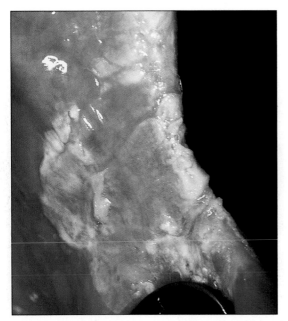

Fig. 10.3 Chronic hyperplastic candidiasis arising at the oral commissure.

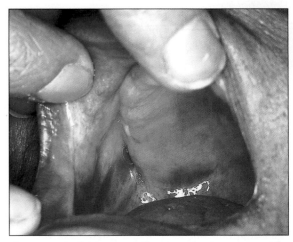

Fig. 10.4 Oral submucous fibrosis arising in a patient who previously chewed betel nut.

These bands progressively contract so that ultimately opening is severely limited, speech becomes hypernasal due to changes in the soft palate and swallowing is disturbed. Tongue movement may also be limited. The condition is almost entirely confined to Asians. Histologically it is characterized by juxtaepithelial fibrosis with atrophy or hyperplasia of the overlying epithelium, which also shows areas of epithelial dysplasia. Paymaster, in 1956, first discussed the precancerous nature of submucous fibrosis (see Langdon and Henk 1995). He noted the onset of a slowly growing squamous cell carcinoma in one-third of such patients. The changes are due to crosslinking of the collagen fibres caused by various alkaloids, particularly arecholine, which leach out of the arecha nut and penetrate the oral mucosa.

The scar bands of submucous fibrosis that result in difficulty in mouth opening can be treated either by intralesional injection of steroids or by surgical excision and grafting, but this has little effect in preventing the onset of squamous cell carcinoma in the generally atrophic oral mucosa. Any aetiological factors should, of course, be eliminated.

Syphilitic glossitis

Before the antibiotic era, syphilis was an important predisposing factor in the development of oral leuko-plakia and oral cancer. The syphilitic infection produces an interstitial glossitis with an endarteritis that results in atrophy of the overlying epithelium. This atrophic epithelium appears to be more vulnerable to those irritants that cause oral cancer or oral leukoplakia. As these changes are irreversible there is no specific treatment, although active syphilis must be treated. Regular follow-up is essential. It should be noted that squamous cell carcinomas may arise in syphilitic glossitis, even in the absence of leukoplakia.

Sideropenic dysphagia (Plummer-Vinson syndrome, Paterson-Kelly syndrome) (Fig. 10.5)

In 1936 Ahlbom showed the relation between sideropenic dysphagia and oral cancer (Langdon and Henk 1995). Sideropenic dysphagia is particularly common in Swedish women, and accounts for the high incidence of cancer of the upper alimentary tract in this group and the higher incidence of women with oral cancer in Sweden. Of women with oral cancer in Sweden, 25% were sideropenic. The pathogenesis of oral cancer in such patients may be similar to that of syphilitic glossitis. The sideropenic dysphagia leads to atrophic epithelium, which is particularly vulnerable to carcinogenic irritants. Although the anaemia will respond to treatment with iron supplements, it is not known whether such treatment reduces the risk of subsequent malignant change.

Oral lichen planus (Fig. 10.6)

Some reports have stated that in erosive or atrophic lichen planus there is a risk of malignant transformation; a 1.2% incidence of malignant change has been found in a series of 570 patients with oral lichen planus followed up for a mean of 5.6 years. If there is an association between lichen planus and oral cancer, the relation exists only with atrophic or erosive lichen planus, and patients with these conditions should be carefully reviewed. Erosive lichen planus should be treated with topical steroids, and in severe cases systemic steroids may be necessary.

Discoid lupus erythematosus

The oral lesions of discoid lupus erythematosus consist of circumscribed, somewhat elevated white patches, usually surrounded by a telangiectatic halo. Epithelial dysplasia may be seen on histological examination and this may lead to malignant transformation, usually on the labial mucosa adjacent to the vermilion border and more often in men than in women. Patients with discoid lupus erythematosus should be advised to avoid bright sunlight and, when in the open air, to apply an ultraviolet barrier cream to the lips.

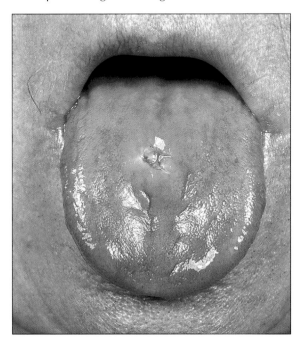

Fig. 10.5 Severe mucosal atrophy in a patient with sideropenic dysphagia.

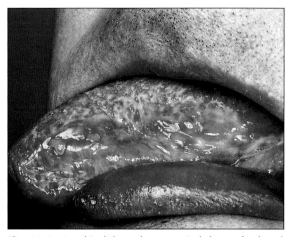

Fig. 10.6 Atrophic lichen planus, particularly on the lateral border of the tongue.
This carries a small risk of malignant change.

Dyskeratosis congenita

This syndrome is characterized by reticular atrophy of the skin with pigmentation, nail dystrophy and oral leukoplakia. Eventually the oral mucosa becomes atrophic and the tongue loses its papillae. Finally the mucosa becomes thickened, fissured and white.

CLINICAL PRESENTATION AND DIAGNOSIS OF ORAL CANCER

> **Indications for urgent referral by general dental practitioner**
>
> - Any ulcer which persists unhealed for more than 2 weeks
> - Any unexplained oral bleeding
> - Any area of induration
> - All unexplained white patches
> - All red or red/white patches

Oral cancer arises from the surface mucosa, and the clinical diagnosis should be easy. Early detection should lead to better outcome. Oral lesions, unlike those at many other sites in the body, give rise to early symptoms. In general, patients become aware of and usually complain about tiny lesions within the mouth and biopsy may be carried out under local analgesia. Yet, despite all the above, between 27 and 50% of patients present for treatment with tumours greater than 4 cm in diameter. Many of these patients are elderly and frail and therefore delay the effort of visiting their doctor or dentist: they are often denture wearers, accustomed to discomfort and ulceration in the mouth and thus see no urgency in seeking treatment. Furthermore, the practitioner may not be suspicious that a lesion is malignant. Not all oral cancers present as classical non-healing ulcers with heaped-up margins: they can start as small areas of ulceration in the depth of fissures in the tongue, as superficial mucosal erosions, as areas of induration in the absence of discernible ulceration or even as gingival hyperplasia mimicking gingival infection. The lesion is often treated initially with antifungal therapy, antibiotics, steroids and mouthwashes, thus causing further delay in the ultimate diagnosis and treatment. Another factor is that oral cancer is not usually painful until such time as either the ulcer becomes secondarily infected or the tumour invades sensory nerve fibres.

The time scale of development of oral cancer is generally weeks to months, by comparison with the scale of a few days seen with acute infective conditions (see p. 88).

> **Presentation of oral cancers**
>
> - Classical ulcer with central necrosis and exophytic margins
> - Small ulcer in the depth of a fissure
> - Superficial mucosal erosion
> - Indurated area within soft tissue
> - Localized area of gingival hyperplasia

The tongue (Fig. 10.7)

Most tongue cancers occur on the middle third of the lateral margins, extending early in the course of the disease onto the ventral aspect and floor of the mouth. Approximately 25% occur on the posterior third of the tongue, 20% on the anterior third and only very rarely on the dorsum.

Early tongue cancer may manifest in a variety of ways. Often the growth is exophytic with areas of ulceration. It may occur as an ulcer in the depths of a fissure or as an area of superficial ulceration

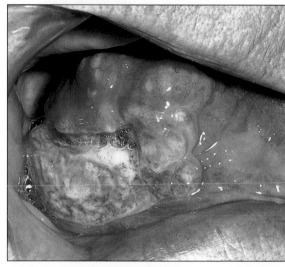

Fig. 10.7 An advanced cancer of the tongue presenting as an ulcer with heaped-up margins and a central area of necrosis.

with unsuspected infiltration into the underlying muscle. Leukoplakic patches may or may not be associated with the primary lesion. A minority of tongue cancers may be asymptomatic, arising in an atrophic depapillated area with an erythroplakic patch with peripheral streaks or areas of leukoplakia.

Later in the course of the disease a more typical malignant ulcer will usually develop, often several centimetres in diameter. The ulcer is hard in consistency (indurated) with heaped-up and often everted edges (Fig. 10.7). The floor is granular, indurated and bleeds readily. Often there are areas of necrosis. The growth infiltrates the tongue progressively, causing increasing pain and difficulty with speech and swallowing. By this stage pain is often severe and constant, radiating to the neck and ears. Lymph node metastases at this stage are common—indeed 50% of patients may have palpable nodes at first attendance. Because of the relatively early lymph node metastasis of tongue cancer, 12% of patients may present with no symptoms other than 'a lump in the neck'.

Floor of the mouth (Fig. 10.8)

The floor of the mouth is the second most common site for oral cancer. It is defined as the U-shaped area between the lower alveolus and the ventral surface of the tongue; carcinomas arising at this site involve adjacent structures very early in their natural history. Most tumours occur in the anterior segment of the floor of the mouth to one side of the midline.

The lesion usually starts as an indurated mass, which soon ulcerates. At an early stage the tongue and lingual aspect of the mandible become infiltrated. This early involvement of the tongue leads to the characteristic slurring of the speech often noted in patients with such cancers. The infiltration is deceptive but may extend to reach the gingivae, tongue and genioglossus muscle. Subperiosteal spread is rapid once the mandible is reached. Lymphatic metastasis, although early, is less common than with tongue cancer. Spread is usually to the submandibular and jugulodigastric nodes and may be bilateral.

Floor of mouth cancer is associated with a pre-existing leukoplakia more commonly than cancer at other sites.

Gingiva and alveolar ridge (Fig. 10.9)

Carcinoma of the lower alveolar ridge occurs predominantly in the premolar and molar regions. The patient usually presents with proliferative tissue at the gingival margins or superficial gingival ulceration. Diagnosis is often delayed because a wide variety of inflammatory and reactive lesions occur in this region in association with the teeth or dentures (Fig. 10.9). Indeed, there will often be a history of tooth extraction with subsequent failure of the socket to heal before definitive diagnosis is made. Another common story is that of sudden difficulty in wearing dentures. Regional nodal metastasis is common at presentation, varying from 30 to 84%, although false-positive and false-negative clinical findings are common.

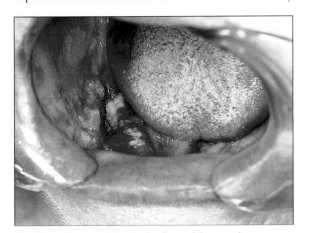

Fig. 10.8 Cancer arising in the floor of the mouth.

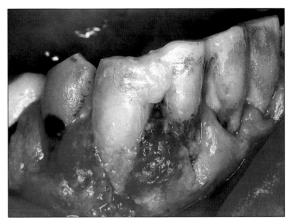

Fig. 10.9 Gingival carcinoma is often initially misdiagnosed as periodontal infection, as in this case.

The buccal mucosa (Fig. 10.10)

The buccal mucosa extends from the upper alveolar ridge down to the lower alveolar ridge and from the commissure anteriorly to the mandibular ramus and retromolar region posteriorly. Squamous cell carcinomas mostly arise either at the commissure or along the occlusal plane to the retromolar area, most being situated posteriorly. Exophytic, ulcerative and verrucous types occur. Tumours are subject to occlusal trauma, with consequent early ulceration, and often become secondarily infected. The onset of the disease may be insidious, the patient sometimes presenting with trismus due to deep neoplastic infiltration into the buccinator muscle. Extension posteriorly involves the anterior pillar of the fauces and soft palate, with consequent worsening of the prognosis. Infiltrating lesions will often involve the overlying skin of the cheek, resulting in multiple sinuses. Lymph node spread is to the submental, submandibular, parotid and lateral pharyngeal nodes.

Verrucous carcinoma occurs as a superficial proliferative exophytic lesion with minimal deep invasion and induration. Often the lesion is densely keratinized and presents as a soft white velvety area mimicking benign hyperplasia. Lymph node metastasis is late and the tumour behaves as a low-grade, squamous cell carcinoma.

The hard palate, maxillary alveolar ridge and floor of antrum (Figs. 10.11, 10.12)

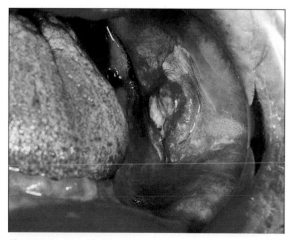

Fig. 10.10 Buccal carcinoma arising in an area of pre-existing leukoplakia.

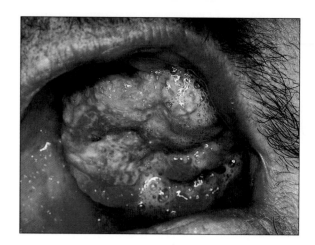

Fig. 10.11 Extensive carcinoma affecting the entire hard and soft palate.

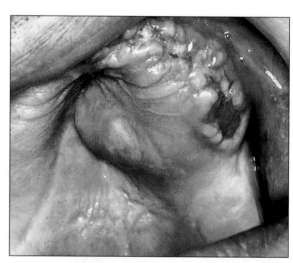

Fig. 10.12 This patient with an antral carcinoma first attended his dental practitioner complaining of loosening of the teeth, which were then extracted. Carcinoma can be seen growing through the sockets from above.

These three sites are anatomically distinct, but a carcinoma arising from one site soon involves the others. Consequently it can be difficult to determine the precise site of origin. Except in countries where reverse smoking is practised, cancer of the palate is relatively uncommon. Most squamous cancers in this site arise in the antrum and later ulcerate through to involve the hard palate (see Ch. 15, p. 225.). The majority of malignant tumours arising from the palatal mucosa are of minor salivary gland origin. Palatal cancers usually present as sessile swellings, which ulcerate relatively late. In contrast to mandibular alveolar tumours, deep infiltration into the underlying bone is uncommon.

Carcinomas arising in the floor of the maxillary antrum often present as palatal tumours. Although an extensive antral carcinoma is difficult to miss, the early symptoms are non-specific and may mimic chronic sinusitis. Patients with tumours of the lower half of the antrum complain of 'dental' symptoms because of early alveolar invasion. The most common features are pain, swelling or numbness of the face. Later symptoms of unilateral nasal obstruction, discharge or bleeding and dental symptoms such as painful or loose teeth, ill-fitting dentures, oroantral fistula or failure of an extraction socket to heal may follow. Lymph node metastasis from carcinomas of the palate and floor of the antrum occurs late but carries a poor prognosis.

DIAGNOSIS

The diagnosis of intraoral carcinoma is primarily clinical, and a high index of suspicion is necessary for all those clinicians seeing and treating patients with oral symptoms. A careful and detailed history, with particular attention to recording the dates of the onset of particular signs and symptoms, must precede the clinical examination. All areas of the oral mucosa should be carefully inspected and any suspicious lesion palpated for texture, tethering to adjacent structures and induration of underlying tissue. Any ulcer persisting for more than 2 weeks, any induration or spontaneous bleeding (particularly in a patient over 50 years who smokes and/or drinks alcohol) requires urgent referral for expert opinion. Dental practitioners should make a full mucosal examination of the mouth and oropharynx part of their routine 'dental inspection'.

INVESTIGATION

Surgical biopsy

A clinical diagnosis of oral cancer should always be confirmed histologically (see Ch. 8), but this should not be undertaken in general dental practice, because a biopsy will alter the appearance of the lesion and make it more difficult for the hospital specialist to assess the tumour. The general dental practitioner should refer the patient with a suspicious lesion immediately to an oral and maxillofacial surgeon.

Within the oral cavity a surgical biopsy can usually be obtained using local anaesthesia: incisional biopsy is recommended in all cases. Whenever possible the patient should be seen at a combined clinic by a surgeon and radiotherapist before even the biopsy is carried out but, provided careful records are made, an initial incisional biopsy is acceptable—and may indeed save time in the planning and initiation of subsequent therapy. The biopsy should include the most suspicious area of the lesion and some normal adjacent mucosa. Areas of necrosis or gross infection should be avoided as they may confuse the diagnosis.

Fine-needle aspiration biopsy

This technique (see Ch. 8), which is often used in hospital, is applicable mainly to lumps in the neck, especially suspicious lymph nodes in a patient with a known primary carcinoma. It consists of the percutaneous puncture of the mass with a fine needle and aspiration of material for cytological examination. The method of aspiration needs no specialized equipment (although devices to enable controlled and prolonged traction on the plunger of the syringe may make it much simpler) and is fast, almost painless and without complications. The accuracy can be improved by using ultrasound to guide the needle into the suspicious mass.

Radiography

Plain radiography is of limited value in the investigation of oral cancer. Only in very advanced lesions involving bone will changes be visible on conventional radiographs: at least 50% of the calcified component of bone must be lost before any radiographic change is apparent. Furthermore, the facial bones are of such a complexity that confusion from overlying structures makes radiographic diagnosis more difficult. However, rotational pantomography of the jaws can be helpful in assessing alveolar and antral involvement provided that the above limitations are understood.

Computed tomography and magnetic resonance imaging

The increasing availability of computed tomography (CT) scanning and magnetic resonance imaging (MRI) has been of great benefit in the investigation of head and neck tumours. For the evaluation of antral tumours, particularly assessment of the pterygoid regions, CT and MRI have superseded plain radiography and conventional tomography. CT is also of value in the investigation of metastatic disease in the lungs, liver and skeleton. Positron emission tomography (PET) scan-ning is a newer modality which relies on the fact that tumours have a higher rate of metabolism of glucose. A radioactive glucose analogue is injected. This is taken up selectively by the tumour and subsequently imaged.

Ultrasonography

Abdominal ultrasound is probably as accurate as CT scanning in detecting liver metastases. It is non-invasive, readily available and cost effective, and is probably the most appropriate technique for assessing the liver.

CLASSIFICATION AND STAGING OF ORAL CANCER

Before starting treatment for a patient with oral cancer the disease must be carefully evaluated. Clinical assessment includes a detailed history, physical examination and laboratory and imaging studies, the purposes of which are to determine the extent of the tumour and the presence or absence of regional lymph node involvement or distant metastasis.

All classification systems have the aim of grouping together homogeneous and comparable elements which share similar prognostic significance. Throughout the world the TNM system is applied. This consists of assessing the size and extent of the primary lesion (T), the presence and condition of associated regional nodes (N) and the presence of distant metastases (M) (Table 10.1).

All gradations of prognosis can be demonstrated by grouping patients together on the basis of T, N and M into groups with similar survival rates. This is tumour staging (Table 10.2).

Table 10.1 Classification of oral cancers

T	N	M
T0: No primary tumour detected	**N0:** No nodes detected	**M0:** No evidence of distant metastases
T1: Tumour less than 2 cm diameter	**N1:** Single ipsilateral node less than 3 cm	**M1:** Distant metastases present
T2: Tumour more than 2 cm but less than 4 cm	**N2:** (a) Single ipsilateral node more than 3 cm but less than 6 cm (b) Multiple ipsilateral nodes not greater than 6 cm (c) Bilateral or contralateral node or nodes not greater than 6 cm	—
T3: Tumour more than 4 cm	**N3:** Any node or nodes greater than 6 cm	—
T4: Adjacent structures invaded by tumour	—	—

Table 10.2 Staging of oral cancers

Stage	T	N	M
I	T1	N0	M0
II	T2	N0	M0
III	T1	N1	M0
	T2	N1	M0
	T3	N0, N1	M0
IV	T4	N0, N1	M0
	Any T	N2, N3	M0
	Any T	Any N	M1

Table 10.3 Prognostic significance of staging of oral cancer

Stage	% 5-year survival
I	57–84
II	49–70
III	25–59
IV	7–47

The prime purpose of staging is that, by knowing the prognosis, an appropriate treatment can be selected which will most favourably affect survival (Table 10.3).

MANAGEMENT OF THE PRIMARY TUMOUR

Role of general dental practitioner before definitive treatment

- Removal of all teeth with a doubtful prognosis:
  - gross caries
  - apical pathology
  - periodontal disease
  - restoration with poor prognosis
  - root filling with poor prognosis
- Elimination of rough cusps, margins, restorations
- Correction of dentures causing discomfort/ulceration
- Thorough scaling and polishing
- Reinforcement of oral hygiene instruction.

Choice of treatment

The principal treatments available for primary tumours remain surgery and radiotherapy. The basic decision to be made is between radical radiotherapy and elective surgery. If the former is chosen surgery is reserved for 'salvage' (i.e. for biopsy-proven recurrent or residual disease). If surgery is chosen, radiotherapy may be used in an adjuvant manner, either before or after surgery, but the operation remains fundamentally the definitive curative procedure. Preferences for one or other policy vary considerably between treatment centres.

Many factors must be considered in deciding the optimum management for each individual patient. These include the site, stage and histology of the tumour and the medical condition and lifestyle of the patient. Ideally every patient should be seen at a joint consultation clinic by a surgeon and radiotherapist, who assess objectively and agree the optimum strategy of management for the particular individual. The following factors influence the decision on treatment policy.

Site of origin

The choice of treatment depends on the part of the mouth in which the tumour arises. The management of primary tumours at the various anatomical sites are discussed later (pp. 140–142). In general, surgery is preferred for tumours arising on or involving the alveolar processes; for other sites surgery and radiotherapy are alternatives.

Stage of disease

A small lesion which can be excised readily without producing any deformity or disability is in general best managed surgically. Surgery is also usually more appropriate for a very large mass or where there is invasion of bone, provided the tumour is operable, because of the low cure rates by radiotherapy in these circumstances. The management of lesions of intermediate stage (larger T1, most T2 and early exophytic T3 tumours) is more controversial, as policies of elective surgery or radical radiotherapy produce generally similar survival rates; hence discussion centres on the likely functional results and morbidity of either approach. When there is involvement of cervical lymph nodes the primary tumour and nodes are usually both treated surgically.

Previous irradiation

It is not advisable to retreat with radiotherapy a tumour arising in previously irradiated tissue. Such a tumour is likely to be relatively radioresistant because of limited blood supply. Also re-irradiation of normal tissue is very likely to result in necrosis of all the tissues in the area.

Field change

Where multiple primary tumours are present, or if there is extensive premalignant change, surgery is the preferred treatment. Radiotherapy in these circumstances is unsatisfactory; irradiation of the entire oral cavity causes severe morbidity and may not prevent subsequent new primary tumours arising from areas of premalignant change.

Histology

The histology report on a biopsy specimen has little influence on choice of treatment. The less common adenocarcinoma and melanoma are relatively radio-resistant and therefore should be treated surgically whenever possible. The histological differentiation of a squamous carcinoma does not usually influence its management, there being little evidence to suggest that a well-differentiated primary should be treated differently from a poorly differentiated one.

Age

The patient's age is often quoted as an important factor which must be taken into account when deciding on a course of management. With a young patient there is the fear that if radiotherapy is given it may induce a malignancy in years to come; in fact this risk is very small compared with the mortality of the disease itself. Elderly patients tend to be poor surgical risks, but on the other hand they also tend to do badly with radiotherapy, especially external radiotherapy, and often deteriorate and may die as a result of the debility and poor nutritional status

---

Factors influencing the decision on treatment

- Site of origin
- Stage of disease
- Previous irradiation
- Field change
- Histology
- Age

---

induced by the irradiation. Chronological age *per se* should not necessarily be regarded as a contra-indication to surgery.

TREATMENT ISSUES SPECIFIC TO SITE OF OCCURRENCE

Carcinoma of the lip

Carcinoma of the lip most commonly arises at the vermilion border of the lower lip, away from the line of contact with the upper lip: only 15% arise from the central third and commissure regions, and 5% from the upper lip. Initially the tumours tend to spread laterally rather than infiltrating deeply; eventually, if uncontrolled, they can spread into the anterior triangle of the neck and invade the mandible. Lymph node metastases occur late. Both surgery and radiotherapy are frequently employed and are highly effective methods of treatment, each giving cure rates of about 90%.

Tongue

Surgery is the treatment of choice for early lesions suitable for simple intraoral excision, for tumours on the tip of the tongue and for advanced disease (when surgery should be combined with postoperative radiotherapy). For intermediate-stage disease surgery and radiotherapy have similar outcomes. When per-forming surgical excision of less than one-third of the tongue, formal reconstruction is not necessary: indeed, the best results are obtained by not attempting to close the defect or to apply a split skin graft. The base of the residual defect should be diathermied and then allowed to granulate and epithelialize spontaneously. Such treatment is relatively pain free and results in an undistorted tongue. When available, a CO_2 laser may be used for the partial glossectomy. The postoperative course is relatively pain free, oedema is minimal and healing occurs with minimal scarring.

Any tongue carcinoma exceeding 2 cm in diameter requires at the very least a hemiglossectomy. Many such tumours will infiltrate deeply between the fibres of the hyoglossus muscle. Extensive tongue lesions often involve the floor of the mouth and alveolus. In any of these circumstances a major resection is indicated. Access is best via a lip split and mandibulotomy. The treatment will involve dissecting the neck in order to remove any lymph nodes that might be harbouring metastatic disease. The tongue defect requires reconstruction, usually with a free-tissue transfer using a radial forearm flap with microvascular anastomosis of the artery and vein.

Role of the general dental practitioner during treatment

- Maintenance of scrupulous oral hygiene
- Irrigation of mouth with 2% chlorhexidine mouthwash
- Use of antifungal agents when indicated
- Use of fluoride mouthwashes

Floor of the mouth

Floor of the mouth cancers spread to involve the under-surface of the tongue and the lower alveolus at a relatively early stage. Therefore surgical excision will nearly always include partial glossectomy and marginal resection of the mandible. The resultant defect must always be reconstructed with either a local or a distant flap. It is unacceptable to advance and suture the lateral margin of the residual tongue to the buccal mucosa because this tethers the tongue, causing severe difficulties with speech and mastication. Small tumours of the floor of the mouth that do not show deep infiltration can be treated by simple excision.

For larger lesions and those involving the ventral tongue and/or the alveolus, surgical access is gained via a midline or lateral (anterior to the mental foramen) mandibulotomy and lip split. As these extensive tumours have a high incidence of nodal involvement the resection must be undertaken in continuity with an ipsilateral neck dissection.

When there is evidence of gross tumour invasion of the bone, resection of the mandible is necessary. In order to avoid functional and cosmetic deformity, immediate primary reconstruction is essential. The choice lies between reconstruction with vascularized bone, a free corticocancellous graft or an alloplastic system usually supplemented with cancellous bone mush.

Buccal mucosa

Lesions confined to the buccal mucosa should be excised with a 2-cm margin, including the underlying buccinator muscle, followed by a split skin graft.

Extensive lesions with complicated three-dimensional shapes—for example, lesions extending posteriorly to the retromolar area, maxillary tuberosity or tonsillar fossa—require reconstruction with a free radial forearm flap; this adapts very well to such shapes and remains soft and mobile postoperatively.

Lower alveolus

In general, surgery is the treatment modality of choice for all alveolar carcinoma, except for patients unfit for surgery. Access is achieved via a lip split approach. Now that the patterns of bone invasion are better understood, the continuity of the mandible can often be preserved by performing a marginal resection. If bone invasion is so extensive that the mandible must be resected in continuity with the tumour, primary reconstruction should always be undertaken, because the results are always better than those of delayed reconstruction.

Several techniques for immediate reconstruction of the mandible are available. Historically, free corticocancellous grafts harvested from the iliac crest or rib grafts have been used. Provided there is a good soft-tissue cover to the graft, results can be very satisfactory, although it is difficult to reconstruct the chin prominence with this technique.

Microvascular tissue transfer is currently favoured for immediate mandibular reconstruction. The radial forearm flap with soft tissue and a section of the radius, the compound groin flap based on the deep circumflex iliac vessels and free fibula flaps have all been advocated. A problem with the radial flap is that the harvested bone, although restoring mandibular continuity, often does not provide sufficient bulk for prosthetic reconstruction. Both the fibula and the groin flap provide sufficient bone stock to allow the insertion of osseointegrated implants (Fig. 10.13) and thus full dental rehabilitation postoperatively.

Retromolar trigone

The retromolar trigone is defined as the anterior surface of the ascending ramus of the mandible. It is roughly triangular in shape, with the base being superior, behind the third upper molar, and the apex inferior, behind the third lower molar. Tumours at this site may invade the ascending ramus of the mandible. They may also spread upwards in soft

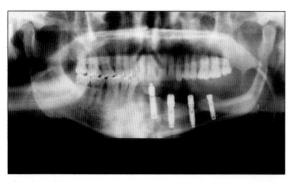

Fig. 10.13 Implants within a reconstructed mandible, following resection for carcinoma.

tissue to involve the pterygomandibular space; this can be difficult to detect clinically or radiologically.

A lip split and mandibulotomy are needed to gain access to the retromolar region. Small defects can often be reconstructed with a masseter or temporalis muscle flap. Larger defects are best reconstructed with a free radial forearm flap, which can be made to conform very well to the shape of the defect at this site.

Hard palate and upper alveolus

These are considered together because they are adjacent and are rare sites of origin of primary squamous carcinoma. A squamous carcinoma presenting at either of these locations is more likely to have arisen in the maxillary antrum than in the oral cavity. An exception is on the Indian subcontinent where carcinoma of the hard palate occurs in association with reverse smoking. Malignant tumours of the hard palate are more likely to arise from the minor salivary glands.

A tumour confined to the hard palate, upper alveolus and floor of the antrum can be resected by a partial maxillectomy. A more extensive tumour confined to the infrastructure of the maxilla requires total maxillectomy. If the preoperative investigations indicate extension of disease into the orbit, pterygoid space or infratemporal fossa, a more extensive procedure is necessary. The chance of obtaining a cure by surgery alone is small and postoperative radiotherapy is essential. If the tumour extends superiorly to involve the dura within the skull then a combined neurosurgical procedure will be required. Following maxillary resection the resulting cavity should be skin grafted to ensure rapid healing and to prevent contracture of the overlying soft tissues.

Malignant melanoma

Oral melanomas are rare. The peak age incidence is between 40 and 60 years; nearly 50% are on the hard palate and about 25% are on the upper gingivae. About 30% of melanomas are preceded by an area of hyperpigmentation, often by many years. Pigmentation varies from black to brown, while rare non-pigmented melanomas (15% of oral melanomas) are red. Oral melanomas may be flat but are usually raised or nodular, and asymptomatic initially but may later become ulcerated, painful or bleed. Because of their rapid growth, most oral melanomas are at least 1 cm across. Approximately 50% of patients have metastases at presentation.

Size and rapid growth, particularly if associated with destruction of underlying bone or presence of metastases, are obvious indicators of a poor outcome. Once the diagnosis has been confirmed, the best hope of cure is provided by the widest possible excision followed by radical radiotherapy. There is no evidence that chemotherapy is of significant value except for palliation. Immunotherapy has been used successfully to prolong survival, sometimes for several years. The 5-year survival rate appears to be about 5%.

MANAGEMENT OF THE NECK

Patients staged N0

The regional lymph nodes, although clinically impalpable, sometimes contain occult foci of malignant cells. It seems reasonable to expect that removal or treatment of regional lymph nodes, even when clinically clear, would improve cure rates. Alternatively, it can be argued that treatment of the regional nodes in all cases is unnecessary, because only a minority have metastases in the nodes. In practice, whenever the surgery for the primary cancer involves opening the neck, a prophylactic neck dissection is undertaken. The submandibular triangle often must be opened as part of the resection of the primary, and therefore a function-sparing elective neck dissection for tumours in the floor of the mouth, lower alveolar ridge and tongue is advocated. In this dissection, structures such as the accessory nerve, internal jugular vein and sternocleidomastoid muscle are preserved.

The operation should preferably be seen as a staging procedure on which is based the decision to give radical postoperative radiotherapy. All patients with two or more positive nodes or extracapsular spread should be treated with postoperative radiotherapy.

Patients staged N1, N2a, N2b

Present evidence suggests that the treatment of choice is a full neck dissection wherever possible sparing the sternocleidomastoid muscle, the accessory nerve and the internal jugular vein, either alone or combined with postoperative radiotherapy if multiple nodal involvement or extracapsular extension is found in the resected specimen. In patients unfit for radical surgery, radical external beam irradiation is indicated.

Patients staged N2c

It is uncommon for patients with oral cancer to present with bilateral nodes. When they do so, there is often a large inoperable primary tumour, which is best treated by external radiation. It therefore seems logical to treat the neck also by irradiation. Occasionally, particularly in a young patient, bilateral neck dissection can be justified. A full radical neck dissection is undertaken on the ipsilateral side and the internal jugular vein is spared if possible on the contralateral side. Most often postoperative radiotherapy will be required for multiple nodal involvement or extra-capsular spread. In such situations, severe post-treatment oedema or congestion of the face and tongue may be anticipated.

Patients staged N3

N3 indicates massive involvement, usually with fixation. Large fixed nodes are often associated with advanced primary disease with a poor prognosis. Surgery is not normally advisable: removal of the common or internal carotid artery with replacement, or extensive resection, of the base of the skull, although technically feasible, is seldom advisable. Treatment is most often by external radiotherapy. In a few younger patients with resectable primaries it is worth rendering a fixed mass in the neck operable by preoperative radiotherapy.

Nodal metastasis appearing after primary treatment

Provided that follow-up at regular intervals is rigorously maintained, it should be possible to detect a lymph node metastasis while it is still relatively small and therefore operable. Ultrasound-guided fine-needle aspiration cytology is particularly useful in this situation to confirm that the palpable node is a carcinoma rather than being enlarged due to reactive hyperplasia. Whenever positive, or if there is any doubt, a radical neck dissection is performed, followed by external irradiation if multiple involved nodes or extracapsular spread are found.

FOLLOW-UP

Approximately 50% of patients treated for oral cancer will die from the disease, approximately 20% of patients will develop a local recurrence at the site of the primary tumour; another 25% will develop nodal metastases. Both of these events are likely to occur within the first 2 years following treatment. A further 20% of patients with oral cancers will develop additional new cancers elsewhere in the upper aerodigestive tract due to field changes resulting from tobacco and alcohol abuse. For all these reasons careful and meticulous follow-up is essential. For the first 12 months following treatment the patient will be seen at the hospital monthly. During the second year the patient is seen at 2- to 3-month intervals and thereafter they are seen every 6 months.

The general dental practitioner has an ongoing role in monitoring and treating dental diseases, which might impact on the tissues treated because of cancer and in observing for any new malignant disease.

Role of the general dental practitioner following treatment

- Regular 6-monthly monitoring for life
- Early attention to all new caries or periodontal disease
- Continuing use of fluoride mouthwash indefinitely
- Urgent referral of patient if any suspicion of recurrence or new cancer
- Absolute avoidance of dental extractions or surgery in patients who have received radiotherapy

---

FURTHER READING

Kramer I. R. H., El-Laban N., Lee K. W. (1978) The clinical features and risk of malignant transformation in sublingual keratosis. *British Dental Journal* 144: 171–180.

Langdon J. D., Henk J. M. (1995) *Malignant tumours of the mouth, jaws and salivary glands*. Edward Arnold, London.

Ord R. A., Blanchaert R. H. (1999) *Oral cancer. The dentist's role in diagnosis, management, rehabilitation and prevention*. Quintessence, Chicago, IL.

Pindborg J. J. (1980) *Oral cancer and precancer*. Wright, Bristol, UK.

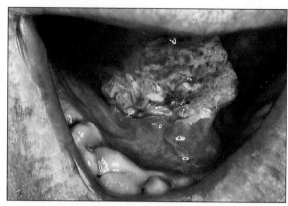

Fig. 10.14 See question 3.

SELF-ASSESSMENT

1. What are the principal risk factors for the development of squamous cell carcinoma of the mouth and oropharynx?
2. How do the following compare with respect to their risk of malignant change?
   (a) Leukoplakia
   (b) Erythroplakia
   (c) Submucous fibrosis
   (d) Lichen planus
3. How are the following cancers likely to be treated?
   (a) A 1-cm diameter squamous cell carcinoma of the tip of the tongue in an otherwise fit 60-year-old person.
   (b) A 3-cm diameter squamous cell carcinoma of the floor of mouth (Fig. 10.14), involving the alveolus and with several positive nodes on the same side of the neck.
   (c) Widespread erythroplakia of both cheeks, floor of the mouth and lips, with multiple early invasive squamous cell carcinomas.
4. What is the role of the dental practitioner following treatment for oral cancer?
5. What are the principal drawbacks of surgery and radiotherapy for the management of oral cancer?

Answers on page 266.

11 | Surgical aids to prosthodontics, including osseointegrated implants

I. R. Matthew

- Preprosthetic surgery is a term for surgical procedures undertaken on the edentulous or partially dentate oral tissues before denture construction.
- The aim of preprosthetic surgery is to provide the ideal denture-bearing area for a prosthesis, having satisfactory stability and retention.
- Preprosthetic surgery is therefore indicated when prosthodontic measures alone are insufficient.
- Preprosthetic surgery procedures are ideally undertaken in consultation with a prosthodontist.

ASSUMED KNOWLEDGE

It is assumed at this stage that you will have knowledge/competencies in the following areas:

- anatomy of the face and jaws
- dental anatomy
- changes in anatomy associated with the extraction of teeth
- the principles of fixed and removable prosthodontics.

If you think that you are not well equipped in these areas, revise them before reading this chapter or cross-check with texts on those subjects as you read.

INTENDED LEARNING OUTCOMES

At the end of this chapter you should be able to:

1. Understand the principles of and indications for preprosthetic surgery
2. Explain the principal advantages and disadvantages of preprosthetic surgery procedures
3. Select suitable cases that might benefit from preprosthetic surgical treatment
4. Recognize which patients require referral for specialist care
5. Suggest a variety of techniques suitable for an individual patient's prosthetic problem.

INTRODUCTION

Although many advances in dental health have been made over the past few decades, it is nevertheless rare for an individual to retain a full complement of natural teeth for life. Teeth are lost for various reasons, notably periodontal disease, dental caries, pathological conditions of the jaws and trauma. Prosthodontics aims to restore not only the function and aesthetics of the dentition after tooth loss but also the aesthetics of the facial form.

A well-constructed removable prosthesis that replaces missing teeth will restore function and appearance. A removable prosthesis should be stable and have adequate retention and stability. To achieve this, the prosthesis should be seated onto well-shaped alveolar ridges with adequate basal bone and a healthy oral mucosa. There will ideally be no major vertical or horizontal skeletal discrepancy, which can compromise denture stability.

Preprosthetic surgery is a term used for surgical procedures that aim to improve the condition of the oral tissues to enable a removable denture to rest on a sound base, free from marked bony protuberances or undercuts, with no interfering muscle attachments, flabby soft-tissue excess or hyperplastic oral mucosa. To achieve the best results, the skills of the oral surgeon and the prosthodontist are combined in a team approach.

Endosseous implants are commonly placed in suitable patients to improve the stability and retention of removable dentures as well as fixed prostheses. Implants may avoid the need for more complex surgery to improve an otherwise unsatisfactory edentulous ridge.

AIMS AND OBJECTIVES OF PREPROSTHETIC SURGERY

The aim of preprosthetic surgery is to prepare the soft and hard tissues of the jaws for a comfortable prosthesis that will restore oral function, aesthetics and facial form.

The objectives of preprosthetic surgery are to help to:

- restore function of the jaws (mastication of food, speech and swallowing)
- preserve or improve jaw structure
- improve the patient's sense of well being (quality of life)
- improve facial aesthetics

by:

- eliminating pain and discomfort arising from an ill-fitting prosthesis by surgically modifying the denture-bearing area
- improving the denture-bearing area for patients in whom there has been extensive loss of alveolar bone
- inserting endosseous implants into the jaws.

Non-surgical options should always be considered first (e.g. remaking a technically unacceptable pros-

thesis, relining, adjusting the occlusal face height or extending the denture flanges to improve retention and stability) before preprosthetic surgery is undertaken.

Preprosthetic surgery may be undertaken to:

- Improve the condition of the residual ridge or the overlying soft tissues before denture construction, and thereby improve the retention and stability of a denture
- Insert endosseous implants within the bone to replace missing teeth or to improve removable denture stability or retention
- Correct skeletal discrepancies in the relationships of the jaws

---

PHYSIOLOGICAL CHANGES IN THE ORAL TISSUES AND MASTICATORY APPARATUS ASSOCIATED WITH AGE

The oral tissues undergo physiological changes with advancing age, some of which may influence the outcome of prosthodontic rehabilitation:

- the effectiveness of mastication decreases
- saliva production sometimes decreases
- blood flow decreases through major blood vessels (e.g. inferior alveolar artery)
- osteoporosis may affect the jaws, particularly in females.

As we age the blood supply to the jaws becomes increasingly dependent on the circulation in the periosteum, rather than from the arteries. This is largely due to age changes leading to narrowing of the lumen of vessels such as the inferior alveolar artery. Consequently, it is important to preserve the periosteum and its blood supply wherever possible, to minimize the risk of ischaemic necrosis of underlying bone.

Physiological changes in the oral tissues are sometimes a consequence of hormonal changes. For example, oral discomfort may occur in women without overt clinical signs, and denture wearing may aggravate the symptoms in some patients. In a few cases, oral discomfort may be attributed to the menopause, and the symptoms may resolve after hormone replacement therapy. It is therefore necessary to obtain a comprehensive history from the patient in order to identify accurately the cause of any oral discomfort associated with denture wearing. Nutrition can also play a part in oral discomfort; some patients with sore mouth may be anaemic.

ANATOMICAL CONSEQUENCES OF TOOTH LOSS

Loss of alveolar bone

Changes occur in the morphology of the jaws after tooth loss (Fig. 11.1). The jaws are composed of alveolar and basal bone. The alveolar bone and periodontium support the teeth, but neither have a physiological function once the teeth are lost, and are therefore resorbed. Alveolar bone changes shape significantly with tooth loss, in both the horizontal and vertical planes, but the overall pattern of resorption is largely predictable. In the maxilla and in the anterior aspect of the mandible bone loss occurs typically in both the horizontal and vertical planes. In the posterior mandible the bone loss is mostly in the vertical plane.

After physiological resorption has occurred, the remaining jaw structure is termed the 'residual ridge'. The bone that remains after alveolar bone has resorbed is termed 'basal bone'. Marked resorption sometimes affects the entire mandible (Fig. 11.2). Basal bone does not change shape significantly unless it is subjected to excessive local forces, for example, in the edentulous anterior maxilla in association with retained natural lower incisors.

Other affected anatomical structures

Other anatomical structures may become more prominent with tooth loss. The genial tubercles and their muscle attachments may become prominent in a patient with extensive resorption of the mandible, sometimes compromising denture stability. Maxillary or mandibular tori may also cause instability of a denture, or may be traumatized by it. A prominent fraenum (Fig. 11.3) can displace a denture during function, and may weaken the denture base so that it fractures through flexing.

Forces transmitted through the teeth during mastication are absorbed by the supporting structures (the

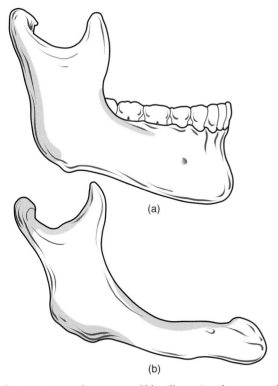

(a)

(b)

Fig. 11.1 (a) A dentate mandible, illustrating the extent of supporting (alveolar) bone around the teeth. (b) An edentulous mandible, illustrating the extent of resorption of alveolar bone that occurs following loss of the teeth. Note also that the angle between the ascending ramus and body of the mandible is more obtuse than in (a), and the mental foramen is also closer to the crest of the edentulous ridge. The shaded areas in this illustration indicate areas of resorption of mandibular bone with advancing age.

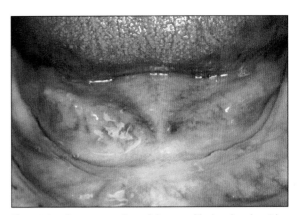

Fig. 11.2 Gross resorption of the mandibular alveolar ridge gives rise to denture instability, due in part to the reduced surface area of the alveolar ridge, but also to the prominence of the mandibular muscle attachments (e.g. genioglossus), which displace the denture during tongue movements.

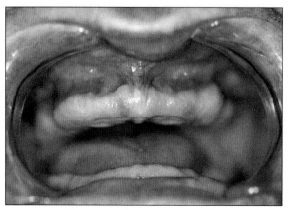

Fig. 11.3 A prominent labial fraenum causes displacement of the denture. If the denture flange is eased to fit round the fraenum, the denture may be weakened. Excision of the fraenum (fraenectomy) is indicated.

Table 11.1 A classification of the edentulous jaws	
Class	Description
I	Dentate
II	Immediately postextraction
III	Convex ridge form, adequate in height and width
IV	Knife-edge ridge form, adequate in height but inadequate in width
V	Flat ridge form, inadequate in height and width
VI	Loss of basal bone, which may be extensive but follows no predictable pattern

From Cawood and Howell (1988)

periodontium and alveolar bone). In an edentulous patient, forces exerted by a denture are transmitted through the oral mucosa to the underlying bone. A denture must therefore fit well if trauma to the oral mucosa overlying an edentulous ridge is to be avoided.

Facial aesthetics are affected by tooth loss. The facial profile collapses (the nose and chin appear too close together) after tooth loss and consequent edentulousness. The loss of face height can be restored with dentures.

CLASSIFICATION OF THE EDENTULOUS JAWS

Cawood and Howell (1988) classified the edentulous jaws according to the state of ridge resorption after tooth loss (Table 11.1). There are other classifications, but this one has been adopted internationally as a means of assisting communication and assessment of a patient's edentulous state.

THE IDEAL EDENTULOUS RIDGE

A removable denture requires a firm bone support with a smooth contour, adequate to provide stability, with access to the vestibule for a peripheral seal, and without any soft-tissue excess (e.g. flabby maxillary tuberosities) likely to cause displacement or weakness of the denture.

Most patients tolerate the loss of their natural teeth and subsequent denture wearing without difficulty. However, there may be extensive loss of alveolar bone after tooth extraction, resulting in an atrophic (flat or knife-edged) edentulous ridge (Fig. 11.4). In some patients this can make denture wearing difficult or uncomfortable. The prosthodontist may be able to modify a denture design to enhance its stability and retention, but this is not always possible. Surgery may therefore be required to enhance retention and stability of the prosthesis.

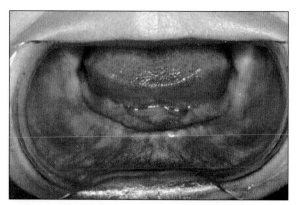

Fig. 11.4 This 32-year-old patient has difficulty in wearing a denture. The alveolar ridge has a 'knife-edge' profile, and there is a loss of sulcus depth.

TREATMENT PLANNING

History

The history will indicate the patient's principal concerns and expectations of treatment. The age and health of the patient influence the treatment plan—a young person with severely resorbed alveolar ridges might tolerate more complex surgery than would a mature patient with similar jaw morphology.

Clinical examination

This will include general extraoral and intraoral assessment of the hard and soft tissues, and specific analysis of the denture-bearing areas.

The height, width and general shape of the alveolar ridges are assessed, with an emphasis on the presence of bony undercuts and the position of anatomical structures such as the mental neurovascular bundle. The depth of the buccal sulci, the position and size of fraenal and muscle attachments and the condition of the alveolar ridges are documented. The dentures should be technically acceptable before considering preprosthetic surgery.

Special investigations

Radiographs are taken to assess the condition of the underlying bone. A panoramic film is useful to assess the overall condition of the edentulous ridges and to identify any retained dental roots or other pathology (e.g. cysts of the jaws). A lateral cephalostat may be taken to demonstrate the anteroposterior skeletal relationship and the height of the alveolar ridges anteriorly. Periapical views are desirable if retained roots are to be removed before construction of a denture.

Articulated study casts facilitate treatment planning and are helpful when explaining the surgical procedure to a patient. A diagnostic wax-up of the prosthesis is desirable to demonstrate the anticipated final aesthetic result to the patient, and as a medico-legal record of the proposed treatment.

PREPROSTHETIC SURGERY PROCEDURES

Various techniques may be used, either alone or in combination, to preserve or improve the denture-

> **Summary of treatment planning**
>
> - Consider the patient's concerns and expectations
> - Assess their medical fitness
> - Examine both extraorally and intraorally
> - Assess the height, width, regularity and relationship of the ridges
> - Consider whether improvement can be achieved by prosthetic means
> - Radiographs may be needed to exclude other pathology and to determine the quantity and quality of bone
> - Study casts and a diagnostic wax-up may be of value

bearing area. There are three broad categories of preprosthetic surgery procedure:

1. Soft-tissue surgery
2. Bone-contouring (or augmentation) procedures
3. Endosseous implant surgery.

Some of the procedures described below may be included in more than one category.

Soft-tissue procedures

Excision of hyperplastic tissue

Hyperplastic oral mucosa under or adjacent to a removable denture usually arises in response to chronic irritation, for example, from an over-extended denture flange or a deficiency in the fitting surface of a denture, trauma from a sharp cusp on an acrylic tooth or an ill-fitting denture clasp. Poor denture design may also cause mucosal hyperplasia (Figs 11.5, 11.6). Surgery may be unnecessary if the cause of the hyperplastic tissue is identified and eliminated; the hyperplastic tissue will then usually diminish in size or resolve completely. Any residual tissue that interferes with denture construction can be removed via an elliptical incision as for an excision biopsy (see Ch. 8, p. 109). Where possible (e.g. in the buccal sulcus or on the cheek), the incision may be closed by suturing the wound edges together (primary closure). On the edentulous ridge, the periosteum is elevated to undermine the edges of the wound, and the edges of the mucoperiosteal flaps can then be advanced to achieve wound closure. A split-thickness skin graft may be required to cover extensive areas of denuded oral mucosa. A keratinized-free mucosal graft may be harvested from the hard palate for smaller areas.

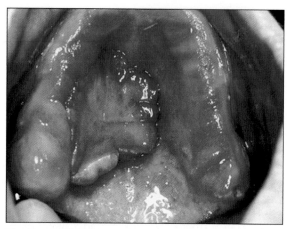

Fig. 11.5 This is an extensive 'leaf fibroma' of the hard palate. The lesion was attached to the hard palate by a small stalk (a peduncle) and resembled the outline of a relief chamber incorporated into the fitting surface of the denture.

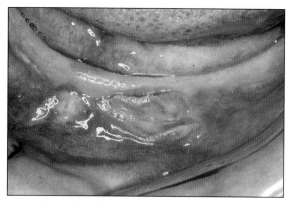

Fig. 11.6 Fibroepithelial hyperplasia associated with the irritant margin of an ill-fitting lower denture.

It is often beneficial to place a temporary soft lining in the existing denture after surgery, to minimize the likelihood of further irritation, prior to remaking the prosthesis.

Prominent labial fraenum

The flange of a denture may traumatize a prominent labial fraenum or muscle attachment (Fig. 11.3). If the fraenum is relatively small, this may be managed by trimming back the labial or lingual denture flange. However, the denture may be weakened and it might fracture if extensive trimming is undertaken to relieve the fraenum. Excision of the fraenum (fraenectomy) may be indicated to avoid this.

For the fraenectomy procedure (also described in Ch. 12) vertical incisions are made parallel to the fraenum, extending into the sulcus from the residual ridge to form a rhomboid-shaped wound (Fig. 11.7). The incisions are widest at the base of the labial sulcus. The insertion of the fraenum into the alveolar ridge is held with either a suture or a pair of toothed tissue forceps and the fraenum is dissected, leaving periosteum covering the surface of the bone. Interrupted sutures are inserted through the mucoperiosteal flap to achieve wound closure. A modification of this procedure incorporates a Z-plasty, to preserve sulcus depth (Fig. 11.8). However, the Z-plasty can be technically more difficult than the fraenectomy technique described above.

Fibrous enlargement of the maxillary tuberosity

Ideally, the maxillary tuberosities are firm for denture support. If they are flabby and mobile, the soft tissues of the tuberosities may displace during impression-taking for a new denture, making denture construction difficult. Fibrous enlargement of a maxillary tuberosity may be reduced (Fig. 11.9) by making two incisions along the crest of the alveolar ridge to form an ellipse, angled towards the centre of the

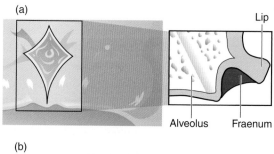

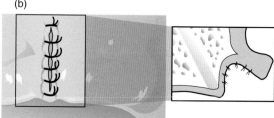

Fig. 11.7 Conventional fraenectomy.
(a, b) With the upper lip everted, a rhomboid-shaped incision is made around the fleshy fraenum, extending through the oral mucosa to the submucosal layer below, preserving muscle fibres of orbicularis oris.

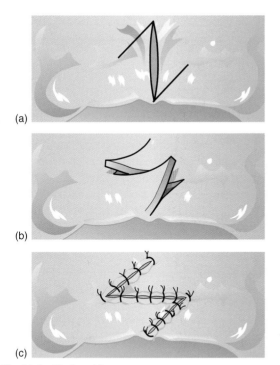

Fig. 11.8 'Z-plasty' fraenectomy.
(a) After the fleshy fraenum has been excised, two oblique incisions are made down to periosteum.
(b) The triangular-shaped flaps are raised to expose underlying bone and the flaps are reversed so that the inferior triangular flap now becomes the most superior.
(c) The wound is closed.

ridge down to bone. A triangular-shaped wedge of tissue is excised, and a 'fillet' of soft tissue is excised from each flap. The wound edges are then sutured together.

Hard-tissue procedures

Dentoalveolar procedures

Care is taken when extracting teeth or dental roots with forceps or via a surgical approach to ensure preservation of alveolar bone and oral mucosa. Buccal bone may fracture and remain adherent to a tooth root after extraction. This is most likely to occur with canine teeth if there has been minimal bone loss through periodontal disease. Use of a dental elevator will minimize the risk of fracture of alveolar bone before delivery of a tooth with extraction forceps. Fracture of the maxillary tuberosity during tooth extraction may result in extensive bone loss leading to poor denture stability.

The periotome (Fig. 11.10) is increasingly being used to extract teeth before implant surgery (cf. extraction instruments described in Ch. 4). This device is composed of a narrow, flat blade which is pushed down into the gingivae, and breaks down the periodontal fibres supporting the tooth. Periotomes preserve the alveolar bone, which is essential when placing an immediate endosseous implant after tooth

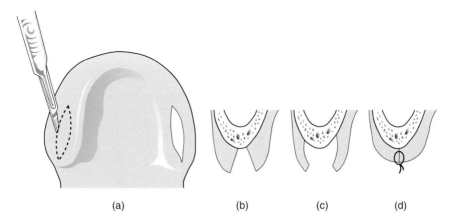

(a)   (b)   (c)   (d)

Fig. 11.9 Reduction of hyperplastic tuberosities.
(a) An elliptical incision is made down to bone and the ellipse of soft tissue is excised.
(b) The scalpel creates an oblique cut, as seen in cross-section.
(c) The underlying submucosa is filleted to reduce the bulk of the tuberosity.
(d) The wound edges are apposed and sutured.

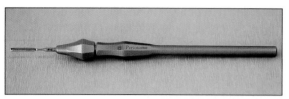

Fig. 11.10 An example of a periotome. The flat blade inserted into the handle is interchangeable with other blades. The blade is inserted into the periodontal ligament and through continuous manipulation, the periodontal fibres are cut around the tooth until it is extracted.

extraction (web sites include http://www.citagenix. com, http://www.klsmartinusa.com/OfficeProducts/ periotome.htm).

If alveolar bone is displaced during tooth extraction, it is repositioned by digital pressure after tooth delivery. Loose fragments of alveolar bone in the socket are removed to prevent delayed healing. Larger fragments with an intact periosteal blood supply are left *in situ*.

Alveoplasty

This procedure is performed to recontour an uneven alveolar ridge. Alveoplasty is undertaken either at the time of tooth extraction (primary) or after the alveolar ridge has healed (secondary). Alveoplasty removes the least amount of bone necessary to achieve a smooth bone contour.

Primary alveoplasty involves the exposure of a tooth socket to allow trimming of bone fragments with bone rongeurs or a bur to create a smooth, rounded socket outline. When several adjacent teeth are removed, alveoplasty may be combined with interseptal alveolotomy to eliminate bony undercuts (Fig. 11.11).

After tooth extraction, a bony protuberance may exist on the edentulous ridge or a bony undercut

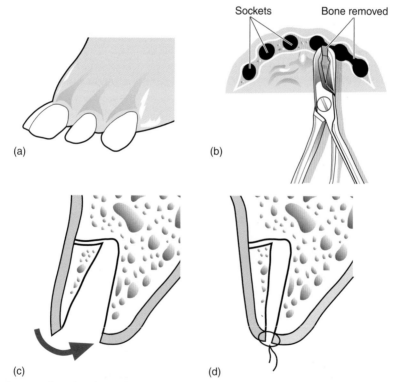

Fig. 11.11 (a) Reduction of an alveolar undercut by removal of the interseptal bone (interseptal alveolotomy). This might be required in the anterior maxilla in a patient with proclined incisor and canine teeth. (b) After extraction, rongeurs (bone nibblers) or bone shears are used to remove the interseptal bone. (c) Using digital pressure the buccal alveolar bone (still attached to the periosteum) is 'in-fractured' to reduce the bony undercut. (d) Sutures are placed to close the wound.

may be present several months later, compromising denture stability. Secondary alveoplasty is then undertaken. An incision is made along the crest of the ridge to expose the alveolar bone surface. The bony prominence or undercut is smoothed with a bur, bone file or a chisel to achieve the desired contour (Fig. 11.12), and after palpating the reshaped ridge to ensure a smooth contour, the wound is closed with sutures.

Excision of a maxillary or mandibular torus

A torus (Figs 11.13, 11.14) is a developmental bone exostosis, present typically either on the midline of the hard palate or on the lingual aspect of the mandible above the mylohyoid ridge (usually bilaterally). Patients are often unaware of their existence. There are other causes of bony expansion of the jaws, some of which may have a history of slow onset and gradual enlargement. A neoplastic lesion (usually of minor salivary gland origin) sometimes develops on the hard palate, and it has been known for a dentist to ease a denture to accommodate an enlarging malignant growth. If there is doubt about the nature of any lesion, the patient is referred for a specialist opinion.

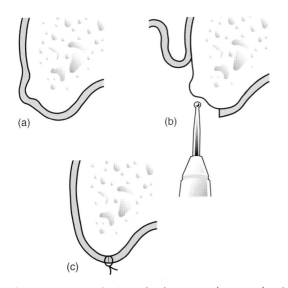

Fig. 11.12 (a) Reduction of a bony protuberance that is interfering with denture fitting. (b) An incision has been made along the crest of the alveolar ridge. A mucoperiosteal flap has been raised, and a round surgical bur is used to smooth the protuberance. (c) The wound is debrided and the flap is sutured back into position.

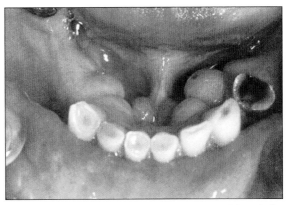

Fig. 11.13 Lingual tori are typically bilateral, although the patient is often unaware of their existence.

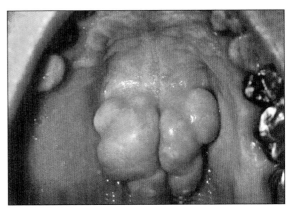

Fig. 11.14 Torus palatinus is typically symmetrical about the midline of the hard palate.

A denture rubbing on a torus may cause ulceration of the overlying oral mucosa and pain. Removal of a torus may therefore be indicated if the denture cannot be constructed to avoid it.

Radiographs are taken before excision of a maxillary torus to examine its structure. If a maxillary torus has an air space within it that communicates with the floor of the nose, then excision of the torus might result in an oronasal fistula, which can be difficult to treat.

Limited surgical access or a pronounced gag reflex might compromise treatment under local anaesthesia. General anaesthesia is sometimes indicated, particularly for maxillary surgery.

Surgical access to a palatal torus is gained via a midline incision over the lesion, with short (avoiding the greater palatine artery) relieving incisions at either end (Fig. 11.15). The flaps are raised to expose

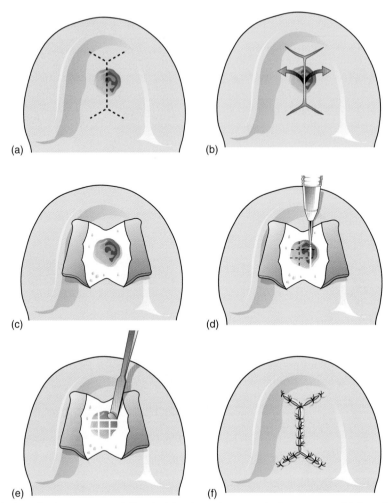

(a)

(b)

(c)

(d)

(e)

(f)

Fig. 11.15 Removal of a palatal torus. (a) A midline incision is made across the bony mass, with lateral extensions anteriorly and posteriorly. (b, c) The mucoperiosteal flaps are reflected to expose the bony mass. (d) A bur is used to divide the torus into small pieces. (e) A chisel is used to elevate the small fragments of bone from the hard palate. (f) The wound is debrided and the bone is smoothed with a bur, then sutures are placed to close the wound.

the torus, and the mass is excised either with a rotary bur, a chisel or both. Destruction of the torus with a rotary bur (e.g. a large acrylic bur) ensures safe, gradual removal of the mass. Alternatively a flat fissure bur is used to section the torus into smaller pieces, which are freed with a chisel and a surgical mallet. After suturing the flaps, an acrylic surgical stent (cover plate) may then be placed to cover the wound, to help prevent haematoma formation.

A mandibular torus is exposed by raising a lingual flap, releasing the gingival margin around any teeth adjacent to the torus. If the patient is edentulous, the incision is along the crest of the alveolar ridge, avoiding the mental neurovascular bundle (Fig. 11.16).

A surgical bur or chisel and mallet may then be used to divide the torus from the surface of the mandible. After removal of the excess bone, the osteotomized surface is palpated to ensure a smooth outline before the lingual flap is replaced and sutured (a surgical stent may be placed to prevent dead space and haematoma formation).

Restoration of grossly deficient denture-bearing areas

Many surgical procedures have been devised to augment atrophic jaw bone. A key problem with bone augmentation is the resorption that follows such surgery, leaving the patient without significant gain

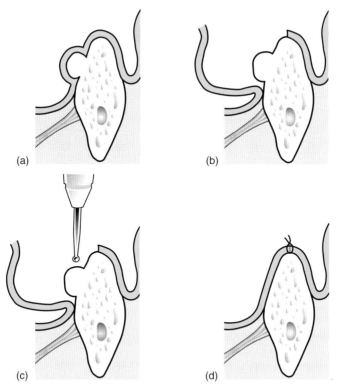

(a)　　　　　　　　　　(b)

(c)　　　　　　　　　　(d)

Fig. 11.16 (a) A lingual torus is covered by thin oral mucosa, and considerable care is required to avoid accidental perforation of the flap. (b) The mucoperiosteal flap is raised to expose the entire bony mass. (c) A surgical bur or chisel may be used to remove the bony torus. Conscious patients may find the sensation of the chisel being used unpleasant, but in experienced hands the technique is quick and safe. (d) The wound is closed with multiple resorbable sutures.

in function. Bone grafting on its own is insufficient to improve a patient's deficiency. When undertaken in combination with endosseous implants, the outcome of bone grafting is often highly encouraging.

OSSEOINTEGRATED (ENDOSSEOUS) IMPLANTS

Endosseous implant surgery offers considerable flexibility in preprosthetic surgery, but the practitioner should gain experience in minor oral surgery procedures before contemplating implant surgery. Further training is required to acquire the additional diagnostic and surgical skills required. Implant companies will not usually sell implant components to a dentist who has not undertaken training in their implant system.

There are three main types of jaw implant:

- **endosseous (literally 'within the bone') implant**: has enhanced both the treatment options and the cost effectiveness of preprosthetic surgery. This type of implant is discussed in detail below
- **subperiosteal implant**: made popular in the 1970s (now rarely if ever used), this device was a custom-made metal frame inserted as an onlay directly onto the surface of cortical bone. The frame was fabricated from impressions taken of the exposed surface of the jaw. The frame was subsequently fitted onto the jaw bone. Abutments that protrude through the oral mucosa supported a denture. Wound dehiscence and infection were common problems with this implant because of mobility between the implant and bone

● **transsosseous implant**: includes the Small mandibular staple implant and the Bosker transmandibular implant. A transsosseous (extending all the way through the bone) implant may be indicated for severe atrophy of the mandible in which endosseous implants are contraindicated, or as an alternative to ridge augmentation.

Endosseous implants

In the past few decades the management of tooth loss has been revolutionized through endosseous implant surgery. Brånemark and colleagues pioneered research on the integration of titanium implants with direct bone contact in the 1960s. Most endosseous implants are constructed from pure titanium because of its ideal biological performance characteristics as an implant material.

Osseointegration is a clinical and histological concept that describes the natural apposition of bone to an implant with a subsequent ability of the implant to sustain loading and transfer the load to and within the adjacent bone (Fig. 11.17). Stringent clinical and technical standards are required to achieve osseointegration. Survival rates for titanium implants in excess of 86% in the mandible and 78% in the maxilla at 15 years have been reported. Recent advances in implant design and surface treatment technology have improved the survival rates.

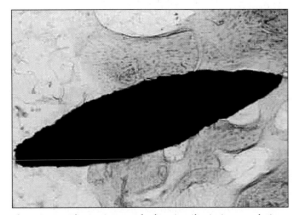

Fig. 11.17 Photomicrograph showing the intimate relationship between newly formed bone and a titanium endosseous implant (shown in black) embedded within cancellous bone of the jaws for 12 weeks.

Factors that influence the success of endosseous implants

These include:

● biocompatibility of the implant material
● design of the implant
● surface characteristics—various surface treatments are applied to enhance the biological response (e.g. titanium plasma spray coating, acid etching, grit-blasting with titanium powder, machined surface finish to improve the gingival attachment)
● physical health of the patient
● quality of bone
● favourable anatomical conditions
● patient's cooperation, oral hygiene status, smoking habits
● operator experience
● loading of the implants after osseointegration.

Implant systems

There are many different implant systems. In selecting a suitable system, manufacturers' claims about the superiority of a particular system should always be supported by laboratory data and published clinical trials. Most are based on a cylindrical or screw design. Implant systems are usually placed as a single-stage fixture (the implant or its healing abutment protrudes into the oral cavity on insertion) or two-stage (the implant is buried beneath the oral mucosa for several months to osseointegrate before it is exposed; a fixture that protrudes into the oral cavity is then inserted). The trend now is for implants to be loaded immediately on insertion or after a relatively short period of osseointegration (a few weeks).

Treatment planning for endosseous implants

A complete history and examination will establish the patient's suitability for implants. A standard proforma for implant surgery will ensure a comprehensive, systematic history and examination. The medical history will identify possible contraindications for implants. An appraisal of the remaining dentition, the periodontal tissues and the standard of oral hygiene is required. Surgical access to the implant site is also assessed (Fig. 11.18). The type of anaesthesia is discussed with the patient at an early stage; intravenous sedation with local analgesia may be preferred in the outpatient or dental practice setting.

Contraindications for endosseous implants

Endosseous implants are not recommended for patients below the age of 16 because of the potential for further growth of the jaws; the implant is anky-losed in the bone, and therefore it will become sub-merged as the jaws grow. There is no absolute upper age limit for endosseous implants.

A patient's medical history will determine their suitability for endosseous implants. For example, a poorly controlled diabetic is at risk of infection and soft-tissue breakdown around an implant, which may contraindicate implant surgery. The patient may have a history of psychosis, or there may be an ongoing history of drug or alcohol abuse. Such patients are unsuitable for implant surgery. Referral for a specialist opinion is recommended if there is doubt about the suitability of a patient with medical problems for implant surgery.

Poor oral hygiene will compromise implant provision because of peri-implant inflammatory disease (which is destructive in a manner similar to perio-dontitis). Patient education can effectively improve oral hygiene status in some patients. A patient must demonstrate consistency in maintaining their oral hygiene over several months; only then can im-plants become a feasible option. Smoking is a rela-tive contraindication, because some smokers are at

increased risk of losing the implant through inflam-mation of the peri-implant mucosa, and increased resorption of peri-implant bone. This manifests clini-cally as an increase in the bleeding index, the peri-implant pocket depth, the degree of peri-implant mucosal inflammation and radiographic evidence of bone resorption mesial and distal to the implant. There is emerging evidence of an increased risk for implant loss in patients on bisphosphonates, though the risk for patients on oral bisphosphonates seems to be less than for patients having intravenous doses (see Ch. 4, p. 42 concerning osteonecrosis follow-ing tooth extraction).

Special investigations

The height, width and overall shape of the residual ridge are evaluated from study models and radio-graphs to ensure adequate bone to support the im-plant. Articulated study casts are required to evaluate the occlusion; there should be no excessive forces on the implant during lateral or protrusive excursions of the jaws. A preliminary assessment of the ideal position and angulation of implants may be made from the study casts, in conjunction with a surgical stent (Fig. 11.19). Radiographs (Fig. 11.20) will deter-mine the quality of the bone and help in assessing suitable sites for implants. The radiographs should

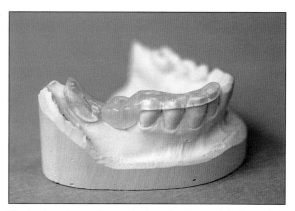

Fig. 11.19 An acrylic stent is placed in the mouth before radio-graphy to evaluate the quality and quantity of bone at the desired site of implant insertion. Gutta percha inserted into a bur hole cut into the acrylic stent will assist in radiographic planning. The dimensions of the gutta percha and the angulation of the bur hole permit accurate assessment of the proposed implant site.

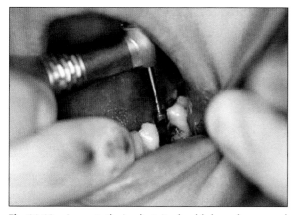

Fig. 11.18 Access to the implant site should always be assessed before embarking on implant surgery. At the beginning of site preparation there is little room to get the drill in a good position.

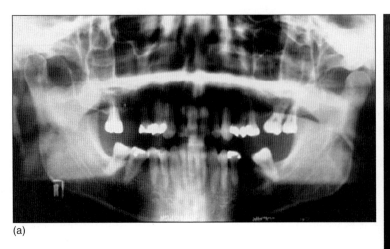

(a)

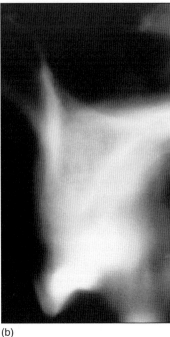

(b)

Fig. 11.20 (a) A panoramic radiograph yields much information about the teeth and jaws, but is unhelpful in determining the suitability of the bone at the proposed site of an implant in tooth 16 position. (b) A tomographic view of the bone in the tooth 16 area gives more information about the quality of the bone and the height of the maxillary sinus.

adequately demonstrate important structures (the inferior alveolar neurovascular bundle, the floor of the nose, the maxillary antrum and adjacent teeth).

It is necessary to establish whether an implant can be placed with the desired stability within bone and satisfactory soft-tissue aesthetics. If there is insufficient bone, then bone grafting must be considered. Bone may be grafted from the patient, e.g. from the chin (Fig. 11.21), tuberosity region or retromolar region in the mandible. Proprietary bone scrapers facilitate the collection of autogenous bone by scraping the cortical surface. Blocks of cortical bone may be taken, or cancellous bone chips may be harvested, depending on the extent of bone deficiency at the implant site.

When the soft tissue is deficient, a connective tissue or mucosal graft might be indicated. Such soft-tissue grafts are taken from the hard palate. Connective tissue grafts e.g. Alloderm (an acellular dermal matrix derived from donated human skin tissue) can also be purchased for use in such situations. The key objective with a soft-tissue graft is to re-establish the gingival contour for aesthetic reasons.

Determining the optimum length of an implant

Most X-ray units do not give 1:1 magnification of the image: this must be borne in mind when planning the optimum dimensions of an implant from the

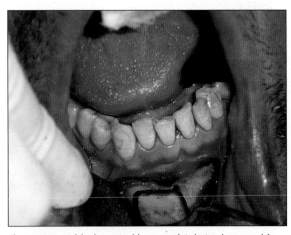

Fig. 11.21 A block cortical bone graft is being harvested from the patient's chin to augment an atrophic upper central incisor socket. The block graft will be fixed with a bone screw at the recipient site.

radiographs. An acrylic stent may be used to determine the planned location of an implant. The stent is fitted over the teeth or edentulous jaw (Fig. 11.19) when the radiograph is taken.

CT scans (Fig. 11.22) are gaining popularity in the assessment of a patient before implant surgery. Cone-beam CT scan units offer improved functionality and convenience over conventional CT scanning units (http://www.imagingsciences.com/pro_iCAT_features.htm). In the above illustration, a patient requesting implants in the right posterior maxillary sextant has undergone an I-Cat scan to assess the bone. There is a deficiency in the buccal bone in sections 34–36, and clearly bone grafting is required before implants can be placed.

Planning the site of the implants from the radiograph

Endosseous implants are positioned within healthy bone, with an adequate height and width of bone. Forces applied to an implant should be axial rather than lateral, to avoid forces that might result in implant failure.

A radiograph is a medicolegal document and should *not* be altered in any way. A copy of the radiograph is therefore made (either a digital copy or a copy made on tracing paper from the original) and

the teeth and other anatomical structures such as the inferior alveolar canal, the floor of the nose and the maxillary antrum are highlighted on the copy. A transparent stencil (fixture guide) is superimposed on the tracing to plan with accuracy the proposed position of the implant. The fixture guide offers various magnifications depending on the X-ray unit used. The tracing may be used to illustrate the treatment plan to the patient.

The morphology of the residual ridge and the thickness of overlying mucosa are determined at the proposed site for the implants. Unless sophisticated CT scanning is available, a suitable implant cannot otherwise be selected reliably, and the procedure might have to be abandoned if there is inadequate bone. The depth of the oral mucosa cannot be assess-ed from a periapical or panoramic radiograph, because the image records the residual ridge only in two dimensions. Ridge mapping (Figs 11.23, 11.24) is simple and reliable, but may cause temporary mucosal trauma and discomfort.

Ridge mapping

Under local anaesthesia, a probe with millimetre markings along its tip is inserted into the oral mucosa overlying the alveolar ridge. The depth of the soft tissue is noted at all sites (Figs 11.23, 11.24). This information is transposed to a study model, and the shape of the residual ridge is recorded by trimming back the model stone to the corresponding depth of soft tissue.

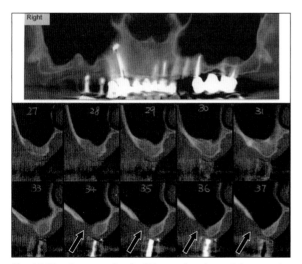

Fig. 11.22 An example of a CT scan showing a right posterior maxillary sextant with an obvious deficiency of bone (arrows), requiring augmentation with a sinus lift before implant placement.

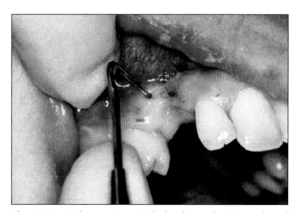

Fig. 11.23 Ridge mapping. Under local anaesthesia, a graduated probe is pushed into the oral mucosa until it contacts bone. The depth of the oral mucosa is measured.

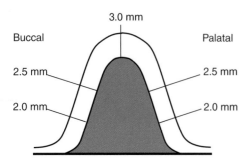

3.0 mm

Buccal   Palatal

2.5 mm   2.5 mm

2.0 mm   2.0 mm

Fig. 11.24   A written record of the ridge mapping readings is recorded in the patient's case notes.

Diagnostic wax-up

Having planned the position of the implants, a diagnostic wax-up (Fig. 11.25) will ensure that the desired aesthetic result can be achieved. If retained roots or other lesions are present, implant surgery must be deferred for 4–6 months after surgical intervention, to ensure satisfactory healing.

Informed consent

A complete discussion with the patient of all aspects of surgery, prior to commencing treatment is a requisite for consent for any operative procedure (see Ch. 2). For procedures which are lengthy, expensive and irreversible, such as implant surgery and subsequent prosthodontic rehabilitation it is doubly important. Only when the patient fully understands what is proposed can they establish realistic expectations of the treatment. Misunderstandings about implant therapy can be avoided when a written outline of the treatment proposed is given to the patient to read and sign. An individual having high (unrealistic) expectations may be disappointed by the outcome of surgery, and litigation may ensue. Written documented evidence of informed consent will help to avoid legal proceedings.

Treatment planning for endosseous implants
• Patient selection: adults, good hygiene, non-smoking, generally healthy • Height, width and shape of ridge, including radiographic examination • Determination of optimal length • Site planning • Ridge mapping • Diagnostic wax-up

SURGICAL PROCEDURE FOR ENDOSSEOUS IMPLANTS

There is a trend towards flapless surgery. The clinician will decide preoperatively whether a flap is required, based on past experience and clinical circumstances.

Flap design

Access is usually gained to the alveolar bone via a broad-based flap to ensure good visibility and reduce the risk of ischaemic necrosis of the flap extremities. The wound will be closed around a single-stage (transmucosal) implant, and the incision should take into consideration the site of the implant. For a two-stage implant the flap is extended palatally, and a rim of soft tissue is preserved around the cervical margin of adjacent teeth. Incisions are placed to avoid friction from a denture during healing.

The mucoperiosteal flap is incised; it may be tightly bound to an edentulous alveolar ridge, and flap elevation is sometimes difficult. Damage to the periosteum may result in postoperative pain and swelling of the tissues and delayed healing. If the flap is perforated, dehiscence or wound infection may result. Extensive exposure of the implant site is usually unnecessary; the blood supply to mandibular bone is dependent on intact periosteum and muscle insertions into the bone.

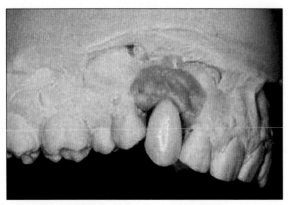

Fig. 11.25   A simple diagnostic wax-up with an acrylic tooth and pink wax.

Insertion of implants immediately after tooth extraction

Immediate implant insertion is gaining popularity, with good outcomes. In some circumstances it may be possible to insert an implant immediately after tooth extraction. Although undertaken by some operators with good results, this technique is not recommended routinely; each case is planned according to clinical circumstances. For example, the prognosis for successful osseointegration is poor in the presence of apical pathology prior to implant insertion. Other problems likely to be encountered include differences between the width of the natural tooth root and the endosseous implant and insufficient bone at the coronal aspect (a bone graft may be required to close the defect). A further disadvantage is that non-keratinized mucosa may have to be advanced to cover the implant.

A solution to the technical problems described above is to remove the tooth or root and insert the implant 4–6 weeks after extraction, when the soft tissues will have healed but the alveolar bone will not have undergone excessive resorption.

Preparation of bone and insertion of the implant

The manufacturer's recommended technique for preparation of the implant site is adhered to at all times. Important factors related to bone preparation are the cutting efficiency and speed of rotation of burs, the use of sterile coolant and the rate of bone cutting. The cutting efficiency of a bur will influence the survival of adjacent bone and the rate of healing. Surgical implant burs (Fig. 11.26) may be designed for single or multiple use; only sharp implant burs are used. Reusable burs are cleaned thoroughly before autoclaving to remove organic debris.

Sterile saline coolant is required at all times during bone cutting. The coolant itself may be refrigerated before use. Even when coolant is used, the temperature adjacent to drills may become excessive without due care; the threshold for tissue damage due to heat from friction during bone preparation is estimated to be 47°C for 1 minute. Gentle pressure is applied to the handpiece when cutting bone, and the bur is removed frequently from the bur hole and allowed to cool. With some implant systems

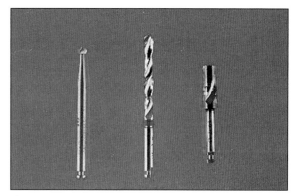

Fig. 11.26 Examples of burs used to prepare bone for an implant. The pilot hole is prepared with the bur on the left; the initial bone preparation is made with the bur in the centre and the cortical bone is cut with the bur on the right.

an internal irrigation system may be used to direct coolant to the tip of the drill.

If the alveolar ridge is uneven where the implant is to be inserted, alveoplasty is undertaken before a pilot hole is created through cortical bone. An acrylic stent, prepared with a bur hole for the proposed site of the implant, is fitted over the teeth and the pilot hole is cut into bone through the hole in the stent. Fine bone shavings are often present in the grooves of the bur. If these are removed and stored in sterile saline, they may be used later as a graft to pack around the implant before wound closure. Bone chips may also be collected via the suction apparatus if a special collecting device is attached.

The pilot hole is progressively widened with burs of increasing diameters. If a self-tapping implant is to be inserted, the hole is prepared (Fig. 11.27) to

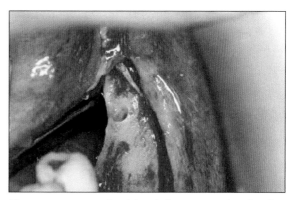

Fig. 11.27 A completed bur hole is irrigated with saline before checking its depth. The lingual aspect of the alveolar ridge should also be checked to ensure that the bur hole has not perforated lingual bone.

accommodate the implant without excessive tightening force; otherwise the screw thread of the implant might shear. Insertion of a self-tapping implant generates heat through friction, and implant insertion is undertaken slowly. The implant is loaded onto its insertion tool (Fig. 11.28) and the surface of the implant is not touched, to avoid contamination. After insertion of the implant, the cover screw is placed (Fig. 11.29). Blood is washed out of the screw threads before a cover screw or healing abutment is placed; it may be difficult to remove later.

Wound closure

The choice of suture material depends on personal preference. If a resorbable suture is used, the suture should remain within the tissues sufficiently long for

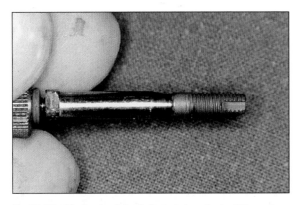

Fig. 11.28　The implant is loaded onto its insertion tool. The surface of the implant should not be touched, to avoid contamination.

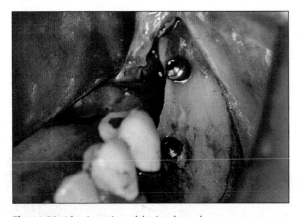

Fig. 11.29　After insertion of the implants the cover screws are placed. Blood is washed out of the screw threads before the cover screw is placed because it can be difficult to remove later.

early wound healing. The ideal retention period for resorbable sutures is 5–14 days.

If single interrupted sutures are placed, care is taken to ensure that the wound edges are approximated accurately without tension. A vertical mattress technique is helpful if the mucosal incision is to be closed near to a muscle attachment (e.g. mentalis muscle), resulting in additional displacement forces on the flap. This will reduce the risk of wound dehiscence, which sometimes occurs in the edentulous mandible after insertion of an implant.

Postoperative care

The patient is reminded of the possibility of postoperative pain, swelling and bruising. There may also be loss of sensation in the oral mucosa, or discomfort relating to a prosthesis. Postoperative antibiotics may be prescribed if a single preoperative dose has not already been given. The patient must refrain from wearing a denture over the implant until the follow-up appointment at 1 week.

The patient will have a soft diet and will keep the wound clean by hot salt-water mouth bath irrigation. The patient should refrain from examining the wound because retraction of the lip may encourage wound dehiscence. A follow-up appointment is made for 7–10 days after surgery. A soft lining (e.g. Coe-Comfort) is recommended when a denture is re-inserted a week after surgery, after extensive trimming of the fitting surface. The patient is advised to remove and clean the denture at night.

The implant is allowed to osseointegrate before physiological loading (after approximately 10 weeks). However, the optimum time for osseointegration is influenced by factors such as the health status of the patient and the quality of the bone around the implant. Therefore, when deciding the most suitable time to load an implant, each case is considered on its own merits.

Second-stage surgery to expose an implant

After the healing phase is complete it can sometimes be difficult to determine the exact location of a two-stage (submucosal) implant. A dental probe can be used to palpate the cover screw through the anaesthetized tissues. Once the cover screw is located, a crestal incision is made to expose it (Fig. 11.30). The

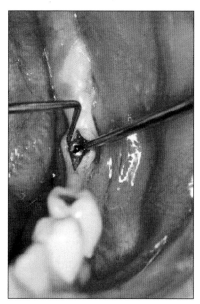

Fig. 11.30 Second-stage surgery. The cover screw is exposed via a small incision.

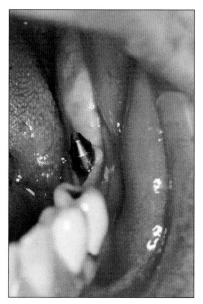

Fig. 11.31 A healing abutment is placed to ensure good healing of oral mucosa to the surface of the abutment.

cover screw is then removed and a healing abutment inserted. If necessary, resorbable sutures are placed to ensure close apposition of the oral mucosa to the healing abutment (Fig. 11.31). After a period of 7–10 days, the healing abutment is replaced with a suitable abutment that will subsequently be loaded.

PROSTHODONTIC REHABILITATION AFTER IMPLANT SURGERY

Prosthodontic rehabilitation typically involves the use of ball attachments, magnets, a retentive bar with clips to support an overdenture, or the construction of a fixed prosthesis (e.g. a crown or bridge as seen in Fig. 11.32). Further discussion of the methods employed may be obtained from a suitable textbook on dental prosthetics.

COMPLICATIONS OF ENDOSSEOUS IMPLANT SURGERY AND THEIR MANAGEMENT

Inappropriate placement of implants may be avoided by meticulous preoperative planning. Haemorrhage is unusual during surgery, but life-threatening haemorrhage has been reported after placement of mandibular implants (through accidental perforation of the lingual cortical plate and rupture of the sublingual

Surgical procedure for endosseous implants
• Incision away from implant site
• Avoid extensive stripping of periosteum
• Site preparation with a bur
• Slow, light pressure, intermittent
• Cooling with saline
• Progressive enlargement of hole with increasing bur sizes
• Slow implant insertion to reduce heating from friction

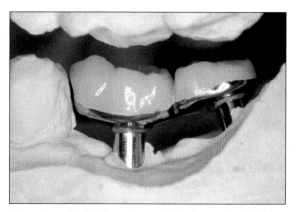

Fig. 11.32 The fixed prosthesis with the free-end saddle fabricated for the patient in Figs 11.27–11.31.

artery). The morphology of the lingual aspect of the mandible is assessed before drilling. Trauma to the inferior alveolar nerve is another distressing complication, and immediate referral is advised to ensure appropriate specialist care.

Wound infection is unusual in the early healing phase, and is controlled with a suitable antibiotic. Chronic peri-implant infection may result from poor oral hygiene. However, the patient's inability to maintain good standards of oral hygiene should have been identified early in the planning stage. Chronic peri-implant infection is difficult to control, and may result in loss of the implant if the patient's oral hygiene standards do not improve.

Mandibular fracture is a rare complication after implant insertion, but can occur in the atrophic mandible. The dental surgeon should be vigilant, both during surgery and in the healing phase, to identify the signs of a mandibular fracture. Immediate referral to an oral and maxillofacial surgeon is appropriate.

MAJOR PREPROSTHETIC SURGERY

Many techniques to augment the edentulous jaws have been developed. However, most have fallen out of favour, principally because of the poor results obtained.

Orthognathic surgery has a role to play in the management of some jaw discrepancies (Fig. 11.33). The surgical techniques employed are described in Chapter 12.

Reconstructive surgery is indicated in a few patients to provide a stable bony base for a fixed or removable prosthesis, particularly after resection of oral cancer. These major procedures are outside the scope of practice of the general dental practitioner— referral to an oral and maxillofacial surgeon is appropriate. Reconstructive surgery for prosthodontic rehabilitation is described in contemporary oral and maxillofacial surgery textbooks.

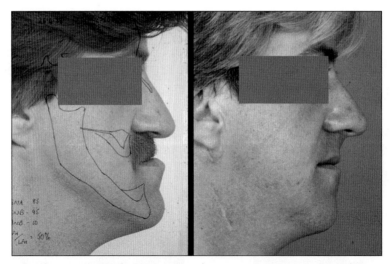

Fig. 11.33 Left: this edentulous patient underwent a vertical ramus osteotomy to correct his mandibular prognathism. Cephalometric tracings have been superimposed over the photograph to aid in planning the surgery. Right: the postoperative profile view. The patient was able to masticate more efficiently after correction of the mandibular prognathism and provision of new dentures.

FURTHER READING

Adell R. (1992) The surgical principles of osseointegration. In: Worthington P. , Brånemark P. I. (eds) *Advanced osseointegration surgery: applications in the maxillofacial region.* Quintessence, Chicago, IL, pp. 94–108.

Adell R., Eriksson B., Lekholm U., et al. (1990) Long-term follow-up study of osseointegrated implants in the treatment of totally edentulous jaws. *International Journal of Oral and Maxillofacial Implants* 5: 347–359.

Berg R., Morgenstern N. E. (1997) Physiologic changes in the elderly. *Dental Clinics of North America* 41: 651–668.

Brånemark P. I., Adell R., Breine U., et al. (1969) Intraosseous anchorage of dental prostheses. I. Experimental studies. *Scandinavian Journal of Plastic and Reconstructive Surgery* 3: 81–100.

Brånemark P. I., Hansson B. O., Adell R., et al. (1977) Osseointegrated implants in the treatment of the edentulous jaw. Experience from a 10-year period. *Scandinavian Journal of Plastic and Reconstructive Surgery* (Suppl) 16: 1–132.

Cawood J. I., Howell R. A. (1988) A classification of the edentulous jaws. *International Journal of Oral and Maxillofacial Surgery* 17: 232–236.

Fiske J., Davis D. M., Frances C., Gelbier S. (1998) The emotional effects of tooth loss in edentulous people. *British Dental Journal* 184: 90–93.

Hildebrandt G. H., Loesche W. J., Lin C. F., Bretz W. A. (1995) Comparison of the number and type of dental functional units in geriatric populations with diverse medical backgrounds. *Journal of Prosthetic Dentistry* 73: 253–261.

Lemons J. E., Laskin D. M., Roberts W. E., et al. (1997) Changes in patient screening for a clinical study of dental implants after increased awareness of tobacco use as a risk factor. *Journal of Oral and Maxillofacial Surgery* 55 (Suppl 5): 72–75.

Norton M. (1996) *Dental implants—a guide for the general practitioner*. Quintessence, Chicago, IL.

Terry B. C., Zarb G. A. (1991) *Report on 4th International Congress on Preprosthetic Surgery*, Palm Springs, FL, 18–20 April 1991. *International Journal of Oral and Maxillofacial Surgery* 20: 314–316.

Verhoeven J. W., Cune M. S., Van Kampen F. M., Koole R. (2001) The use of the transmandibular implant system in extreme atrophy of the mandible; a retrospective study of the results in two different hospital situations. *Journal of Oral Rehabilitation* 28: 497–506.

Wardrop R. W., Hailes J., Burger H., Reade P. C. (1989) Oral discomfort at menopause. *Oral Surgery* 67: 535–540.

Wedgwood D., Jennings K. J., Critchlow H. A., et al. (1992) Experience with ITI osseointegrated implants at five centres in the UK. *British Journal of Oral and Maxillofacial Surgery* 30: 377–381.

SELF-ASSESSMENT

1. In general terms, in which circumstances would you consider undertaking preprosthetic surgery?
2. What may be done at the time of tooth extraction to improve the success of subsequent dentures?
3. How do the three main types of jaw implant differ?
4. What factors may influence the success of endosseous implants?
5. What may be done to reduce bone damage while preparing sites to receive implants?

Answers on page 267

12 | Surgical aids to orthodontics and surgery for dentofacial deformity

C. M. Hill
D. W. Thomas

- Some orthodontic procedures require surgical assistance.
- Unerupted or impacted teeth are the most common reason for surgical intervention but, occasionally, soft-tissue surgery is indicated.
- Some cases cannot be treated simply by orthodontics alone and require surgery to the mandible and/or maxilla—orthognathic surgery (osteotomies). Such cases require a combined approach and careful planning to ensure optimal results.
- Although treatment of facial deformity is not within the scope of general dentistry, the dentist has an essential role to play in the general dental care of such patients. This is especially important in cleft patients.
- Dentists must be able to give accurate advice to patients who may be considering surgery for facial deformity and their relatives.

THE ORTHODONTIC/ORAL SURGERY INTERFACE

Oral and maxillofacial surgery, in the context of this chapter, includes a wide spectrum of procedures ranging from the removal and exposure of unerupted teeth to bimaxillary osteotomies. In planning these procedures, it is essential to involve the specialist orthodontist and the patients themselves from an early stage.

Surgery in the orthodontic patient will often be an integral part of a protracted treatment programme which may, especially in the case of adult fixed-appliance therapy, take 2 years or more to complete. It is essential, at the planning stage of the dentoalveolar surgery, that patients understand (and are willing to comply with) the extent and duration of the proposed therapy.

This prolonged treatment may relate either to the creation of space for eruption or to the application of external mechanical force to stimulate/induce the eruption of malpositioned teeth. Patients with dental indicators of poor motivation such as irregular attendance, high caries rates and inadequate oral hygiene should have appropriate treatment plans. The treatment administered should be simplified as far as possible to reflect the anticipated extent of cooperation from the patient and to expedite any prescribed treatment. Whilst in the past orthodontics has principally been undertaken in adolescents, adult orthodontics is becoming increasingly popular. Any relevant medical history will influence the type of treatment the patient is offered and the mode of anaesthesia.

The interface between oral surgery and orthodontics is difficult to define accurately but relates to those patients whose treatment decisions lie within both specialties. There will always be cases where choices must be made—to recommend orthodontics alone, surgery alone, a combination of the two or whether no intervention should be recommended. Decision-making in complex cases requires a combination of skill and experience and must be taken with the patient's best interests as the fundamental starting point.

> **The orthodontic/oral surgery interface:**
>
> The area of clinical decision-making where treatment can legitimately involve either oral surgery, orthodontics, both or neither

MANAGEMENT OF UNERUPTED AND IMPACTED TEETH

Nowhere is the practice of dentoalveolar surgery and orthodontics more closely related than in the management of unerupted and impacted teeth. The teeth most frequently affected by failure of eruption are generally the last to erupt in a particular series—wisdom teeth, canines and second premolar teeth. The management of third molar teeth is discussed in Chapter 5.

Assessment of unerupted teeth—clinical

In orthodontic cases it is unusual for patients to suffer any symptoms from unerupted teeth; they are far more frequently noted after clinical examination or as incidental radiographic findings. Careful monitoring of the eruption of the dentition is essential and the general dental practitioner is best equipped to perform this task. The combined oral surgery and orthodontic treatment options for unerupted teeth are threefold: extraction, exposure ± orthodontics and autotransplantation (most frequently of canines). In some cases (e.g. mesiodens when no orthodontics is planned) unerupted teeth may be left *in situ*. The autotransplantation of teeth is performed far less frequently than it was in the past due to unpredictable results and the reliability of osseointegrated implants and adhesive bridgework.

The timing of extractions or exposure is dependent on the age of the patient and the stage of development of the dentition. The principal treatment decision in the management of unerupted teeth is whether to extract. In general terms the rationale for removal of unerupted/malpositioned teeth resembles that for wisdom teeth (see Ch. 5). The principal indications for extraction are:

- space creation
- pathology associated with the unerupted tooth (e.g. caries or cyst formation)
- evidence or risk of root resorption of adjacent teeth
- malformation of the crown and/or root of the unerupted tooth, which would impede eruption or render the tooth useless cosmetically and functionally if it were to erupt.

There is some evidence that timely extraction of deciduous teeth may prevent later impaction, particularly in the case of upper canines.

The surgical and radiographic assessment of unerupted teeth in orthodontic cases is based upon determining:

- the position of the teeth
- factors which may impede conventional surgical removal (or indeed eruption), such as dilaceration, hooked roots, proximity to adjacent teeth
- the proximity of the teeth to important anatomical structures—e.g. the mental nerve, maxillary sinus or adjacent unerupted teeth.

Whilst the crowns of these teeth are frequently in communication with the oral cavity, even where the teeth are not directly visible, clinical examination and palpation of the alveolus will often demonstrate a bulbosity associated with crowns of unerupted teeth, thereby giving an indication of their position. Additionally, the inclination of adjacent teeth may give some important clue to the position of the crown of an unerupted tooth. Radiographic analysis, however, is essential to determine the apex position, morphology and pathologies associated with unerupted teeth.

Assessment of unerupted teeth—radiographic

Radiographic assessment of the unerupted tooth will provide several valuable pieces of information in planning its management: stage of tooth development, crown/root morphology and angulation and the presence or absence of local disease. Most orthodontic assessment will include an orthopantomogram (OPT) and a lateral cephalometric view. Intraoral views are essential, however, for the management of unerupted maxillary anterior teeth due to the poor definition of the OPT in this region. In this situation, the OPT will usually be supplemented with periapical and/or upper anterior occlusal films. The use of 'parallax' analysis, in which two periapical views of the same area are taken from different angles (see Ch. 5), can be useful in determining whether the impacted teeth are buccal or palatal and therefore in planning the surgical approach to the teeth. In radiographic analysis, the stage of tooth

development must also be carefully considered because it is inappropriate to expose teeth whose development is incomplete.

Exposure of unerupted teeth

The assessment of whether unerupted teeth are suitable for exposure is beyond the scope of this text and should be undertaken in conjunction with an orthodontic specialist. The decision to expose or not, however, is principally based on three factors: the angulation of the unerupted tooth, the depth of impaction and the relationship to other teeth. In general terms there are four treatment options:

- extraction
- autotransplantation
- simple exposure
- exposure with the application of direct mechanical force to the tooth.

The principles of treatment planning are discussed below in relation to the anterior maxillary region but can equally be applied in relation to unerupted teeth at other sites (most commonly mandibular second premolar teeth or even wisdom teeth).

The objective of exposing an unerupted tooth is to move it into a good functional and aesthetic position. In assessing teeth for exposure one of the prime considerations is the available space into which the tooth can erupt. This may be estimated by comparing the crown width of the unerupted tooth with the available space, either directly from the radiograph (with reference to the magnification in the system) or by measurement of the crown width of the contralateral corresponding tooth.

Unerupted and impacted teeth

A decision must be taken as to whether they should be:
- left *in situ*
- exposed
- transplanted
- removed

Surgical technique

Exposure at its simplest consists of removal of the soft tissues overlying the crown of an unerupted tooth under local anaesthetic. The exposure of teeth in this fashion has major disadvantages:

- removal of the attached keratinized gingiva
- the possibility of re-epithelialization and healing of the defect before the tooth has time to erupt
- the loss of an acceptable mucogingival contour.

Attempts should be made to retain the keratinized tissues by employing displacement of the attached gingiva with apically or, occasionally, laterally repositioned flaps. The apically repositioned flap retains the mucogingival collar around the tooth and is displaced apically and sutured into place. The bunched gingiva will remodel as wound healing occurs (Fig. 12.1). If the tooth is misaligned, a bracket and gold chain may be etched to the canine to direct its eruptive path appropriately (Fig. 12.2).

Although simple exposure is satisfactory for superficially placed teeth situated close to the surface and impacted in soft tissue alone, most unerupted teeth are located more than 3–4 mm from the oral mucosal surface and the crown cannot be seen completely after raising a flap (Fig. 12.3). As impaction of unerupted teeth usually involves hard tissue as well as soft tissue, all bone covering the tip of the crown as far as the maximum width of the tooth should be carefully removed. If the tooth is superficial and covered by thin bone this can often be undertaken using a scalpel blade. Where bone coverage of the unerupted tooth is more extensive, a small rose head bur or hand-held chisel may be used to clear overlying bone from the crown. Extreme caution must be taken to avoid damaging the tooth crown and the roots of the adjacent teeth. Unnecessary removal of bone should also be avoided. Whilst soft- and hard-tissue exposure of unerupted teeth is in some instances successful, most commonly (and especially in the case of deeply impacted teeth) the created surgical defect will become re-epithelialized if patency is not maintained. The defect is, therefore, packed with an antiseptic gauze dressing or a glass-ionomer cement bonded to the tooth crown in order to inhibit contraction and re-epithelialization (Fig. 12.4). Postoperative antibiotics are seldom indicated unless there is a known increased risk of wound infection, e.g. patients with insulin-dependent diabetes mellitus.

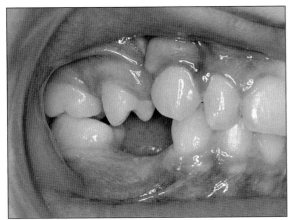

Fig. 12.1 An erupted canine 3 months after exposure using an apically repositioned flap. The irregular gingival contour will gradually diminish with the passage of time.

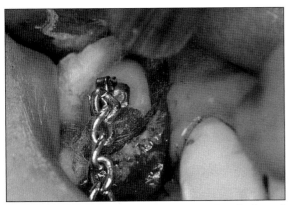

Fig. 12.2 A bracket and gold chain bonded to the buccal surface of an exposed canine. The chain can be attached to a fixed appliance to direct the tooth into the correct location.

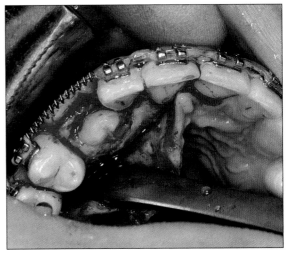

Fig. 12.3 Raising a palatal flap reveals a totally embedded canine that will require bone removal to expose it.

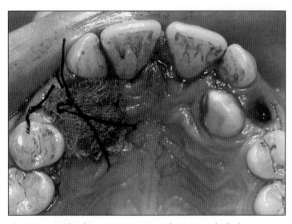

Fig. 12.4 Palatal exposure requires the removal of a large piece of palatal mucosa. The ability of the mucosa to regenerate should not be underestimated, hence the use of some form of packing such as Whitehead's varnish on half-inch ribbon gauze (shown) or glass-ionomer cement.

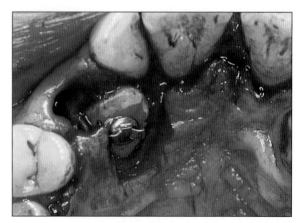

Fig. 12.5 A bracket bonded to the palatal surface of an unerupted canine. Either wires or elastics can be attached to the cleat.

Mechanical traction and unerupted teeth

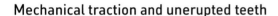

The application of mechanical force to stimulate and guide eruption of buried teeth is frequently necessary because the angulation of the root of an unerupted tooth is frequently unfavourable. This mechanical force may be employed in a number of ways: gold chains, steel or elastic ligatures and even magnets attached to an orthodontic appliance have all been used to induce the eruption. Mechanical traction is indicated:

- for unerupted teeth with angulation that will inhibit spontaneous eruption
- where buried teeth are obstructed from erupting by other teeth
- where teeth are exposed long after their root development is complete.

If the crown tip of a maxillary canine is beyond the midline of the lateral incisor root, spontaneous eruption will not usually occur and mechanical traction will be necessary. Bonding of the bracket to the tooth following its exposure (Fig. 12.5) involves a sequence of etching, washing, drying and bonding similar to that employed in conventional adhesive dentistry. Bonding is best performed in collaboration with an orthodontist to ensure the angulation and position of the bracket is appropriate in relation to the force to be applied to the tooth. During the procedure maintenance of a meticulously dry field

is essential and this is facilitated by careful suction and local infiltration of epinephrine-containing local anaesthetic.

Following the bonding, the flap is apically repositioned (see earlier) or may simply be closed as both compare favourably if external traction is to be applied. If traction is not to be applied immediately, the ligatures or chains may be sutured to the mucosa or orthodontic appliance using non-resorbable material. This minimizes any discomfort from the loose chain.

Although bonding could be undertaken as a second procedure following exposure, this results in greater inconvenience and discomfort to the patient. Whilst simple exposures can typically be undertaken under local anaesthesia, bonding (where the procedure is more protracted and requires excellent moisture control in the operative site) is generally best performed under general anaesthesia.

Autotransplantation and surgical repositioning of teeth

In the past, autotransplantation was a popular treatment for unerupted canine, premolar and even molar teeth but there are some considerable biological problems associated with the technique to be overcome. Although individual studies have suggested clinical and radiographic success rates as high as 80% for the transplantation (at 1–5 years following surgery), most transplanted teeth will develop evidence of root resorption or even ankylosis if they are not root-treated. The success rate of transplantation can be maximized by careful handling of the tooth and preparation of the socket with minimal trauma. Resorption is directly influenced by the extent of trauma to the periodontal tissues on the root surface and care must be taken to minimize this during the removal of the tooth. For this reason, transplantation should be undertaken only on young, medically fit patients and should exclude all teeth which will be difficult to extract or those with hooked apices which will preclude simple elevation.

During the removal of the unerupted tooth only the crown of the tooth should be manipulated with instruments and whilst the socket is being prepared the tooth is 'stored' in the buccal or palatal sulcus beneath the flap. When preparing the 'socket', bone removal should be undertaken very carefully, with particular reference to not generating heat. A slow-running, well-irrigated bur is the preferred option to achieve this, although some surgeons use small chisels or osteotomes to remove the bone or expand the socket.

The repositioned tooth should be secured free from occlusion and splinted in place, usually by direct bonding using orthodontic brackets or wire and composite. Alternatively a thin vacuum-formed splint can be constructed and cemented in place. Following removal of the splint (usually after 3 weeks) the tooth should be root-filled with calcium hydroxide and reviewed clinically and radiographically at regular 3-month intervals for at least 1 year to check for resorption or ankylosis. Although the technique appears to be reasonably successful in the short term, the advent of adhesive bridgework and osseointegrated implants offers far more reliable, less inconvenient alternatives to management of missing maxillary canines. These techniques also avoid the inexplicable 'late loss' of transplanted teeth, which may occur after 10–15 years.

SUPERNUMERARY TEETH AND ODONTOMES

Supernumerary teeth may occur as teeth with normal morphology (supplemental) or with abnormal or rudimentary form. Supplemental teeth may be left *in situ* if they are cosmetically and functionally acceptable.

Supernumerary teeth and odontomes often must be removed as they can delay eruption or impede orthodontic tooth movement, particularly of maxillary incisors. If supernumerary teeth are removed from the path of eruption, the underlying teeth will often erupt given sufficient space. It has been estimated that this will occur spontaneously in approximately 60% of cases. If the underlying teeth fail to erupt, a second operation will be required to expose the teeth and apply mechanical traction. To avoid this risk some clinicians advocate the application of mechanical traction to the underlying permanent teeth when the overlying supernumerary teeth are removed. It is increasingly being recognized, however, that deeply buried supernumerary teeth in fully developed dentitions can be left *in situ* (Fig. 12.6) and require nothing more than occasional radiographic review. If these teeth are to be removed then careful surgical technique is essential to minimize risk of damage to adjacent unerupted teeth or the roots of erupted teeth (see Ch. 5).

Odontomes are less common than supernumerary teeth, although the differentiation between the two is considerably blurred. Odontomes may be simple

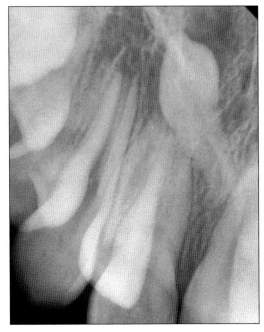

Fig. 12.6 An inverted supernumerary tooth—usually referred to as a mesiodens if it occurs in the incisor region. It should only be removed if there is a genuine clinical indication.

(tooth-like), compound (multiple tooth-like) or complex composite (containing elements of the tooth germ in a disorganized fashion). All true odontomes are benign, do not grow and are not true tumours. Like unerupted teeth, odontomes need only be removed if there are clinical indications (infection, they are obstructing eruption of other teeth, etc.).

FRAENECTOMY

Fraenectomy—the surgical removal of fraenal attachments (usually in the midline) in the upper or lower jaw—may be a valuable surgical adjunct to orthodontic therapy (its use is also discussed in Ch. 11). Its use has been questioned over recent years and certainly the case for early surgical intervention has largely been dismissed. However, there are some instances when surgery is indicated; these are discussed below.

Labial fraenectomy

Upper labial fraenectomy aims to remove or reposition the entire labial fraenum, including its attachment to bone, and to remove all interdental tissue. It must be remembered that spacing of the incisors in children is a normal developmental process and is present until the eruption of the permanent canine teeth in adolescents. Labial fraenectomy should usually be delayed until after orthodontic treatment, unless the labial fraenum prevents closure of a diastema or displays evidence of trauma. The technique is usually performed if the fraenum extends to the incisive papilla and contributes to post-treatment stability of the orthodontically closed diastema. The pronounced fraenal attachment extending into the palate may often be viewed radiographically as a V-shaped depression. There are differing surgical techniques to remove the labial fraenum; one is outlined in Fig. 12.7 (see also Figs 11.7, 11.8).

Under local anaesthesia the upper lip is firmly retracted, demonstrating the extent of the fraenal attachment. If the fraenum is particularly fibrous, its whole length is outlined and excised with a scalpel using an elliptical or rhomboid incision. The remaining fibres attached to the exposed bone can be curetted or gently removed with a bur but care must be taken not to damage the roots of adjacent teeth. The mucosa is then undermined and the defect

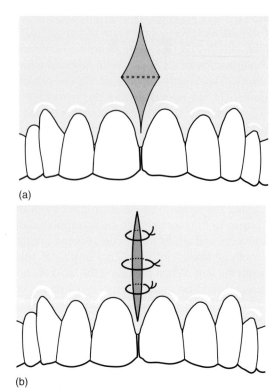

(a)

(b)

Fig. 12.7   The surgical technique for a labial fraenectomy:
(a)   incisions;
(b)   closure.

closed with simple interrupted sutures. Patients are normally reviewed in 5–7 days.

Lingual fraenectomy

Lingual fraenectomies are occasionally recommended in younger children to assist in phonetic development or to avoid functional embarrassment. In older patients it may also be undertaken if tongue movement is so restricted that patients cannot lick the buccal surfaces of their upper molars to aid oral hygiene.

The procedure is usually performed under local anaesthesia. The surgical technique is similar to that of a labial fraenectomy although minimal tissue removal, if any, is required. The tongue is grasped and pulled upwards and the fraenal attachment is released using a single horizontal incision. The defect may be closed with two or three simple, interrupted, resorbable, 3/0 catgut sutures. Care must be taken to avoid damaging the submandibular salivary duct openings, either in the incision or when suturing

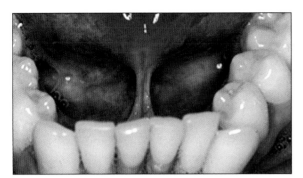

Fig. 12.8 Periodontal problems associated with a high lingual fraenum, resulting in direct trauma and poor oral hygiene.

the wound. Rarely, failure to undertake a lingual fraenectomy leads to periodontal problems in later life (Fig. 12.8).

ASSESSING THE NEED FOR SURGERY FOR DENTOFACIAL DEFORMITY

The development of the dentition and the facial skeleton is a series of complex and inter-related processes, beginning with the early embryological formation of the branchial arches and continuing through life with the growth of the skull, mandible and maxilla and the eruption of two dentitions. Between the ages of 6 and 12 years, the dentition is mixed and it is during these years that many of the problems of facial disproportion and malocclusion become apparent.

In addition, the cranium grows more rapidly than the rest of the skeleton and its pattern of growth (as is that of the facial skeleton) is highly complex. As such, it is perhaps surprising that in the vast majority of individuals harmonious growth occurs in three dimensions, resulting in broadly symmetrical faces with functional occlusions. Despite this, however, there is an enormous variability in forms and dimensions between sexes, individuals and cultures. Since such variation is universal, it is impossible to consider any particular pattern of growth—either the process or the end result—as 'normal'.

Assessing the need for any surgical intervention must be on the basis of understanding the technical requirements and considering the relevant cultural, racial and ethical issues. Distinguishing between normal and abnormal variations is not always possi-

ble. However, it is possible in general terms to categorize the different types of anomalies as:

- mandibular
- maxillary
- bimaxillary
- craniofacial.

In each of these cases the variations may be symmetric or asymmetric, congenital or acquired. Treatment planning may be affected accordingly, although the general principles of treatment are not just dependent on aetiology. In all cases, however, the assessment of the need for surgical intervention must be based on a variety of factors, the principal one being the patient's own desire for some form of treatment. Assuming this is the case, it is important to be able to recognize which cases are treatable with orthodontics alone and which will also require surgical intervention.

In general terms, orthodontics alone is unlikely to be adequate in patients:

- who cannot retrude into an edge-to-edge occlusion (prognathism—Class 3 occlusions)
- who cannot protrude into an edge-to-edge occlusion (retrognathism—Class 2 occlusions)
- with anterior open bites due to skeletal causes (i.e. not due to thumb- or finger-sucking habits)
- with true asymmetry
- with marked discrepancies in the vertical dimension.

This list is not exhaustive and does not preclude some patients from having treatment that may, at least in technical terms, be a compromise. However, most patients with any of the above problems will require surgery, and it then becomes important to determine the diagnosis of their anomalies. These will be considered in the same order as listed at the start of this section. Many technical terms have been devised to describe the jaw relationships which are useful in considering orthognathic surgery; these are italicized.

Mandibular anomalies

In relation to a normal upper jaw, the lower jaw can be too big or too small. When the mandible is too large the condition is referred to as *prognathism*; when it is too small it is termed *retrognathia*—literally, backwards positioning of the jaw. A genuinely diminutive mandible is probably better referred to as *micrognathic* although this term is usually reserved for cases where there is a failure of the ramus to develop. Such cases are often associated with various syndromes of the face including Apert's and Treacher-Collins' syndromes.

Prognathism is usually due to excessive growth of the mandible between the ages of 8 and 17 years but occasionally becomes apparent after an adolescent growth spurt. Features of prognathism include reversal of the mandibular/maxillary relationship, a reverse overjet and a diminished or absent overbite. The lower incisors tend to be retroclined and the upper incisors proclined, although they are also less visible on smiling. In addition to the increased horizontal length of the mandible there may be an increase in the vertical length. This vertical excess can be very variable and its management may be addressed by either mandibular shortening or maxillary impaction osteotomies. In addition to the simple excessive developmental growth there are other causes of prognathism, including hormonal disturbances such as would be found in cases of acromegaly. In all cases the enlargement of the mandible is basically symmetrical, although some lateral difference is always possible and the variation in the vertical dimension can be considerable.

It is also possible to have a normal skeletal base relationship (i.e. the teeth in a normal occlusal relationship) and yet have a marked protrusive or retrusive appearance in profile. This is caused by the failure of the chin to develop in proportion to the skeletal bases, excess development being termed *progenia* and underdevelopment *retrogenia*. An inadequate depth of bone between the apices of the anterior teeth and the base of the mandible is correctly termed *microgenia* but the term is frequently confused with *retrogenia*. The opposite condition, *macrogenia*, is also seen on occasion and all these conditions can be treated with different types of genioplasty (surgical sectioning and repositioning of the chin).

In some cases the jaw forms an asymmetric excess; this occurs commonly in *condylar hyperplasia*. This idiopathic condition is usually seen in patients between the ages of 20 and 40 years although it is not restricted

to any age. Asymmetric loss of bone can also occur, for example, as a result of trauma or as a result of certain pathological conditions such as *hemifacial microsomia*, Still's disease (juvenile rheumatoid arthritis) or severe *hemifacial atrophy*. Fortunately such conditions are relatively rare; they should be treated in a specialist unit. It should also be noted that asymmetry can be the result of soft-tissue changes such as masseteric hypertrophy, fibrous dysplasia or benign tumours such as neurofibromata.

Maxillary anomalies

The mid-face actually comprises some 23 bones, of which the two maxillae are fused to form the major part. The articulation of the mid-facial skeleton is complex and for many years orthognathic surgery was directed towards the mandible when the problems were really maxillary (mid-facial). Modern orthognathic surgery addresses the concept of the whole facial skeleton and the need to achieve a balance of the hard and soft tissues in three dimensions—lateral, vertical and anterior-posterior. Additionally, in developmental terms, the formation of the maxillary hard and soft tissues is complex and it is of little surprise that congenital defects in the form of cleft lip and/or palate are the world's second most common congenital defect (see later).

Maxillary abnormalities can be classified thus:

- protrusion or retrusion and intrusion or extrusion
- dental arches that are normal, widened or narrowed (in relation to the bony skeleton)
- dental arches that slope to one side, a condition usually referred to as a *cant*.

Abnormal vertical development of the posterior maxilla

Increased posterior facial height may result in the anterior teeth failing to meet (i.e. a reverse overbite, which is commonly referred to as an *anterior open bite*). A similar condition may result from suppressed eruption of the incisors, such as that caused by thumb-sucking, but the two conditions are treated completely differently with only the former requiring surgical intervention. Isolated instances of reduced vertical dimensions of the maxilla are less common but they often accompany maxillary retrusion.

Bimaxillary anomalies

Bimaxillary anomalies are the most common type of facial variation because the growth of one jaw is always, to some extent, dependent on the other. This is clearly demonstrated in children who have cleft lips and palates. Inadequate surgical repair of the cleft in infants often inhibits growth of the maxilla in later years. This may then allow excessive growth of the mandible, resulting in a pronounced class 3 occlusion.

However, it is difficult to justify performing bimaxillary osteotomies when only small movements of two jaws are required; it is therefore sometimes necessary to operate on one jaw and compromise on which jaw is likely to give the best result. Conversely, single-jaw operations when movements in excess of 10 mm are required are more prone to significant relapse. Bimaxillary surgery, when indicated, usually gives more aesthetically and functionally pleasing results and it is always better to avoid compromise when at all possible (Figs 12.9, 12.10).

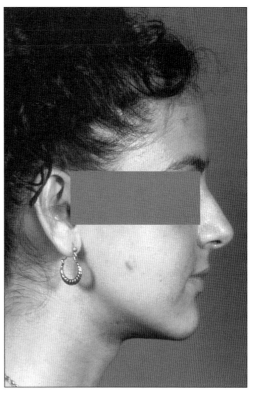

Fig. 12.10   Postoperative view of the patient shown in Fig. 12.9.

Craniofacial anomalies

The details of craniofacial anomalies are outside the scope of this book, but it is important for the dental profession to be aware of the rare conditions such as Crouzon's syndrome and Apert's syndrome, which can result in severe facial deformity.

Much of the pioneering work on these groups of patients was carried out by Paul Tessier. It is now possible to perform complex craniofacial reconstructions to ameliorate the worst of the anomalies.

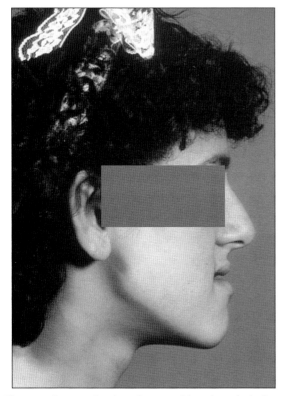

Fig. 12.9   Preoperative view of a prognathic patient who is about to undergo bimaxillary surgery to correct her facial proportions.

Assessing the need for surgical intervention
• Patient choice
• Class 3 or severe class 2 occlusion
• Anterior open bite (skeletal)
• Asymmetry
• Abnormal vertical relationship
• Accurate diagnosis

THE PLANNING OF OSTEOTOMIES, IN THEORY AND PRACTICE

Treatment planning for orthognathic surgery is a process that must take account of the wishes of the patient in relation to the whole of the facial complex—the facial skeleton, the occlusion and the soft tissues which they support. The tissues must be considered both individually and collectively in relation to the patient, whose wishes and aspirations are of fundamental importance. The general principles of collecting data through history, clinical examination and special investigations should be followed. The patient's medical and social history and psychological profile are also important in considering surgery that will significantly change their facial appearance.

A detailed history should reveal the patient's principal complaints and the extent to which they concern him or her. These can generally be classified as functional or, more usually, aesthetic—although a combination of the two (in variable proportions) is common. It is important to try to grasp the true concerns of a patient because surgical intervention aimed at addressing the wrong issue carries obvious risks. Patients' perceptions of their appearance are heavily influenced by upbringing, culture, race and their own psyche. If there is any doubt about a patient's real motive for requesting surgery, a psychiatric assessment should be sought.

Surgical interventions should ideally, therefore:

- address the patient's real requirements
- improve the occlusion and therefore the function
- improve the skeletal relationship and therefore the soft tissues.

In addition to the history of the problem, a detailed medical and social history should be taken. Patients considering orthognathic surgery undertake a major personal commitment and require as much support as possible. Any relevant medical condition or social pressure point should be assessed in relation to the overall treatment plan.

Clinical examination should be undertaken thoroughly but systematically—beginning with the general and working towards the specific. Examination of the face requires considerable experience in being able to categorize anomalies. For example, maxillary hypoplasia and mandibular prognathism are often difficult to distinguish, even to the trained eye. Similarly, asymmetric development is not always easy to define unless it results in a marked midline shift; and even in such cases the dentition can be the result of excessive or inadequate growth. For example, condylar hyperplasia on the left side of the jaw results in a midline shift of the mandible to the right side; a similar displacement also occurs in right-sided condylar hypoplasia or ankylosis.

Generally, certain features of the face are relatively constant (Fig. 12.11). Horizontally, a line drawn between the pupils bisects the head and will cross the upper insertion of the ear. Vertically a line drawn perpendicularly to the midpoint of the interpupillary line will pass through the middle of the nose, the columella, the philtrum, the upper and lower central

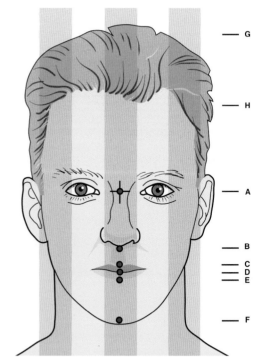

Fig. 12.11 The ideal proportions of the head and face. The vertical lines shown divide into fifths (alternatively vertical lines bisect each pupil to create thirds). The following lengths also correspond: AF = AG; AD = BF; CD = DE; AH = AD = DF. In addition, BD = 0.5 × DF and BF = 0.55 × AF. In reality, very few people fit the exact figures shown, yet the degree of overall conformity is extremely high despite the multiplicity of facial forms.

incisors and the midpoint of the chin. Various other relationships which define anterior and posterior facial height exist.

In all cases, it is essential that the face is viewed as a three-dimensional structure even though virtually all the analyses currently available are two dimensional. It is important to realize that 'moving' one part of the face affects the whole facial balance. For example, reducing the length of the mandible in a case of prognathism invariably results in the nose appearing larger. The converse is true for a forward-sliding maxillary osteotomy.

Special investigations relevant to orthognathic surgery include a full orthodontic assessment, radiology of the craniofacial skeleton and photography. Historically, matched cephalometric radiographs and photographs were used to 'predict' the desired outcomes of surgery. The radiographs and photographs were made as full-size transparencies and were cut to shape. They were then related to plaster models on which the desired movements were assessed. The method was crude and not always effective but it gave a rough idea of the expected profile after surgery. Nowadays, such analyses are undertaken by computer, using digitized cephalometric radiographs and photographs, with sophisticated software (Fig. 12.12). This enables the surgeon to 'try out' a variety of treatment options, including possible operations and orthodontic movements. The 'occlusal fit' still must be assessed on models but the accuracy of the predictions is fairly dependable. It is, however, still only an assessment of the profile and many have questioned the value of this from the patients' viewpoint because this is a view they would rarely see. Full-face predictions will undoubtedly be possible but the software for this is not yet commercially available.

In the future, three-dimensional analyses and laser images that can be manipulated may well become the norm. Pseudo-three-dimensional images can already be created using computed tomography, and this can easily be extended to milling machine technology, allowing the construction of prostheses, models or attachments which can assist in both the planning and the surgery itself.

The detail of orthognathic surgery is outside the scope of this book and readers are advised to study the textbooks listed at the end of the chapter for further information.

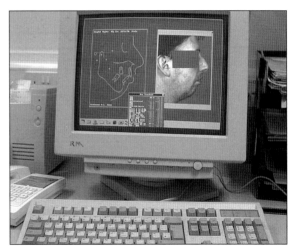

Fig. 12.12 The use of the 'Dentofacial planner'—computerized software which enables predictive projections for various surgical and orthodontic options.

Planning for orthognathic surgery

- Full history
- Clinical examination
- Radiographs and photographs
- Study models
- Detailed analysis

THE NATURE OF THE BASIC OSTEOTOMY PROCEDURES, INCLUDING THEIR MANAGEMENT, RISKS AND COMPLICATIONS

Surgery to the mandible

As orthognathic surgery began on the lower jaw it is perhaps not surprising that a variety of procedures have been described and many of them modified as time has passed. There are several basic principles that should be observed in all orthognathic procedures.

- The results of surgery should be anatomically and functionally stable and acceptable.
- The surgical procedure should carry no undue risk in terms of morbidity and mortality.
- The procedure should be predictable in nature and not subject to relapse.
- The end result should be likely to fulfil the realistic expectations of the patient.

- Any side effects (particularly long-term ones) should be fully explained and acceptable to the patient.

Surgery of the mandible can be applied to any point on the ramus, body or the dentoalveolar segment, although ramus surgery is the most common. The two classical operations—the sagittal split osteotomy (SSO) and the vertical subsigmoid (VSS)—have been adapted and modified in various ways from those originally described.

Sagittal split surgery—where the ramus and posterior part of the mandible are sectioned between the buccal and lingual surfaces—can be used to treat both the severe class 2 and class 3 malocclusion, whereas the VSS is used only to correct relatively mild prognathism. The sagittal split is performed via an intraoral approach (Figs 12.13, 12.14). The lingual tissues are retracted posteriorly and retained using one of the special retractors developed for this purpose. Buccally, the periosteum is retracted to the lower border of the mandible in the second molar region. The lingual bone cut is made horizontally, through the cortical plate, above the level of the lingula; in the past it was extended to the posterior margin of the ramus but this degree of extension is not necessary and may contribute towards relapse. The sagittal cut is made as lateral as is practicable on the external oblique ridge and extended as far forwards as necessary to ensure adequate contact of the split surfaces after repositioning. Finally the buccal cut is made vertically to the lower border. Bone cuts can be undertaken with burs but reciprocating and

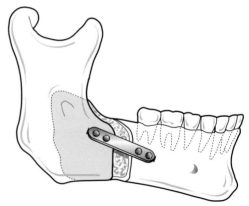

Fig. 12.14 Forward-sliding sagittal split osteotomy. Fixation with miniplates improves stability, and reduces morbidity and the risk of relapse.

oscillating saws are more efficient and less likely to cause soft-tissue damage. Once the cuts have been completed the mandible is carefully split using ultra-fine osteotomes. The inferior dental nerve should be identified (usually towards the buccal aspect) during this process and gently dissected away from its canal.

On completion of both sides the jaw can be repositioned using an acrylic wafer to locate the mandibular teeth accurately into the maxillary arch. The mandible is then stabilized with intermaxillary fixation and plates and/or screws are used to stabilize the fragments in their new position.

The other common mandibular osteotomy (the VSS) can be approached intraorally or extraorally. A carefully performed VSS carries little risk of damage to the inferior dental nerve because the bone cuts are made distal to the lingula, unlike the SSO, which frequently results in neuropraxia (and occasionally neurotmesis), causing profound anaesthesia in the distribution of the nerve distal to the point of trauma.

Other mandibular osteotomies using different cuts have been described but are beyond the scope of this book. Surgery of the dentoalveolus alone was popular for a short time in the 1970s and 1980s but its use has diminished considerably because 'dentoalveolar' surgery was often undertaken to correct an anomaly in the opposing jaw (or of apparently abnormal tooth position) and did not, therefore, really address the underlying problem in the basal bone adequately.

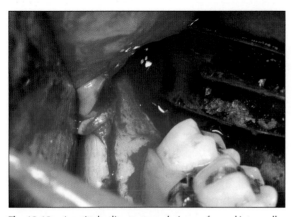

Fig. 12.13 A sagittal split osteotomy being performed intraorally. The cuts can be made with a bur or a reciprocating or oscillating saw.

Surgery to the maxilla

When orthognathic surgery was first developed, surgical procedures on the maxilla were very limited, usually being restricted to anterior dentoalveolar procedures. The first attempts at total maxillary osteotomies at the Le Fort I level (see Fig. 13.2) were carried out through small multiple vertical incisions because of concern for the vascularity of the maxilla and the presumed risk of total exfoliation of the osteotomized segment. In reality this has not proved problematic and the Le Fort I osteotomy is now a common operation. Higher-level osteotomies at Le Fort II or III level can also be carried out using bicoronal flaps for access. The latter are only necessary for complex cases such as Crouzon's and Apert's syndromes (where intracranial surgery may also be necessary), and most simple orthognathic surgery on the maxilla can be carried out via a Le Fort I osteotomy. As with the mandible, surgery restricted to the alveolus has lost its popularity and anterior segmental osteotomies (such as the Wassmund and Wunderer procedures) are becoming uncommon.

The Le Fort I osteotomy is a versatile procedure, which can be performed at different levels above the apices of the teeth, entering the nasal cavity at the base or higher up on the lateral wall. The only limiting structure of note is the infraorbital nerve, which must be avoided. Posteriorly, care must be taken in separating the pterygoid plates from the posterior wall of the maxilla because any improper use of the chisel may damage the maxillary artery, the consequence of which may be profuse bleeding. Rarely, it is necessary to transfuse a patient because of excessive blood loss, although the likelihood of this can be minimized by careful surgical technique, local anaesthetic with vasoconstrictor and general anaesthesia with induced hypotension.

The actual technique involves a horizontal incision from molar to molar regions. The height of the incision can be varied but there is some evidence that there is less relapse when the incision is made well above the level of the apices. Anteriorly, the floor of the nose, the septum and lateral walls all need to be exposed carefully so as not to tear the nasal mucoperiosteum. The buccal bone cuts are normally made with a bur or reciprocating saw, whilst the septum, the lateral nasal walls and the pterygoid plates are detached with specifically

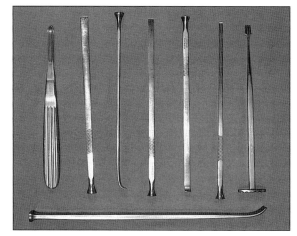

Fig. 12.15 A selection of special chisels and osteotomes designed for use in orthognathic surgery. Many more designs exist, each with a special function.

designed chisels and osteotomes (Fig. 12.15). After mobilizing the fractured bones, as in mandibular osteotomies, an acrylic wafer between the upper and lower teeth should be used with intermaxillary fixation to establish the new position of the jaw. Care must be taken to avoid unwanted rotational movements before stabilizing the maxilla in its new position with titanium miniplates. Maxillary osteotomies with at least four miniplates *in situ* are relatively stable and intermaxillary fixation can be replaced with elastic fixation postoperatively. Any cyanosis of the buccal tissues should rapidly resolve at this stage, before the wounds are closed with interrupted or continuous sutures.

The basic osteotomy procedures

- Osteotomies are controlled fractures
- Surgery should only be undertaken if it offers a realistic chance of fulfilling expectations
- Procedures should be stable with minimal relapse expected
- Sagittal split operations are the most common mandibular osteotomies and Le Fort I osteotomies the most common in the maxilla

CLEFT LIP AND PALATE

The incidence of cleft lip and palate varies considerably around the world but is estimated by the WHO to be the second most common birth defect. It is, however, difficult to classify since it could refer to anything from a bifid uvula to a complete bilateral cleft affecting the upper lip, nasal floor and whole of the palate. Cleft lip and palate are extremely important because:

- they are visually disturbing especially for new parents and children are often stigmatized or even excluded in some societies
- they affect the muscular function of the mouth
- they affect the ability to thrive
- speech (and sometimes hearing) can be significantly affected
- jaw and tooth development is affected by both the cleft and as a result of some types of surgery.

Details of the surgical management of cleft patients are outside the scope of this book but it is important to be aware of the stages of treatment so that parents can be reassured and in order to encourage dental development as normally as possible. Previous generations have sought to repair clefts at the earliest possible opportunity but much of our current thinking has been based on the work of two French surgeons (Malek and Delaire). The latter particularly promoted the concept of functional repairs—establishing normal anatomy insofar as was possible which was never the purpose of the original surgical techniques such as the Millard lip repair. This is probably best achieved once a baby has reached the age of 4–6 months but it requires considerable support for parents who (for obvious reasons) wish to pressurize surgeons into earlier intervention.

Surgery to the palate is usually completed by the first birthday and, for the next few years, further surgery should be avoided giving more attention to speech, social and educational development. Alveolar clefts in the canine region respond well to bone grafting and, when this is required, it should be undertaken well before the canine is due to erupt—usually around the age of 9–10 years.

Finally, when the child reaches the age of 14–15 years he/she should be assessed with a view to orthodontic treatment + orthognathic surgery. Orthodontic treatment in severe cases can take in excess of two years and so should be timed for completion once growth of the facial skeleton can be expected to have finished (17–18 years of age). Recent improvements in the care of cleft babies and children have focused on the establishment of regional centres with teams of specialists and sub-specialists. This, and the much closer attention to research and outcomes, has undoubtedly raised the standards of care available to cleft patients in the UK.

FURTHER READING

Becker A., Shpack N., Shteyer A. (1996) Attachment bonding to impacted teeth at the time of surgical exposure. *European Journal of Orthodontics* 18: 457–463.

Epker B. N., Stella J. P., Fish L. C. (1995) *Dentofacial deformities*, 2nd edn. Mosby, St Louis, MO.

Henderson D. (1985) *A colour atlas of orthognathic surgery.* Wolfe Medical, London.

McBride L. J. (1979) Traction—a surgical/orthodontic procedure. *American Journal of Orthodontics* 76: 287–299.

Schatz J. P., Joho J. P. (1992) Long-term clinical and radiologic evaluation of autotransplanted teeth. *International Journal of Oral and Maxillofacial Surgery* 21: 271–275.

Vermette M. E., Kokich V. G., Kennedy D. B. (1995) Uncovering labially impacted teeth: apically repositioned flap and closed eruption techniques. *Angle Orthodontist* 65: 23–32.

SELF-ASSESSMENT

1. The tooth shown in Fig 12.16 is unerupted, asymptomatic and impacted.
   (a) At what age does this tooth most frequently erupt?
   (b) Describe three possible sequelae of leaving this tooth *in situ*.
   (c) How could the position of the tooth be determined more accurately before surgery?
2. The patient in Fig. 12.17 presents with failed eruption of the permanent upper central incisor.
   (a) At what age should this tooth have erupted? List four causes of delayed eruption.

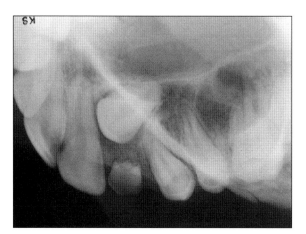

Fig. 12.16   See question 1.

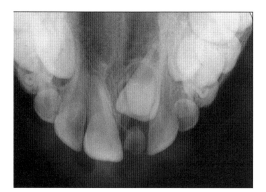

Fig. 12.17   See question 2.

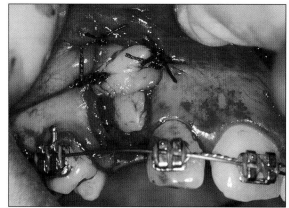

Fig. 12.18   See question 3.

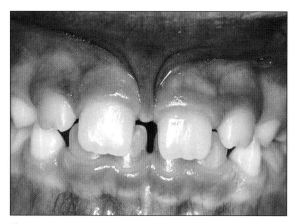

Fig. 12.19   See question 4.

(b) List three local complications of surgery in this region to expose the tooth.

(c) What is the radio-opacity overlying the tooth crown?

3. In Fig. 12.18 the upper right canine tooth has been surgically exposed.

(a) Describe the type of flap that has been used.

(b) Why has the excess tissue not been surgically excised at the same time?

(c) What other technique can be used to prevent the defect healing?

(d) What else could be done at the time of surgery to encourage eruption of the tooth?

4. The patient in Fig. 12.19 presents with a pronounced labial fraenum and a median diastema.

(a) How else might the extent of the fraenum be visualized?

(b) What are the indications for lingual fraenectomy?

5. The patient in Fig. 12.20 presents complaining about the appearance of her lower jaw.

(a) What is this jaw relationship termed?

(b) Describe two inherited conditions in which abnormal jaw relationships may occur.

(c) Describe three typical features of prognathism.

(d) If surgery were to be considered, list three further investigations that would be essential in planning the surgery.

(e) List three complications of the sagittal split osteotomy.

6. The parents of a baby, 6 weeks old with a cleft lip and palate, ask what operations will be needed in his lifetime.

(a) List the possible operations.

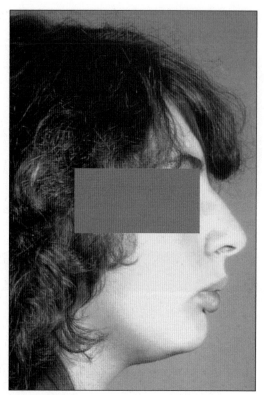

Fig. 12.20 See question 5.

(b) What ages will they be required?
(c) Why is alveolar bone grafting advisable?
(d) Give three reasons why the cleft lip is not repaired in the first week or two of life.

Answers on page 267.

13 | Maxillofacial trauma

J. P. Shepherd

- A major component of maxillofacial trauma is trauma of the teeth and jaws.
- Even when the teeth themselves are not affected, they are of key importance in treating patients who have sustained facial injuries.
- Most injuries encountered by dentists are relatively minor: broken teeth, fractures of alveolar bone, bruising and minor lacerations of the face and oral mucosa and single fractures of the mandible.
- Although most dentists will not be involved in the management of patients with serious or life-threatening maxillofacial trauma, they are involved in the rehabilitation once the patient leaves hospital.
- There are important medicolegal and psychological aspects of the treatment of maxillofacial injuries, particularly as violence is a common cause.
- This chapter is about injuries that are more serious than those confined to the teeth.

ASSUMED KNOWLEDGE

It is assumed that at this stage you will have knowledge/competencies in the following areas:

- anatomy of the cranial base, face and jaws
- principles of the management of fractures
- principles of resuscitation
- pharmacology of analgesics and antimicrobials.

If you think that you are not well equipped in these areas, revise them before reading this chapter or cross-check with texts on those subjects as you read.

INTENDED LEARNING OUTCOMES

At the end of this chapter you should be able to:

1. Recognize clinical features typical of:
   (a) injuries of the soft tissues of the face and oral mucosa
   (b) injuries of the jaws including dentoalveolar fractures
   (c) injuries of the zygomas, orbits, nose and cranial base
   (d) injuries of the contents of the orbits which are associated with orbital fractures
   (e) and distinguish between such injuries
2. List the causes of facial injury and the principles of primary and secondary prevention
3. Describe the clinical and radiographic evaluation and diagnosis of maxillofacial trauma
4. Distinguish between cases requiring surgical intervention and those that do not

5. Describe the emergency care of patients with acute maxillofacial injuries
6. Understand the principles of surgery for facial bone and soft-tissue injury, building upon knowledge of the principles of treatment of fractures in general; select appropriate drug therapy, particularly in relation to antimicrobials and analgesics; plan and provide rehabilitation after repair has been carried out
7. Recognize the complications associated with maxillofacial trauma and the features of psychological disturbance and psychiatric illness associated with maxillofacial trauma
8. Describe medicolegal responsibilities associated with managing those injured in violence, road accidents and other trauma.

INTRODUCTION

Facial injury can occur in isolation or in combination with injuries elsewhere. Regardless of the site of injury, there are local and systemic effects. Trauma causes physical injury to soft or hard tissues and this gives rise to an inflammatory response, resulting in pain, tenderness, swelling and reduced function. Loss of physical integrity at the sites of injury is also common: the skin may be abraded, lacerated or lost and bones and teeth may be stressed to the extent that they fracture or dislocate. Indirect soft-tissue injury is rare, but can occur through traction to the skin due to blunt trauma and tearing at distant sites. Indirect trauma is a more common cause of fracture: for example, a blow to the mandibular symphysis can cause a distant subcondylar fracture.

As well as the inflammatory response and local effects of trauma, systemic effects involving biological and psychological stress reactions occur. Biological stress reactions include release of endogenous catecholamines (the 'fight, flight and fright reaction') and associated psychological stress reactions often comprise feelings of shock, fear, an increased sense of vulnerability and sometimes denial (inability or failure to appreciate that the injury has actually occurred). Metabolic changes are similar to those which follow administration of high doses of steroids. Oxygen consumption, carbon dioxide production and protein breakdown increase.

An understanding of the cause of injury is important for several reasons. It helps to focus on the need for injury prevention; it may help identify typical patterns of injury (e.g. the blow to the symphysis associated with a condylar fracture or head injury), and it may raise awareness of the risk of future injuries (for example, in cases of domestic violence). There are many unique features of injuries of the face because it is responsible for the senses of sight, smell, taste and hearing. In addition, eating, drinking, speech and communication through facial expression depend on the integrity of maxillofacial structures. Disruption of the maxillofacial skeleton can hazard the airway.

In those with maxillofacial injuries it is also necessary to consider the possibility that there may be injury to the base of the skull, cranial vault and brain, the cervical spine and the upper aerodigestive tract. Indirect effects on the upper aerodigestive tract may include airway obstruction or partial obstruction because of blood, saliva and fragments of teeth or bones. Airbag injuries may affect the neck and face together. The presence and extent of brain injuries influences the risk of distant effects on the aerodigestive tract where, for example, coma may predispose to the inhalation of fragments of teeth and blood.

There is some evidence that the face acts as a 'crumple zone' (in the same way as the front of an automobile absorbs impact which might otherwise be transmitted to the passenger compartment) and therefore has a protective effect in terms of brain injury. Facial injuries and brain injuries are often seen together simply because they share the same anatomical region. Overall, the more serious the facial injury, the more likely is brain injury.

THE CAUSES AND PREVENTION OF MAXILLOFACIAL INJURY

The causes of maxillofacial injury reflect the culture in which it is sustained. The most frequent cause of serious maxillofacial injury in the developed world in the past century has been the motor vehicle, the only exception being epidemics of injury sustained in two world wars. Overall, incidence of maxillofacial injuries has reflected death rates on the roads such that, for example in the UK, incidence reached a peak in the 1960s and the 1970s and has been falling since. Violence has become a more common cause of maxillofacial fracture, on both sides of the Atlantic, since the late 1960s.

The causes of historical increase in road trauma include progressive industrialization and expansion of the motor industry leading to steadily increasing numbers of vehicles, lack of focus on safety during the first 60 years of automobile and motorcycle development and lack of investment in motorways until the 1970s. Determined efforts to reduce risks have led to drink-drive and seat-belt legislation, construction of safer roads and increased safety of the vehicles themselves. Increases in violence have been caused by numerous factors, including low levels of social control of young people in families and in the workplace, unemployment, the development of a drug culture, decline in real alcohol prices and more leisure time. Surveys of maxillofacial injuries in Middle-Eastern countries demonstrate much lower incidence of injury overall and a lower incidence of alcohol-related trauma.

The most effective approach to prevention of maxillofacial injury has been attention to the particular circumstances of injuries in particular environments (secondary prevention). Thus, wearing a cycle helmet has been shown to prevent upper facial injury, gum shields prevent many sports injuries and toughened or plastic glassware reduces the risk of facial injury in assault in licensed premises. Educational interventions, for example in schools, have had much less effect. Preschool education together with early family support (primary prevention) has been shown to reduce later assault as well as other forms of delinquency such as truanting, drug abuse and early pregnancy.

THE MANAGEMENT OF MAXILLOFACIAL TRAUMA

Management of the acutely injured patient

The management of the acutely injured patient in the accident and emergency department depends on organized, well-practised teamwork, under the direction of a team leader. However, whenever a seriously injured, perhaps unconscious patient is encountered, the presence of a cervical spine injury should be assumed until proved not to exist and neck movements should therefore be kept to a minimum. Obvious bleeding should be controlled using pressure, wire ligatures around teeth adjacent to fractures, ligature of vessels (such as the facial artery) and inserting ribbon gauze packs into, for example, intraoral lacerations of the sulci. The airway must be established and maintained by altering posture, by aspiration and, if necessary, by means of endotracheal intubation. Tongue control, by means of oropharyngeal or nasopharyngeal tube airways, may be useful. Where there is total upper airway obstruction, a laryngotomy through the cricothyroid membrane may be necessary. Chest radiography and analysis of blood loss are necessary early in the case of chest emergencies. Ventilation to keep the arterial pO_2 above 10 kPa and pCO_2 below 5.5 kPa can be achieved by a bag valve mask. To support the circulation, the insertion of the largest possible cannula into an antecubital vein is usually the best option for intravenous infusion.

This focus on **A**irway, **B**reathing, **C**irculation, in this order, together with the assessment of cervical spine integrity, disability and neurological state, comprise the primary survey and resuscitation phases, which are key to life support for trauma patients. This facilitates the logical progression to secondary injury surveys and the definitive care phase.

Practical skills in resuscitation are essential for all clinicians and these can be learnt and maintained only by attending recognized practical courses.

History of injury

Accurate verbatim accounts of injury are important because this medical evidence may be of great relevance to investigations by the police, insurance companies and researchers. Although it is not usually necessary to record the cause of injury in detail, a short summary is always helpful. In relation to assault, for example, this should include the type of weapon, how many assailants were reportedly involved and where precisely the assault took place. For car occupants, seat-belt wearing and position in the car should be recorded. An essential part of the history relates to tetanus prophylaxis: the year of the most recent 'booster' should be established and prophylaxis administered if necessary.

Dental surgeons are often asked to see the injured person after their general condition has been stabilized. Occasionally this is not the case, however, and a dental practitioner may be the first to the scene of a serious accident or assault. If injuries are life-threatening, the history should be dispensed with until airway, cervical spine, breathing and circulation have been stabilized.

It is often said that records about alcohol are important, but at the initial consultation it can be extremely difficult without objective measurement to assess its effects. It is a mistake to blame people for their injuries just because they have been drinking. Nevertheless, if alcohol abuse is to be investigated then breath analysis is appropriate for acute intoxication. Pure ethyl alcohol, reflecting its volatile nature, may be smelt on the breath, but almost all alcoholic drinks contain other volatile components (congeners), which make smell alone an unreliable measure of alcohol consumption.

The Glasgow Coma Scale

First described by two Glasgow neuroscientists, the Glasgow Coma Scale (GCS) is an internationally recognized method for measuring coma. It cannot discriminate between causes of coma, such as brain injury or alcohol intoxication, but it provides an excellent means of assessing the need for hospital admission and recovery (Table 13.1).

Diagnostic information sought in the history

- Alteration in the way the teeth meet
- Pain site(s), aggravating, relieving factors, severity
- Numbness of skin, mucosa and teeth
- Alteration in ability to speak, swallow, chew, open mouth
- Disturbances of vision: blurring, double vision
- Reduced patency of oral and nasal airway
- Hearing disturbance
- Abnormal sounds from the jaw joints
- Neck problems.

Examination

Very often, by the time a dental practitioner is called to see an injured person, some radiographs have

Table 13.1 The Glasgow Coma Scale

	Score
Eyes open:	
Spontaneously	4
To speech	3
To pain	2
Never	1
Best motor response:	
Obeys commands	6
Localizes pain	5
Flexion withdrawal	4
Decerebrate flexion	3
Decerebrate extension	2
No response	1
Best verbal response:	
Orientated	5
Confused	4
Inappropriate words	3
Incomprehensible sounds	2
Silent	1

Scores for the three components can be added together (< 8 is defined as coma; maximum score = 15) or listed separately.

already been obtained. Looking at these before seeing the patient is a mistake. An enormous amount can be missed from focusing first on radiographs. For example, they do not show soft-tissue injuries and superimposition often makes primary diagnosis of mandibular, symphyseal and cranial base fractures difficult or impossible. Much information can be gained simply by observation of the patient. Although dental practitioners will usually not be responsible for managing injuries outside the maxillofacial region, examination should always start with an overall assessment of injuries.

Pay particular attention to signs of bleeding or other discharge from the ears, eyes, nose and mouth. In seriously injured patients there may be leakage of cerebrospinal fluid from the ears or nose. Look for signs of impact, including on the scalp. Abrasions (Fig. 13.1) or haematomas often signal the sites of underlying bone injury. There is often little swelling in the immediate aftermath of injury. However, within 6 hours mandibular angle fractures, for example, are often associated with swelling over the angle (Fig. 13.1) and subcondylar fractures with preauricular swelling.

Always take a systematic approach to the examination of the maxillofacial region. As with occipitomental radiographs, start superiorly and work down the face in a series of arcs to reduce the chances of an injury being missed.

An examination may follow this order:

- start by considering the scalp
- then the frontal bones and supraorbital ridges
- then the orbits and nasoethmoidal region (traumatic telecanthus and a saddle nose deformity)
- then the external auditory meati, zygomatic arches and infraorbital margins
- then the zygomatic buttresses, alar regions and upper teeth
- finally the temporomandibular joints, mandible and lower teeth.

Having carried out a thorough inspection of the mouth and face, the facial skeleton should be palpated in the same systematic manner, paying particular regard to:

- asymmetry—to help identify bruising, oedema or fractures
- step defects—to help identify bone fractures
- discontinuity—to help identify bone fractures
- crepitus—to help identify the presence of air in the tissues
- tenderness
- neurological deficit—cranial nerves V and VII; also III, IV, VI if there are signs of orbital injury—to identify nerve injury
- missing and mobile teeth
- mobility of the mid-face—to help identify a mid-face fracture.

Stand behind and above the patient when assessing facial asymmetry, particularly in relation to suspected zygomatic fractures. In this position place an index finger on the maximum convexity of the zygoma on both sides equidistant from the tip of the nose. Then compare the overlap of the index fingers with the supraorbital ridges.

Mobility of the middle third of the face, such as that brought about by Le Fort I, Le Fort II and Le Fort III pattern fractures (Fig. 13.2) is best assessed by placing the patient's head securely against a head rest,

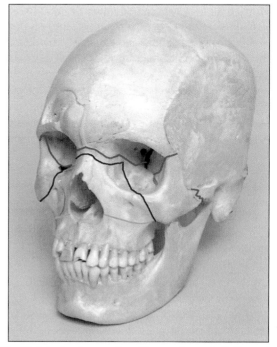

Fig. 13.2 Le Fort fracture lines illustrated on a skull. Green, Le Fort I; blue, Le Fort II; red, Le Fort III.

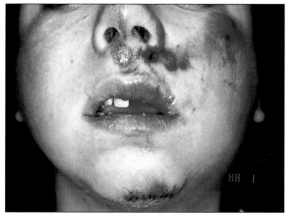

Fig. 13.1 Abrasion of the mid-face that might overly a fracture.

grasping the upper teeth and alveolus and moving them gently, but purposefully, laterally, superiorly and anteriorly. Simultaneous palpation of the nasal bones has often been advocated but this can give rise to false-positive findings because of the mobility of the scalp and skin in this region. A 'cracked cup' sound when the upper teeth are percussed can be diagnostic of a Le Fort pattern fracture.

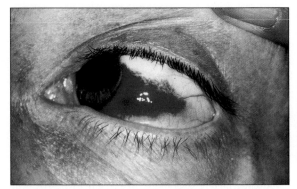

Fig. 13.3 Subconjunctival ecchymosis.

Le Fort pattern fractures

- Le Fort I: Horizontal fracture of the maxilla immediately above the teeth and palate
- Le Fort II: Pyramidal fracture extending from the zygomatic buttresses through the infraorbital margins to the bridge of the nose
- Le Fort III: Detachment of the facial bones, including the zygomas, from the skull base

NB: These extensive mid-face fractures rarely present in classic form. Most involve comminution (fragmentation) and there is frequently a different combination of injuries on the two sides of the face.

A good test for a mandibular fracture is to exert gentle but purposeful backward pressure on the symphysis. The patient will indicate discomfort at the angles or condyles if there are fractures in these regions. If there is symphyseal injury or injury of the overlying skin, then gentle medial pressure on both mandibular angles simultaneously may provide evidence of mandibular fracture in or near the mandibular midline.

Although a comprehensive examination of cranial nerve function is not usually necessary, hearing loss may be investigated by rubbing the thumb and forefinger together 1–2 cm from the patient's external auditory meatus. Hearing loss may be caused by blood in the external auditory meatus or, exceptionally, may be associated with a cranial base fracture or neurological dysfunction. Whatever the cause, hearing deficit should prompt referral to an otolaryngologist.

Examination of the orbits and eyes should focus first on visual acuity, diplopia in the various directions of gaze and evidence of bleeding into the surrounding skin, under the conjunctiva (Fig. 13.3), or into either chamber of the eye. Anterior or posterior displacement of the globe gives rise to exophthalmos and enophthalmos respectively and is most important in relation to the diagnosis of retrobulbar

haemorrhage (because this condition can give rise to irreversible blindness if left untreated), or a 'blow-out' fracture of the orbital floor or medial wall. Examination of the canthi is important for eliminating the possibility of traumatic telecanthus (widening of the distance between the inner canthi due to detachment from sound bone). Corneal abrasions, conjunctival tears and eyelid laceration or loss need to be sought by careful examination of the eyes and charted thoroughly. Diplopia (double vision) is most often caused by haemorrhage or oedema in or adjacent to extraocular muscles, but can be caused by mechanical tethering of muscle attachments or by injuries to the third, fourth or sixth cranial nerves.

Thorough examination of the nose is an aspect of maxillofacial examination often neglected and includes attention to:

- symmetry
- deformity in all three dimensions
- bilateral or unilateral epistaxis (bleeding from the nose)
- possible leak of cerebrospinal fluid (identity may be confirmed by high sugar and low protein content)
- septal haematoma or disruption
- anosmia or paranosmia (absent or altered sense of smell)
- crepitus (grating sound) associated with mobile nasal bones
- unilateral epistaxis, often associated with an ipsilateral (same sided) fracture of the zygoma, secondary to bleeding into the maxillary antrum.

Examination of the mouth with a good light, paying attention to the junction of the hard and soft palate (Le Fort pattern fractures cause haematomas here), dental arches and the sulci, is important. The teeth should be charted, noting particularly broken teeth and retained roots, especially those that are very mobile and which may cause airway embarrassment. Gentle but purposeful pressure should be applied to all teeth to detect possible dentoalveolar fractures, a split palate and fractured teeth. Patients with fractures of the mandible between the mental foramen and the mandibular foramen often have reduced levels of sensation in the distribution of the inferior alveolar or lingual nerves and patients with zygomatic fractures often have areas of reduced sensation in the distribution of the infraorbital and anterior superior alveolar nerves. Any such areas of altered sensation should be recorded. Intraoral soft-tissue injuries are usually obvious and some extensive lacerations of the hard and soft palate may be present—for example, if a child has impacted a toy or other object into the mouth during a fall. Sublingual haematomas and tears at the gingival margin can be diagnostic of mandibular fractures (Fig. 13.4).

Examination of jaw function should include meas-urement in millimetres of maximal comfortable mouth opening from the tips of the central incisors on one side; this should be recorded clearly in the medical records. Abnormalities of jaw function should be sought and recorded: these include deviation on opening, abnormal joint sounds and disrupted occlusion (Fig. 13.5). Temporomandibular joint dislocation is rarely a result of injury but traumatic effusions can give rise to temporary mild posterior open bite. Crucially, anterior open bite can be a feature of Le Fort pattern fractures in which the middle third of the facial skeleton moves backwards

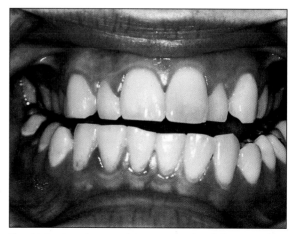

Fig. 13.5 Anterior open bite associated with fracture of the mandible.

and downwards on the cranial base or of bilateral fractures of the mandibular condyles in which the pterygomasseteric sling shortens the ascending rami.

It is important to carry out a thorough examination of the skin of the face, including the pinnae, the scalp and the neck. Areas of numbness or partial numbness should be assessed by means of touch testing, comparing sides and two-point discrimination and recorded. Careful attention needs to be paid to all facial orifices, in particular to discontinuity of eyelids, external nares, the external auditory meati and the vermilion border of the lips. High-quality soft-tissue reconstruction depends on accurate repositioning of the oral mucosa, musculature and skin in these areas.

SPECIAL INVESTIGATIONS

Special investigations should only follow thorough clinical examination: many fractures have been missed by ordering radiographs first. Radiographic examination forms the basis of special investigations of maxillofacial injury and should be specific to the areas of concern. Radiographs should be obtained according to the following categorization:

- skull views: posteroanterior and lateral
- mid-face: two occipitomental views at different angles (Fig. 13.6)
- nasal bones: soft tissue lateral

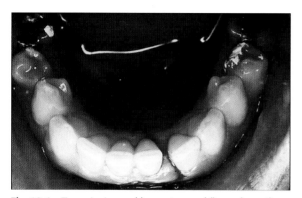

Fig. 13.4 Torn gingiva and haematoma of floor of mouth.

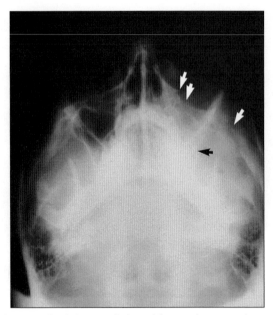

Fig. 13.6 Occipitomental view of fractured zygoma. Arrows indicate fractures at the infraorbital rim, zygomatic arch and zygomatic buttress areas.

- tooth-bearing areas of the jaws: orthopantomogram and posteroanterior (Figs 13.7, 13.8)
- nasoethmoidal region and orbits: coronal computed tomography
- teeth: periapical and occlusal.

Radiographs may be necessary not only to reach a diagnosis but also to inform treatment decisions, for example, about where bone plates should be applied. They also commonly reveal injuries which

may not need treatment, for example, undisplaced or minimally displaced fractures, medial blow-out fractures of the orbit and comminution of the midface. Radiographs provide much more detailed information on hard-tissue injuries than the clinical examination so they may, for example, show fractures of the roots of teeth and signs of associated soft-tissue abnormality, such as herniation of orbital contents into the maxillary antrum (Figs 13.9, 13.10).

Additional tests may include hearing tests (though these are almost always performed by audiologists or otologists), tests for monocular and binocular single vision such as Hess testing (by orthoptists) and various other ophthalmological tests. The management of patients with multiple maxillofacial injuries relies on teamwork, and it is preferable for specialist ear, eye and neurosurgical tests to be ordered by the relevant specialists so that treatment can be comprehensive and coordinated.

SURGICAL INTERVENTION IN THE MANAGEMENT OF MAXILLOFACIAL INJURY

Many facial injuries require no active treatment and heal spontaneously. Examples include small haematomas, clean abrasions, small lacerations, undisplaced stable fractures and some displaced fractures, such as those of the mandibular condyle where the occlusion is not deranged or where the occlusion settles spontaneously. As with any surgical

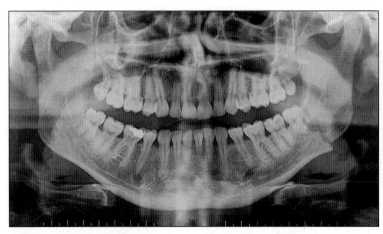

Fig. 13.7 Orthopantomogram of fractured mandible.

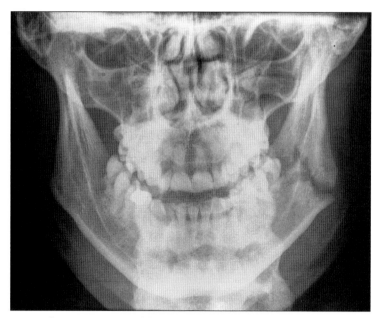

Fig. 13.8 PA view of the jaws, showing a fractured mandible.

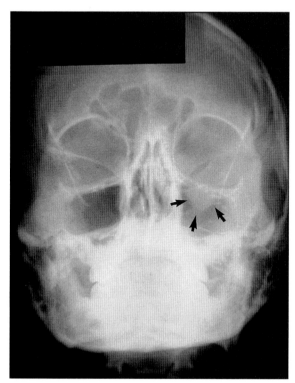

Fig. 13.9 Occipitomental view of a fracture of the left orbital floor. Note the herniated orbital contents, outlined by the arrows.

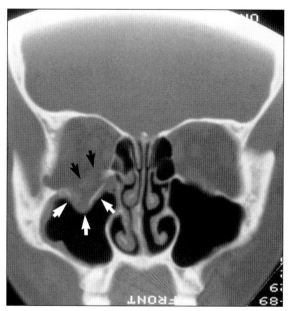

Fig. 13.10 CT scan showing herniation of orbital contents (white arrows) through an orbital floor fracture. The inferior rectus muscle is highlighted with black arrows.

intervention, a crucial decision is whether operative treatment will benefit the patient. Given there are few randomized controlled trials, and given the recorded clinical experience of generations of oral and maxillofacial surgeons, the management of maxillofacial trauma is more of an art than a science. It is possible to overtreat or undertreat. For example, one may overtreat mandibular condyle fractures if it is not appreciated that many displaced fractures of the neck of the condyle heal spontaneously without complications. Similarly, neglect of grossly displaced condylar fractures can give rise to long-term occlusal derangement.

Indications for surgery and brief descriptions of appropriate operative procedures are set out below.

As in orthopaedics, the principles of treatment are:

- reduction—repositioning fragments of bone to their anatomical positions
- fixation—making sure fragments remain in position until fractures have healed
- immobilization—preventing the broken bone from moving during the healing period
- rehabilitation—returning the patient to normal function after the fracture has healed.

Although these principles remain the cornerstone of management of fractures, immobilization is now much less important than it has been historically. This is because research has demonstrated that complications such as long-term jaw stiffness, airway restrictions and psychological problems are greater if the jaws are immobilized (traditionally by wiring them together). Furthermore, the advent of small bone plates provides a method of fixing many fractures precisely and with a degree of stability which makes immobilization unnecessary.

Surgery for fractures of the zygomatic complex

Indications for surgical intervention include:

- flattening of the zygomatic prominence or externally obvious zygomatic arch depression
- tethering of the eye secondary to orbital floor fracture
- mechanical interference of the coronoid process by the overlying zygomatic body.

Trismus often resolves spontaneously because it is often not caused by mechanical interference but by haemorrhage into the masseter or temporalis muscles.

The basis of treatment for zygomatic fractures remains the Gillies' procedure. This depends upon the anatomical relationship of the temporalis fascia, which is attached to the superior aspect of the zygomatic arch, and the temporalis muscle, which passes beneath the zygomatic arch and body and is attached to the coronoid process and anterior aspect of the ascending ramus. Thus, if an elevator is passed between temporalis fascia and muscle, it can be used to elevate the displaced bone from underneath (Fig. 13.11). Access is achieved by making a 2-cm incision in the temporal scalp, above and in front of the ear and incising through temporalis fascia. If the elevated bone is unstable then it is necessary to stabilize the zygoma with mini-plates across the fracture lines in the zygomatic buttress region, the zygomaticofrontal suture (Fig. 13.12) (particularly if

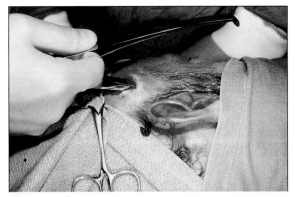

Fig. 13.11 Elevation of the zygoma.

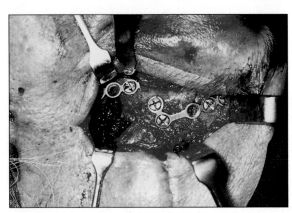

Fig. 13.12 Mini-plate across a frontozygomatic fracture.

the frontal process of the zygoma is displaced medial to the zygomatic process of the frontal bone) and the zygomaticomaxillary region. Surgical approaches to the orbital floor are necessary to retrieve orbital contents from the maxillary antrum and prevent recurrence by the insertion of a graft of either bone or synthetic material. Transconjunctival (with or without lateral canthotomy) and transcutaneous (lower lid or infraorbital) approaches to the orbital floor are in use. The principal objective is limitation of scarring in this most visible and socially important area of the face while gaining sufficient access to the fracture site. Minimizing skin scarring has to be balanced against risks of corneal and subconjunctival injury.

Isolated fractures of the zygomatic arch are much less common than fractures of the zygomatic complex (separation of the entire zygoma) but operative intervention is sometimes necessary because untreated fractures give rise to cosmetic problems or arch/coronoid interference, resulting in restriction of mandibular movement. Again the Gillies' approach is the basis of treatment. As the zygomatic arch is not a substantial bone, reductions are sometimes unstable and splinting is occasionally necessary. There are a number of ways of doing this—for example, using a Foley catheter inflated under the arch for 48 hours, or using external splinting by means of transcutaneous circumzygomatic sutures.

In extensive or panfacial (multiple fractures of all or most regions of the facial skeleton) trauma, it may be necessary to gain access to craniofacial sutures at a number of sites; in these cases, the coronal scalp flap can be invaluable. In this approach, a coronal scalp incision is made above the hairline, allowing the scalp to be turned down over the face to expose the nasoethmoidal and zygomatic regions. Thus, for example, by such an approach it is possible to reduce a complex nasoethmoidal fracture, repair a cerebrospinal fluid leak and reduce and fix bilateral zygomatic or Le Fort pattern fractures. The basis of the surgical treatment of nasoethmoidal fractures is reduction of the canthal attachment and reduction of the nasal bones. Very often, the medial canthal ligaments are not simply detached from the bone, but rather the ethmoid bone to which they are attached fractures from the rest of the nasoethmoidal skeleton. The basis of treatment is usually the reduction of intercanthal distance to normal by approximating the medial canthal ligaments using a wire suture.

The basis of treatment of fractures of the nasal bones is reduction of each nasal bone and the nasal septum using instruments inserted into the anterior nares. Nasal splinting is often inadequate, particularly with T-plasters, which simply compress haematoma and oedema rather than stabilize the reduced nasal fracture. It is therefore often necessary to provide intranasal splinting using, for example, expansive flexible splints or tulle gras (paraffin wax impregnated gauze) to prevent the nasal bones from falling medially. Occasionally, nasal trauma gives rise to bilateral septal haematoma, which should be drained early to avoid necrosis of the cartilaginous septum.

Operative procedures for Le Fort pattern fractures

These fractures are sometimes undisplaced or minimally displaced, resulting in minimal occlusal derangement, which corrects itself with masticatory function during the first week. Indications for operative intervention are asymmetry, displacement, comminution and sustained occlusal derangement. As with almost all fractures of the mid-face, immediate surgical intervention is rarely necessary. Exceptions include haemorrhage and the need to take the patient to the operating theatre for surgery for other injuries. There are many advantages in leaving definitive treatment until 5–7 days have elapsed. These include resolution of soft-tissue swelling that makes operative assessment and access difficult, resolution of any brain injury or other systemic trauma and resolution of any acute intoxication with alcohol or other drugs.

The basis of treatment for these fractures is direct visualization of the fracture sites and fixation with mini-plates, paying particular attention to achieving the correct occlusion. Postoperative intermaxillary fixation (IMF) is rarely necessary, although retention of arch bars (metal bars wired to the teeth facilitating wiring the jaws together) (Fig. 13.13) may assist if there are mandibular fractures that have not been fixed directly and for which elastic traction (pulling the teeth into the correct position using elastic bands) may be necessary to settle the occlusion.

Operative procedures in the treatment of fractures of the mandible

Most fractures of the teeth-bearing part of the mandible require operative intervention to restore

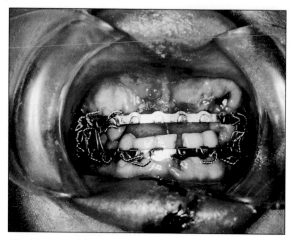

Fig. 13.13 Arch bars.

occlusion and minimize pain due to mobility. Undisplaced fractures, especially in children, may, however, not require operative intervention. Open reduction and fixation with mini-plates is the treatment of choice for displaced fractures of the teeth-bearing aspect of the mandible. Mini-plates are usually applied intraorally to the external oblique ridge in the case of angle fractures or to the midline in the case of symphyseal fractures. The placement of plates is critical in relation to:

- avoiding close proximity to the oral mucosa
- use of two parallel plates where the use of only one may lead to a fulcrum about which the healing mandible may become mobile
- the anatomy and distribution of the roots of the teeth
- the course of the inferior dental nerve
- comminution, where non-linear and multi-hole plates may be necessary.

As with the use of implants at other sites, for example in hip replacement, biocompatibility is not as important as it is in dental implantology. Thus, success has been achieved in terms of biointegration with stainless steel, cobalt-chrome alloy and titanium mini-plates and screws, the costs of which are generally great. There are numerous types of mini-plates currently on the world market and there are clear opportunities for cost savings if a generic rather than a proprietary approach is adopted, as with drugs. Disadvantages of the use of plates include the need

for access to the fracture sites and potential for infection and plate mobility leading to plate loss.

Teeth in fracture lines should normally be retained to assist in the accurate reduction of both fractures and the occlusion. They act as spacers and their loss can lead to poor reduction. However, if teeth are fractured, displaced from the socket or terminally diseased in relation to periodontal disease or caries they should be removed.

Fractures of the ascending ramus and condyle of the mandible are almost always of the condylar neck. The most important distinction to be made is between condylar fractures that involve the articular surface and those which do not. Because the occlusion and masticatory function tend to maintain the dimensions of the ascending ramus, operative intervention is normally necessary only when the occlusion does not return to normal within the first 10 days after trauma. All intracapsular fractures should be mobilized immediately and solitary intracapsular fractures are unlikely to affect the occlusion unless there is a traumatic effusion. The majority of sub-condylar fractures heal with no long-term occlusal disturbance: the support provided by the occlusion is akin to the weight of the arm, which is normally sufficient to maintain a fractured humerus in a satisfactory position without recourse to surgical intervention. Condylar fractures that may benefit from open reduction and internal fixation are those where:

- there is gross displacement with wide separation of the bone ends
- there is little or no sign of the occlusion settling by 10 days
- bilateral fractures are causing anterior open bite
- it is necessary to reconstruct the condyle to establish the integrity of the mandible before fixation of central mid-face fractures
- there is a fracture dislocation.

Fractures of the condyle may be reduced and fixed using mini-plates or transfixion screws and the app-roach may be intraoral or extraoral. Precision at operation is critical because errors may be magnified in the tooth-bearing part of the mandible.

The nature of fixation

Most mini-plates provide slight flexibility and are therefore forgiving of minor errors in fixation. Slight movement at the fracture area during the healing period is an advantage because it promotes osteogenesis through the 'fixator' effect, first described in orthopaedics, which accelerates healing through periods of slight, controlled, movement of a fracture. Rigid fixation with substantial 'reconstruction' plates requires very precise surgical techniques but is more often successful in the presence of infection.

Wire fixation has too much in-built flexibility, leading to deformation in function. Traditional means of immobilizing the jaw with intermaxillary fixation are eyelet wires and arch bars. Both provide wire loops, through or around which tiewires are passed. Arch bars, intraosseous screws or orthodontic brackets may be used if elastic traction is necessary, for example, to maintain the occlusion after bilateral sub-condylar fractures. With mini-plates, intermaxillary fixation is usually not required, apart from intra-operatively to maintain occlusion while mini-plates are applied.

Infection and maxillofacial fractures

Although most maxillofacial fractures are compound into (communicate with) the mouth or paranasal sinuses, the incidence of infection is low in otherwise healthy patients. Bone surgery and grafting increase the chances of infection but this risk can be reduced by giving broad-spectrum antibiotics during the operation, using the intramuscular or intravenous routes and postoperatively using the oral route.

Stabilization of middle-third fractures with antral packs is associated with more infection than other means of stabilization. Small fragments of bone, particularly in the mid-face, rarely become infected.

Gross infections of non-united mandibular fractures usually require sequestrectomy and rigid fixation with reconstruction plates.

Repair of facial lacerations

It is important not to neglect soft-tissue injuries because of too sharp a focus on underlying fractures.

These injuries usually comprise abrasions, contusions and lacerations but deep, penetrating injuries and loss of soft tissue may also occur, particularly in firearm wounds. Many of the principles of management have been set out above but, in summary, skin, oral mucosa and intervening musculature should be repaired accurately in layers, especially at the margins of the eyes, nose and lips. Account should be taken of the orientation of the muscles of facial expression. Inaccurate repair of a laceration of the vermilion border can lead to an ugly step defect and the need for scar revision.

Even minor scars can be constant reminders of the original trauma as well as socially embarrassing. Resorbable suture material should be used for the oral mucosa and musculature and it is important that the oral mucosa is allowed to heal before muscle sutures resorb. Continuous sutures are often useful for linear mucosal lacerations and can be useful externally. Accurate repositioning of irregular wounds nearly always necessitates the use of interrupted sutures. Infection rates are lower with monofilament suture material (like nylon) than with multifilament or braided suture material (like silk).

Tips for soft-tissue repair

- Look for and remove all foreign bodies: skin tattoos are preventable. Fragments of glass, wood, road grit and gun projectiles can often be identified using radiographs. Copious irrigation can be used to flush out multiple small fragments.
- When repairing lacerations of the eyelids or vermilion border tack the mucosa/ skin borders accurately together before proceeding with muscle repair.
- Excise obvious cyanotic skin tags; otherwise they will become necrotic and cause a lumpy scar.
- Apply a broad-spectrum antibiotic preparation to the skin after repairing lacerations; infection of minor wounds is surprisingly common.
- Do not shave the eyebrow when suturing this area.
- Use magnification routinely when suturing facial lacerations; this aids precision.
- Suturing all but the simplest facial lacerations takes time: children and some adults need

general anaesthesia/sedation to give time for a high standard of repair.
- Operate on fractures before soft-tissue injuries: traction of the lips during fixation of fractures can ruin soft-tissue repairs.

Psychological injury

About one-third of adults with maxillofacial skeletal injury and lacerations more than 3 cm long develop post-traumatic stress disorder (PTSD). This may be defined as acute or chronic, depending on the basis of persistence after 6 months. A diagnosis of PTSD requires the presence of flashbacks to the trauma that produced injury, depression, sleep disruption and irritability/hyperarousal ('jumpiness'). The risk of developing PTSD is increased for patients with a previous history of psychiatric illness, patients who are upset immediately after their injury and people who have been injured in assaults. It has been shown that house surgeons/residents can predict accurately, on the basis of how shocked the patient appears to be initially, who will go on to develop PTSD. The symptoms of PTSD can be reduced by early intervention, for example cognitive-behavioural therapy, for those at risk, who should be referred early to relevant mental health professionals. Liaison psychiatrists are becoming important members of trauma teams. However, non-targeted, blanket mental health interventions, such as 'critical incident debriefing', are now known to do more harm than good.

Psychological problems are not limited to PTSD and may include anxiety, fear of further injury or depression. The prevalence of these conditions is very high in people with facial injuries, and dental practitioners need to be alert to them and have routes of referral to appropriate mental health professionals and voluntary agencies such as Victim Support. It is important not to separate the physical effects of trauma from the psychological effects: the two are often interlinked and minor physical symptoms such as lack of ordinary sensation in the lip can trigger the flashbacks of PTSD.

Dental injuries

Thoroughly chart all dental injuries, including those of the enamel/dentine, root fractures and displaced or avulsed teeth. Account for all the major fragments. Minor damage to the enamel usually requires no immediate intervention. Exposed dentine should be dressed to control sensitivity and prevent loss of vitality. Use thermal rather than electrical pulp testers: pulp reactions can be misleading in the acute phase. Monitor pulp vitality closely but remember that non-responding teeth may reflect neurological rather than pulpal injury.

Fractures of the coronal third of the root of a single-rooted tooth usually necessitate extraction. Undisplaced fractures of the middle and apical third of the root may repair without recourse to treatment. Wire loops can be used to temporarily stabilize mobile teeth or a fracture between two teeth. Reimplanted teeth require calcium hydroxide root-filling at 1–2 weeks to prevent later resorption. Avoid splints that involve the gingival margins.

REHABILITATION

Return to normal function and appearance is the goal of all clinical management. In many cases, particularly of pan-facial trauma, definitive repair of soft-tissue injuries and fractures is only the first step in rehabilitation. Since mini-plates and direct fixation have largely replaced intermaxillary and internal wire fixation, there is great opportunity for early mobilization of the mandible. This reduces the risk of permanent limitation of jaw movement. Many patients with jaw fractures require restorative dentistry as part of their rehabilitation from either family dentists or specialists in restorative dentistry. Lacerations should be reviewed for at least 12 months to assess the need for scar revision, which should not normally be done earlier because scars change in shape, bulk and colour over that time.

Rehabilitation may include the need for the services of an ophthalmic optician to replace spectacles or contact lenses or provide them for the first time if there are permanent effects on vision. Advice from a dietitian may help patients whose nutrition has been compromised through associated injuries of the digestive tract and for those who have postoperative intermaxillary fixation.

In relation to psychosocial rehabilitation it is important to be aware of the level and quality of support at home and to involve the voluntary sector if support is lacking. In many parts of the developed world victim support organizations exist to provide social support, help with practical difficulties (such as those that may follow a robbery), support with police investigations, appearances in court as prosecution witnesses and help with completing applications for criminal injuries compensation.

Family dental practitioners are responsible for ongoing restorative care, and therefore have opportunities to monitor a patient's psychological state and refer if there is evidence of depression or more serious psychiatric problems such as PTSD.

Alcohol misuse predisposes to maxillofacial trauma. In both hospital and primary care settings, effective treatments are available. Patients with maxillofacial trauma should be screened for alcohol problems with a standard test, such as AUDIT (Alcohol Use Disorders Identification Test) and appropriate treatment instituted.

MEDICOLEGAL MANAGEMENT

Practitioners who treat patients with facial injury are often asked to provide factual statements about the injuries and treatment and may be called upon as expert or professional witnesses to interpret the causes and effects of such injuries. A medical report should be completed promptly according to solicitors' instructions but practitioners should ensure that confidential information about a patient is disclosed only with their written consent. All practitioners who treat patients with maxillofacial injuries should be prepared to give written reports and oral evidence in court. Remember that it is not usually the standard of treatment or the possibility of negligence which is important to the courts, but the causes, nature and effects of injury.

FURTHER READING

Ali T., Shepherd J. P. (1994) The measurement of injury severity. *British Journal of Oral and Maxillofacial Surgery* 32: 13–18.

American College of Surgeons (1998) *Advanced trauma life support (ATLS) course*. American College of Surgeons, Chicago, IL.

Andreason J. O., Andreason F. M., Bakland L. K., Flores M. T. (1999) *Traumatic dental injuries: a manual*. Munksgaard, Copenhagen, Denmark.

Bisson J. I., Shepherd J. P., Dhutia M. (1997) Psychological sequelae of facial trauma. *Journal of Trauma* 43: 496–500.

Bisson J. I., Shepherd J. P., Joy D., Probert R., Newcombe R. G. (2004) Early cognitive-behavioural therapy for post-traumatic stress symptoms after physical injury. *British Journal of Psychiatry* 184: 63–69.

Brickley M. R., Shepherd J. P. (1995) The relationship between alcohol intoxication, injury severity and Glasgow Coma Score. *Injury* 26: 311–314.

Evans T. R. (ed) (1989) ABC of resuscitation. *British Medical Journal*, London.

Harrison M. G., Shepherd J. P. (1999) The circumstances and scope for prevention of maxillofacial injuries in cyclists. *Journal of the Royal College of Surgeons of Edinburgh* 44: 82–86.

Omovie E. E., Shepherd J. P. (1997) Assessment of repair of facial lacerations. *British Journal of Oral and Maxillofacial Surgery* 35: 237–240.

Shepherd J. P. (2005) Victim services in the NHS: combining treatment with violence prevention. *Criminal Behaviour and Mental Health* 15: 75–81.

Shepherd J. P., Farrington D. P. (1995) Preventing crime and violence. *British Medical Journal* 310: 271–272.

Shepherd J. P., Qureshi R., Preston M. S., Levers B. G. H. (1990) Psychological distress after assaults and accidents. *British Medical Journal* 301: 849–850.

Ward L., Shepherd J. P., Emond A. M. (1993) Relationship between adult victims of assault and children at risk of abuse. *British Medical Journal* 306: 1101–1102.

Williams J. L. (ed) (1994) Rowe and Williams'. *Maxillofacial injuries*, 2nd edn. Churchill Livingstone, Edinburgh.

SELF-ASSESSMENT

1. A 16-year-old boy is brought to the dental surgery by a teacher, concerned about bleeding from the mouth following a collision on the football field. How would you proceed?
2. How may extraoral inspection help in the diagnosis of maxillofacial injuries?
3. What do you understand by the term 'fixation', and how is this applied?
4. A 13-year-old girl fell off her bicycle onto a gravel path and sustained a 1-cm ragged laceration of the lower lip, extending through onto the oral mucosa. How should definitive treatment proceed?
5. You are providing routine dental care for a 35-year-old woman who you know has sustained a cheekbone fracture from her violent partner in the last year. She appears listless. How would you decide whether she was suffering from psychological problems and what help might she need?

Answers on page 268

14 Salivary gland disease

J. D. Langdon

- Salivary gland disease is an important consideration in the differential diagnosis of facial swelling.
- Viral parotitis (mumps) is the most common cause of parotid swelling.
- Although a complaint of dry mouth is common, it is rarely due to disease of the salivary glands.
- A large number of benign and malignant neoplasms may affect the major and minor salivary glands but of these 75% are benign pleomorphic adenomas of the parotid gland.

ASSUMED KNOWLEDGE

It is assumed that at this stage you will have knowledge/competencies in the following areas:

- anatomy of the oral cavity
- anatomy of the parotid gland and the infratemporal fossa
- anatomy of the submandibular gland and the submandibular triangle
- the role/functions of saliva
- factors influencing salivary flow rate and composition
- the classification of disorders of the salivary glands.

If you think that you are not competent in these areas, revise them before reading this chapter or cross-check with relevant texts as you read.

INTENDED LEARNING OUTCOMES

At the end of this chapter you should be able to:

1. Distinguish the clinical features of infections of the salivary glands from those in other structures
2. Differentiate on clinical grounds between infection, obstruction, benign and malignant neoplasms of the salivary glands
3. Plan and evaluate the results of the investigation of disorders of the salivary glands
4. List the important/relevant information to be elicited from patients with salivary gland disorders
5. Select cases which require referral for a specialist opinion
6. Describe the causes of a dry mouth and be able to distinguish between organic and functional causes.

APPLIED ANATOMY

Parotid gland

The parotid gland is the largest of the salivary glands. There is considerable variation in size between individuals but for any individual both sides are similar. Although embryologically the parotid consists only of a single lobe, it is convenient to speak of a superficial lobe (superficial to the plane of the branches of the facial nerve) and a deep lobe (deep to that plane). The superficial lobe of the parotid is limited laterally by the preparotid fascia and overlying fat and skin. The zygomatic arch and temporomandibular joint is superior, the masseter muscle is anterior and posteriorly are the cartilaginous external auditory meatus, the mastoid process and the sternocleidomastoid muscle. The isthmus of the parotid gland is bounded by the ramus of the mandible anteriorly and the posterior belly of the digastric behind. The deep lobe is related to the medial pterygoid anteriorly, the styloid apparatus posteromedially and the internal jugular vein. Its deep surface lies immediately superficial to the tonsillar fossa and neoplasms arising from the deep lobe often present as tonsillar masses. The trunk of the facial nerve arises from the stylomastoid foramen just behind the styloid process. It enters the posterior parotid and becomes rapidly more superficial before dividing into two divisions, the superior larger zygomaticotemporal and the smaller buccocervical division. The facial nerve then further divides into five main branches—temporal, zygomatic, buccal, mandibular and cervical—as it passes forwards in a plane separating the superficial and deep lobes. The main collecting duct arises within the superficial lobe and passes horizontally forwards, parallel to the buccal branch in a direction corresponding to a line joining the tragus to a point midway between the alar and the commissure. The duct crosses the masseter muscle horizontally, then turns at right angles to pierce the buccinator muscle and enters the oral cavity at the parotid papilla opposite the second upper molar.

Submandibular gland

The submandibular gland consists of two lobes—superficial and deep—which are folded over each other posteriorly around the posterior free border of the mylohyoid muscle. The larger superficial lobe lies within the submandibular triangle covered by deep cervical fascia, platysma, fat and skin. The mandibular branch of the facial nerve loops down below the lower border of the mandible. It usually lies on the deep surface of the fascia but may lie between the fascia and the overlying platysma. The deep lobe of the submandibular gland is 'suspended' from the lingual nerve and sublingual ganglion by

the parasympathetic secretomotor fibres, which must be carefully divided without damaging the sensory fibres of the lingual nerve when removing the gland. The hypoglossal nerve lies in the bed of the deep lobe. The submandibular duct arises from the anterior pole of the deep lobe and runs forwards in the floor of the mouth, crossing the lingual nerve as it passes medially to innervate the tongue.

Sublingual gland

The sublingual gland is a complex of major and minor salivary glands, which occupies much of the submucosa of the floor of the mouth extending posteriorly to the second molar region. It lies partly within the sublingual fossa of the mandible above the mylohyoid line. Up to 20 small ducts open directly in the floor of the mouth. Some open directly into the submandibular duct.

When considering the many and various conditions and disorders that can affect the salivary glands, it is useful to classify the various conditions according to the standard 'surgical sieve' (see Ch. 2).

DEVELOPMENTAL DISORDERS

Developmental disorders such as accessory lobes, ectopic development, agenesis, duct atresia and congenital fistula are rarely a problem to the dental practitioner.

INFLAMMATORY DISORDERS

Viral

Mumps (Fig. 14.1) is the most common cause of acute painful parotid swelling affecting children. It is endemic in urban areas and spreads via airborne droplet infection of infected saliva. The disease starts with a prodromal period of 1 or 2 days, during which the child experiences feverishness, chills, nausea, anorexia and headache. This is typically followed by pain and swelling of one or both parotid glands. The parotid pain can be very severe and is exacerbated by eating or drinking. Symptoms resolve spontaneously after 5–10 days. In a classical case of mumps the diagnosis is based on the history and

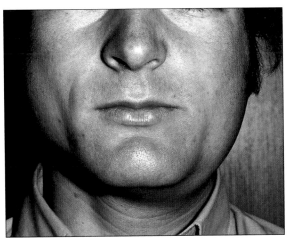

Fig. 14.1 Mumps can affect not only the parotid glands but also the submandibular glands.

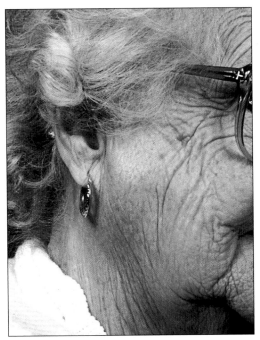

Fig. 14.2 Ascending bacterial parotitis often affects fit young patients as well as the elderly, without obvious predisposing risk factors.

clinical examination: a history of recent contact with an affected patient and bilateral painful parotid swelling is sufficient. However, the presentation may be atypical or sporadic or have predominantly unilateral or even submandibular involvement. In this situation mumps-specific IgM can be identified in the serum as early as 11 days following original exposure to the virus. This antibody is also detectable in the saliva. One episode of infection confers lifelong immunity.

The treatment of mumps is symptomatic. Regular paracetamol and encouragement to maintain fluid intake is important. Complications such as orchitis, oophoritis, meningoencephalitis, pancreatitis and sensorineural deafness are uncommon in children but are more likely in adults. The incidence of mumps is becoming less common as, increasingly, children are receiving the mumps, measles and rubella vaccine at an early age. However, it is important to bear it in mind as a diagnosis whenever a febrile fretful child presents with salivary gland enlargement.

A number of other viral agents—Coxsackie A and B, parainfluenza 1 and 3, ECHO and lymphocytic choriomeningitis—can all cause identical signs and symptoms. Cytomegalic inclusion disease affects mainly newborn infants and children. It is believed to be an intrauterine infection which becomes manifest after birth.

Bacterial

Acute ascending bacterial sialadenitis affects mostly the parotid glands (Fig. 14.2). Historically, it was described in dehydrated, cachectic patients often following major abdominal surgery when the patient was on a 'nil by mouth' regime. The reduced salivary flow and oral sepsis resulted in bacteria colonizing the parotid duct and subsequently involving the parotid parenchyma. With current hospital practice and improved oral hygiene, patients are rarely allowed to become dehydrated and this clinical pattern is uncommon. The typical patient presenting with an acute ascending bacterial parotitis now is an otherwise fit young adult with no obvious predisposing factors.

Clinical presentation is of the onset of tender, red, painful parotid swelling over a few hours. There is associated malaise, pyrexia and often regional lymphadenopathy. Pain is exacerbated on attempting to eat or drink. The parotid swelling may be diffuse but often it is localized to the lower pole of the gland, presumably because the infection tends to localize under the effect of gravity.

If the gland is gently 'milked' by massaging the cheek cloudy turbid saliva can be expressed from the parotid duct; this should be cultured. The infecting organism is usually *Staphylococcus aureus* or *Streptococcus viridans*. Sialography must never be undertaken during the acute phase of infection as the retrograde injection of infected material into the duct system will result in bacteraemia. Ultrasound imaging shows the characteristic dilatation of the acinae.

If the patient presents at an early stage before abscess formation, the infection can usually be controlled with antibiotics. The clinician should not delay waiting for the results of bacterial culture: in a patient not allergic to penicillin a combination of a broad-spectrum penicillin (ampicillin) and a penicillinase-resistant agent (flucloxacillin) is usually effective. In patients allergic to the penicillins, clindamycin is a good alternative. This antibiotic is actively secreted in saliva. The levels in the saliva exceed those in the circulating serum. If the gland becomes fluctuant, indicating abscess formation, the pus must be drained. Occasionally it is possible to drain the abscess by aspirating the pus through a large-bore hypodermic needle, but usually it is necessary to undertake formal surgical drainage under general anaesthesia.

Care must be taken when making the incision not to damage a branch of the facial nerve. Only the skin should be incised and the operation continued with blunt dissection using sinus forceps. A small drain is inserted for 24 hours. Surprisingly, following removal of the drain, the incision heals uneventfully and a salivary fistula does not occur.

Chronic bacterial sialadenitis is far more common in the submandibular salivary gland and usually occurs secondary to chronic obstruction (see below). Unfortunately the submandibular gland has a poor capacity for recovery following infection and in most cases, following control of any acute symptoms with antibiotics, the gland itself must be removed. The operation is performed in hospital under general anaesthesia. Great care must be taken not to damage the mandibular branch of the facial nerve when making the incision, the lingual nerve when mobilizing the gland and clamping the duct and the hypoglossal nerve when separating the gland from the floor of the submandibular triangle.

Chronic sclerosing sialadenitis is a condition that can affect the submandibular gland after a long period of chronic bacterial infection. Progressive atrophy and fibrosis eventually results in a small hard mass, which may undergo dystrophic calcification. This then presents in the submandibular region as a

Kuttner tumour (the word tumour being used in its literal sense as a lump and not as a neoplasm).

Acute bacterial sialadenitis

- Never perform sialography in acute phase
- Culture saliva from duct orifice
- Start broad-spectrum and penicillinase-resistant antibiotics
- Refer for surgical drainage if gland is fluctuant
- Encourage intake of fluids
- Sialography following resolution of symptoms to assess function

---

Recurrent parotitis of childhood

Recurrent parotitis of childhood exists as a distinct clinical entity but little is known regarding its aetiology and prognosis. It is characterized by the rapid swelling of usually one parotid gland, accompanied by pain and difficulty in chewing, as well as systemic symptoms such as fever and malaise. Although each episode of parotid swelling is usually unilateral, the opposite side may be involved in subsequent episodes. Each episode of pain and swelling lasts for 3–7 days and is followed by a quiescent period of a few weeks to several months. Occasionally episodes are so frequent that the child loses a considerable amount of schooling. The onset is usually between 3 and 6 years, although it has been reported in infants as young as 4 months. The diagnosis is based on the characteristic history and is confirmed by sialography, which shows a very characteristic punctate sialectasis often likened to a snow storm against a dark night sky (Fig. 14.3).

Traditionally the episodes of parotitis have been treated with antibiotics and symptoms settle within 3–5 days on such a regimen. Occasionally, recurrent episodes are so frequent that prophylactic antibiotics are required for a period of months or years. Symptoms seem to resolve spontaneously at puberty but some of these patients go on to develop chronic bacterial parotitis later in life.

'Specific infections' (granulomatous sialadenitis)

Swelling of the salivary glands may occasionally be caused by mycobacterial infection, cat-scratch develops progressively after the radiation has been completed and results in xerostomia.

HIV-associated sialadenitis

Chronic parotitis in children is almost pathognomonic of HIV infection. In adults a sicca syndrome and lymphocytic infiltration of the salivary glands are more usual. The presentation of HIV-associated sialadenitis is very similar to classical Sjögren's syndrome (see later). Dry mouth, dry eyes and swelling of the salivary glands together with lymphadenopathy suggests the diagnosis. Histologically the condition closely resembles Sjögren's syndrome and differentiation may be difficult. However, autoantibodies—including antinuclear, rheumatoid factor, SS-A and SS-B—are absent unless the patient coincidentally has a connective tissue disorder. AIDS-associated lymphoma presenting as salivary gland swelling has also been described.

Another presentation of salivary gland disease in HIV-positive patients is multiple parotid cysts causing gross parotid swelling and significant facial disfigurement. On imaging with CT or MRI the parotids have the appearance of a Swiss cheese, with multiple large cystic lesions (Fig. 14.4). The glands are not painful and there is no reduction in salivary flow rate. Surgery may be indicated to improve the appearance.

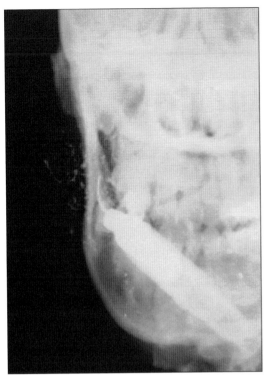

Fig. 14.3 Characteristic punctate sialectasis seen in recurrent parotitis of childhood: the 'snow storm' appearance.

disease, syphilis, toxoplasmosis, mycoses, sarcoid, Wegener's and other granulomatous disease.

Allergic sialadenitis

A variety of potential allergens causing acute parotid swelling have been identified. Some foods, drugs (most frequently chloramphenicol and tetracycline), metals such as nickel and pollens have been incriminated.

Radiation sialadenitis

Following the start of therapeutic irradiation, when the parotid glands are within the radiation field the patient develops an acute parotitis, usually after 24 hours. The glands are swollen and tender, there is a marked rise in salivary amylase and the salivary flow rate is reduced. The reaction is self-limiting and resolves after 2 or 3 days, even though the radiotherapy continues. This reaction is quite distinct from the permanent radiation atrophy that occurs with therapeutic doses above 40 Gy, which

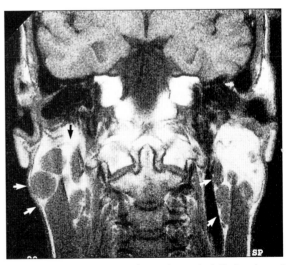

Fig. 14.4 This MRI scan shows the typical 'Swiss-cheese' appearance of multiple large cysts within the parotid glands.

Sialadenitis of minor salivary glands

Whenever the major salivary glands are involved, the same histological changes will be present in the minor glands. Similarly, Sjögren's syndrome invariably involves the minor glands—and indeed the diagnosis is often confirmed on the basis of a minor salivary gland biopsy.

Stomatitis nicotina is a chronic inflammatory disorder of the minor salivary glands of the palate, seen in heavy smokers. The appearance is of multiple small target lesions in which the central opening of the gland is inflamed and bright red, but the surrounding halo of palatal mucosa is white as a result of hyperkeratosis. The condition does not carry a risk of malignant change and is reversible, if the patient can be persuaded to stop smoking.

Acute necrotizing sialometaplasia is an unusual condition, which was first described in 1973. It occurs only on the hard palate in the molar region in the vault of the palate midway between the midline and the gingival margin. It is seen only in heavy smokers. It has a characteristic appearance, which resembles a carcinoma with central ulceration and raised erythematous margins. The ulcer may be as much as 3 cm in diameter. As it so closely resembles a carcinoma the diagnosis is often made on the basis of surgical biopsy. The lesions are self-healing, but often take 10–12 weeks to resolve. As they are extremely painful it is helpful to construct a removable cover plate for the patient to wear, particularly during meal times.

OBSTRUCTION AND TRAUMA

Papillary obstruction

Occasionally a rough upper molar tooth or an overextended denture flange will irritate the parotid papilla. If this is sufficient to cause ulceration with consequent inflammation and oedema salivary flow might be obstructed, particularly at meal times when the flow rate is increased significantly. In this situation the patient suffers rapid-onset pain and swelling at meal times. Rarely, an aphthous ulcer on the parotid papilla will cause the same symptoms.

If the trauma to the parotid papilla continues there will be progressive scarring and fibrosis in the soft tissues and permanent stenosis of the papilla can occur. Once this is established even removal of the original factor causing the irritation will be unlikely to resolve the problem, and a papillotomy will be required. This is a simple procedure performed under local anaesthesia. A probe is inserted into the orifice of the papilla and with a scalpel blade the papilla is split open by incising down onto the probe. This lays open the papilla and divides the stenosis, allowing free drainage of saliva.

Stone formation (sialolithiasis)

As many as 80% of all salivary stones occur in the submandibular gland or duct (Fig. 14.5), 10% occur in the parotid, 7% in the sublingual gland and the remainder occur in the minor salivary glands. Most stones occur in the submandibular glands because their secretions contain mucus and the viscosity is

Summary of inflammatory disorders

- Mumps, the most common cause of acute parotitis
- Acute bacterial ascending infection, which may be associated with dehydration or cachexia
- Recurrent parotitis of childhood
- 'Specific infections'
- Allergies to foods, drugs and metals, which are rare
- Radiation
- HIV-associated

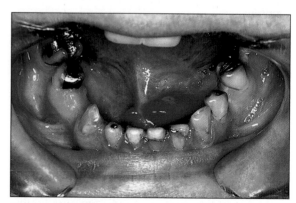

Fig. 14.5 A stone in the left submandibular duct can be seen ulcerating through the duct wall.

higher. Of submandibular stones 80% are radio-opaque and can be identified using plain radiographs. Occlusal views are particularly helpful because the image of a small stone must be projected away from other radio-opaque structures such as the teeth and jaws (Fig. 14.6). By contrast the majority of parotid stones are radiolucent and cannot be detected on plain radiography.

The typical presentation of a submandibular calculus is acute pain and swelling at meal times. Onset is rapid, within a minute of starting the meal, and the swelling resolves over a period of about 1 hour, after the meal is completed. However, this classical picture occurs only when the stone causes almost complete obstruction, often when it is impacted at the opening of the submandibular duct. More often the stone causes only partial obstruction and is lying either within the hilum of the gland or within the duct in the floor of the mouth. In this situation the patient may complain of occasional swelling, often with minimal discomfort, or of a chronically enlarged mass in the submandibular triangle with episodes of dull aching pain. This results from chronic bacterial infection, usually due to *S. viridans*, arising in an obstructed gland with salivary stasis

and poor emptying. Often a salivary stone is totally asymptomatic and is discovered coincidentally during radiography for other reasons.

If a stone is identified on plain radiographs, no other investigation is necessary. If the symptoms suggest a diagnosis of a stone, but the stone cannot be seen on routine radiographs, sialography will be needed. However, this procedure does carry the risk of displacing the stone more proximally in the duct system, to a position where it may be difficult to remove. A radiolucent stone will show as a filling defect in the column of contrast medium and the emptying film will show retained contrast medium proximal to the site of the stone.

A submandibular stone often impacts at the papilla or lies in the floor of the mouth, where it is usually palpable. Less commonly, the stone lies partially within the substance of the gland at the hilum where the duct leaves the gland. If the stone is trapped at the duct papilla, it can often be released by gently probing and dilatation of the papilla. It may be necessary to slit the duct in order to release the stone. If the stone is lying in the submandibular duct in the floor of the mouth, anterior to the point at which the duct crosses the lingual nerve (second molar region), the stone can be released by opening the duct longitudinally. It is important to pass a large suture around the duct posterior to the stone so that during the operative procedure the stone cannot be displaced backwards in the duct. Once the calculus has been released, the wall of the duct should be sutured to the mucosa of the floor of the mouth to maintain an opening for the free drainage of saliva. No attempt should be made to repair the duct wall as this will lead to stricture formation. A parotid stone located at the confluence of the collecting ducts can be released surgically by raising a preauricular flap, exposing the parotid duct and incising it longitudinally to release the stone. Salivary stones can sometimes be retrieved endoscopically or under fluoroscopic X-ray control using small wire baskets or angioplasty balloons.

Obstruction in and around the duct wall

Scarring and fibrosis in the duct will result in stricture formation and obstruction to salivary flow. It often presents as a complication of long-standing sialolithiasis but may occur as a result of trauma,

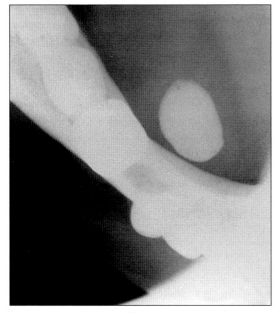

Fig. 14.6 Occlusal radiograph, showing the typical appearance of a submandibular stone.

particularly to the floor of the mouth. In patients with masseteric hypertrophy the parotid duct may be stretched around the anterior border of the muscle and this may cause obstruction of salivary flow at meal times.

Salivary neoplasms usually develop within the substance of the salivary gland and grow slowly, compressing and displacing the adjacent normal gland tissue. On occasion, the enlarging tumour presses on an adjacent collecting duct and the subsequent obstruction leads to the appearance of a sudden increase in size of the tumour, suggesting malignant change. It is important to recognize that this is not necessarily so.

Mucoceles

Mucous retention cysts and mucous extravasation cysts arise in the minor salivary glands as a result of mechanical damage to the gland or its duct. The common sites are on the mucosal aspect of the lower lip (Fig. 14.7), particularly in patients with a deep overbite, and in the buccal mucosa posteriorly where an upper wisdom tooth is erupting buccally. Typically the patient presents with a history of recurrent swelling that develops over days or weeks, ruptures and then recurs after a few weeks. The cysts rarely exceed 1 cm in diameter and are tense, bluish, sessile swellings. The treatment is not to the cyst alone but the underlying minor gland, which must also be excised under local anaesthesia.

A ranula is a large mucocele arising from the sublingual gland, and typically presents as a large tense bluish swelling in the anterior floor of the mouth, often displacing the tongue (Fig. 14.8). However, the ranula may push its way through the midline mylohyoid dehiscence in the floor of the mouth and enter the submental space presenting as a midline swelling in the upper neck. This is the 'plunging ranula'. The swelling may be entirely in the neck or the ranula may take on an hourglass shape with both submental and intraoral swelling. The treatment of a ranula must include excision of the sublingual gland.

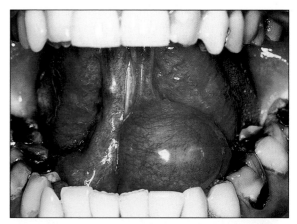

Fig. 14.8 Ranulae are large mucoceles arising from obstruction of a sublingual gland.

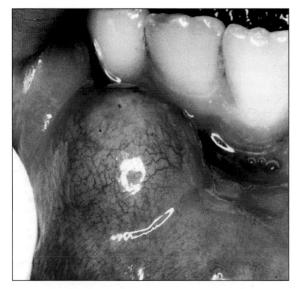

Fig. 14.7 The most common site for mucoceles is the mucosal aspect of the lower lip.

Obstruction and trauma

- Papillary obstruction secondary to trauma: papillotomy
- Stones—80% submandibular: remove stone if in the duct, remove gland if stone is within the gland
- Strictures due to trauma: excise the affected gland
- Mucoceles, most commonly found in the lower lip: excise the cyst and underlying minor gland

SALIVARY NEOPLASMS

Salivary neoplasms comprise 1.2% of all neoplastic disease. The WHO classification of salivary gland tumours, published in 1991, categorizes the tumours according to the tissue of origin as being of epithelial or non-epithelial origin. In addition, there is a group of unclassified and allied conditions, which, although not strictly neoplastic, can present as a localized swelling that clinically may mimic a neoplastic condition.

Clinical presentation

Nearly all salivary neoplasms present as slowly growing masses which have often been present for several years (Fig. 14.9). Usually, even malignant salivary tumours grow slowly. Unfortunately, pain is not a reliable indication of malignancy. Certainly if a malignant salivary neoplasm is invading a sensory nerve, pain or paraesthesia can occur. Similarly, if the facial nerve is invaded, paralysis can occur. Frequently at surgery a nerve that has been functioning normally preoperatively is seen to be invaded by tumour. Furthermore, benign tumours often present with pain and aching in the affected gland, presumably due to capsular distension and possibly also due to an element of outflow obstruction. Therefore the only reliable clinical indication of malignancy is facial nerve palsy in the case of the parotid, induration and/or ulceration of the overlying skin or mucosa and regional lymphatic metastasis.

Investigation

For parotid and submandibular tumours, CT scanning or MRI are the most helpful imaging techniques (Fig. 14.10). They will confirm that the mass being investigated is indeed intrinsic to the gland; they accurately image the borders of the tumour and show if it is well circumscribed (and likely to be benign) or diffuse and invasive (and likely to be malignant). In addition, scans show the relationship of the tumour to other anatomic structures and help with the planning of subsequent surgery. Unfortunately, in the case of parotid tumours, these scanning techniques cannot reliably image the facial nerve and therefore reliably determine whether the tumour is superficial or deep to the plane of the nerve. However, this plane can usually be inferred, as the course of the facial nerve is constant from the stylomastoid foramen, becoming more superficial and passing forwards over the masseter muscle.

Conventional sialography has very little to offer in the investigation of neoplastic salivary disease. Apart from demonstrating the presence of a space-occupying lesion, it does not reliably differentiate benign from malignant tumours and is extremely poor at distinguishing between deep lobe and superficial lobe parotid tumours. Ultrasound scanning is a readily available, inexpensive and non-invasive technique that is useful in imaging the

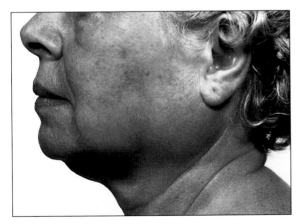

Fig. 14.9 Nearly all salivary neoplasms—both benign and malignant—present as slowly growing painless masses.

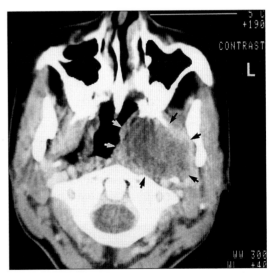

Fig. 14.10 A large pleomorphic adenoma arising in the deep lobe of the parotid gland.

parotid. The two most common tumours have very characteristic echo patterns and often an accurate diagnosis can be suggested. Isotope imaging with technetium pertechnetate gives inconsistent results.

Open surgical biopsy of intrinsic neoplasms of the major glands is absolutely contraindicated. At least 75% of all parotid tumours and more than 50% of all submandibular gland tumours will prove to be benign pleomorphic adenomas. This tumour, which is only poorly encapsulated, is very tense and if an incision is made into it the contents escape into the surrounding tissue planes—and it is almost impossible to eradicate the microscopic spillage of tumour cells. If this happens the patient will be at risk of developing multiple local tumour recurrences over many years. However, if there is overt skin infiltration or ulceration an open biopsy is essential to establish a preoperative diagnosis upon which to plan surgery. For tumours of the minor salivary glands, particularly in the palate, there is a much higher chance of the tumour being malignant and, as it is not necessary to open up other tissue planes to gain access to the tumour, open incisional biopsy is important.

Fine-needle aspiration (see Ch. 8) is a safe alternative to open biopsy of a major gland. Evidence suggests that provided the needle gauge does not exceed 18 G there is no risk of seeding viable tumour cells. Although advocates of this technique claim high accuracy and specificity there is inevitably a high risk of sampling error. Many salivary neoplasms are not homogeneous and, following excision, the entire tumour mass often must be sectioned to find the one critical diagnostic area of the mass.

EPITHELIAL TUMOURS

Of all salivary epithelial tumours 75% arise in the parotid glands and of these only 15% are malignant; just over 10% occur in the submandibular glands and approximately one-third are malignant; about 15% of tumours occur in the minor salivary glands and nearly half of these will be malignant. Tumours arising in the sublingual glands are very rare (0.3%) but nearly all will be malignant.

Both benign tumours (adenomas) and malignant tumours (carcinomas) occur.

> **Clinical features of salivary tumours (WHO classification of 1991, simplified)**
>
> - **Pleomorphic adenoma:** any age; M:F = 1:1; 75% of parotid tumours; 50% of submandibular tumours
> - **Warthin tumour:** over 50 years; M:F = 4:1; occurs only in parotid
> - **Acinic cell carcinoma:** often low grade
> - **Mucoepidermoid carcinoma:** often low grade
> - **Adenoid cystic carcinoma:** invariably fatal, *but* good 5- and 10-year survival; perineural spread and pulmonary metastases
> - **Adenocarcinoma, squamous cell carcinoma, undifferentiated carcinoma and carcinoma in pleomorphic adenoma:** all have a poor prognosis
> - **Lymphoma and non-epithelial tumours:** less frequent

Adenomas

Of the variety of benign adenomas that have been described only two, the pleomorphic adenoma and Warthin tumour, arise with any frequency.

The pleomorphic adenoma occurs at any age (mean 42 years) and has an equal sex incidence. It accounts for at least 75% of parotid tumours and more than 50% of submandibular tumours but for rather less than 50% of minor gland tumours. Clinically the tumour has the texture of cartilage and has an irregular and bosselated surface. In the palate, the overlying mucosa is rarely ulcerated. Rarely, after a number of years the tumour may undergo malignant change, so all patients presenting with pleomorphic adenomas should be advised to undergo surgical removal of the tumour.

The Warthin tumour occurs only in the parotid gland, where it accounts for approximately 15% of all neoplasms. It is a disease of the elderly, with a mean age of presentation of 60 years. Historically it had a male:female ratio of 4:1 but is now becoming increasingly common in women. Recent evidence suggests that this tumour is related to cigarette smoking. It is also unusual in that in 10% of cases it arises either bilaterally in the parotids or is multicentric in the one gland. It does not undergo malignant change.

Carcinomas

The acinic cell carcinoma and the mucoepidermoid carcinoma, although undoubtedly malignant tumours with a potential for local invasion and metastatic spread, are frequently very low grade histologically and do not require the radical treatment needed for more aggressive tumours. Together they account for only 5% of all tumours at any site.

The adenoid cystic carcinoma, adenocarcinoma, squamous cell carcinoma and undifferentiated carcinoma are all aggressive malignant tumours that carry a poor prognosis regardless of treatment. The adenoid cystic carcinoma is characterized by inevitably killing the patient, by relentless perineural spread along the cranial nerves and into the brain. However, it grows extremely slowly and, although invariably fatal, the 5- and 10-year survival figures are 70% and 40%, respectively. It is also unusual in having a predilection for distant metastasis to the lungs, where it often produces multiple 'cannon ball' tumours, which can remain symptomless for many years. The other carcinomas mentioned above have 5-year survival figures of around 35–40%. Carcinoma arising in a pleomorphic adenoma carries a very poor prognosis, with a 5-year survival rate of only 25%.

Management of epithelial tumours

Both benign and malignant tumours arising in the parotid or submandibular glands are treated surgically, by excision with wide margins. In the parotid gland, excision is by either superficial or total parotidectomy, according to the location of the tumour. Unless the patient presents with facial nerve palsy (indicating a malignant tumour) the facial nerve should be preserved (Fig. 14.11). In the submandibular gland treatment is by excision of the gland. If the definitive pathological diagnosis is of a high-grade malignancy, then the patient should receive radical postoperative radiotherapy. In those cases when the tumour involves skin or other adjacent structures, or where there is lymphatic metastasis, the patient should undergo radical excision, including a neck dissection and sacrificing any structures invaded by tumour, and treated with postoperative radiotherapy.

Pleomorphic adenomas arising in the minor salivary glands can be treated by local excision with a 5-mm margin. They do not invade periosteum

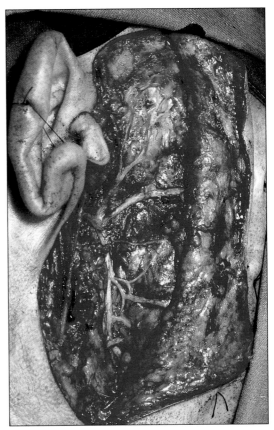

Fig. 14.11 The facial nerve is exposed following a superficial parotidectomy.

and so in the hard palate they should be excised subperiosteally without removing any underlying bone. Mucoepidermoid carcinomas and acinic cell carcinomas require rather more radical excision, with a 10-mm margin, and when they are situated in the palate palatal fenestration should be undertaken. Postoperative radiotherapy is indicated only for high-grade tumours or if the margins are not clear. For the remaining carcinomas arising in the minor salivary glands, radical surgical excision and postoperative radiotherapy is indicated. In the palate this will be by maxillectomy.

Salivary tumours

- Refer urgently any mass arising in the parotid or submandibular region, in the palate or the lips
- Imaging best with CT or MRI
- Never perform incisional biopsy on parotid or submandibular tumours

---

Complications of parotidectomy

In experienced hands permanent damage to the facial nerve should not occur in conservative parotidectomy when the facial nerve is being preserved. However, various degrees of transient weakness, lasting typically 6 weeks, are common, occurring in approximately 33% of cases. This is due to demyelination as a result of handling the nerve and ischaemia in the nerve following surgery. This demyelination reverses spontaneously. Surprisingly, postoperative salivary fistula formation is uncommon. More common is the formation of recurrent collections of saliva under the flap (sialoceles); although these are often aspirated to reassure the patient, they recur initially for a period of a few weeks and then resolve without active intervention.

Gustatory sweating (Frey's syndrome) is a complication that occurs in at least a third of patients following parotid surgery. Symptoms first develop 12–18 months following surgery and the patient complains of redness of the overlying skin and sweating of the skin at mealtimes. Usually the symptoms are mild but the sweating can be so profuse that at mealtimes the patient must drape a towel over the shoulder on the affected side to absorb the perspiration. It is claimed that the condition occurs as a result of the regeneration of secretomotor parasympathetic nerve fibres along the myelin sheaths of the sympathetic nerve fibres of the sweat glands in the overlying skin. The condition is difficult to treat surgically, but subcutaneous infiltration of botulinum toxin into the affected area controls the symptoms very well.

NON-EPITHELIAL TUMOURS

A variety of non-epithelial tumours arise in the salivary glands. Haemangiomas and lymphangiomas (cystic hygromas) occur in childhood. Haemangiomas occur mostly in the parotid, appearing shortly after birth and growing progressively for several months. The majority undergo spontaneous regression by 2 years of age. Females are more frequently affected than males. Lymphangiomas are less common. They may affect any of the salivary glands, and form spongelike multicystic lesions: 50% are manifest by 12 months and 90% will be evident by the end of the second year. Lymphangiomas do not undergo spontaneous involution. They frequently extend into the neck and mediastinum and can undergo dramatically rapid growth, causing respiratory obstruction. Treatment is by complete surgical excision but this may be technically very difficult.

Neurofibromas and neurilemmomas are the most common non-epithelial tumours arising in adults. Clinically they are not distinguishable from other salivary tumours and are diagnosed only following surgery for a presumed epithelial tumour. Lipomas occur only in the parotids, particularly in adult males. They are treated by surgical excision.

MALIGNANT LYMPHOMAS

True extranodal lymphoma arising in the salivary glands, usually the parotids, is rare. It occurs as a manifestation of a mucosa-associated lymph tissue (MALT) lymphoma. More common is lymphoma arising from the lymph nodes, either on the surface of the glands or within the parenchyma of the gland. Lymphoma also arises in the salivary glands as a complication of HIV disease, in the benign lymphoepithelial lesion, and Sjögren's syndrome (see below). The peak incidence for non-Hodgkin's lymphoma is the sixth and seventh decades and women are twice as likely to be affected, largely due to lymphomatous change in Sjögren's syndrome, which is more common in women. By contrast Hodgkin's disease arises in the juxta-glandular nodes rather than within the salivary gland parenchyma. Its peak incidence is the third and fourth decades and males predominate in the radio of 4:1.

Salivary gland lymphomas usually present as firm painless swellings and more than 90% occur in the parotids. If the lymphoma is confined to the parotid, treatment is by parotidectomy with postoperative radiotherapy. If there is evidence of spread beyond the salivary gland, treatment is by polychemotherapy according to the accepted protocols, based on histological characterization.

UNCLASSIFIED AND ALLIED CONDITIONS

Sialosis is an uncommon, non-inflammatory cause of salivary swelling, usually affecting the parotid glands symmetrically. It is usually associated with conditions such as alcohol abuse, diabetes mellitus, pregnancy, malnutrition and some drugs (usually sympathomimetics). It typically affects middle-aged and elderly patients, who present with bilateral soft parotid swellings which are usually painless. Biopsy of the glands reveals extensive fatty replacement but otherwise normal tissues. No treatment is known to be effective but sometimes parotidectomy is required to correct the disfigurement.

Necrotizing sialometaplasia, benign lympho-epithelial lesion (see later), salivary duct cysts, Kuttner tumour and cystic lymphoid hyperplasia of HIV disease can all mimic salivary gland neoplasia. Similarly, branchial cysts and dermoids can cause diagnostic confusion on occasion.

DEGENERATIVE CONDITIONS

Sjögren's syndrome

Sjögren's syndrome is an autoimmune condition causing progressive destruction of the salivary and lachrymal glands. In 1933 Sjögren, a Swedish ophthalmologist, first described the association of keratoconjunctivitis sicca (dry eyes) and xerostomia (dry mouth). Shortly thereafter he noted that these symptoms frequently occurred in patients with rheumatoid arthritis. It has since been realized that Sjögren's syndrome can occur in association with any connective tissue disorder: indeed, the association is more common in many connective tissue disorders than it is with rheumatoid arthritis. Only 15% of patients with rheumatoid arthritis develop Sjögren's syndrome, whereas 30% of patients with systemic lupus erythematosis and nearly all patients with primary biliary cirrhosis do so. This combination of dry eyes, dry mouth and a connective tissue disorder (most often rheumatoid arthritis as this is by far the most common connective tissue disorder) is called secondary Sjögren's syndrome. The same combination of dry eyes and dry mouth but without associated connective tissue disorder is known as primary Sjögren's syndrome. Primary Sjögren's syndrome also differs from secondary Sjögren's syndrome in that xerostomia and xerophthalmia are more severe, dysfunction of other exocrine glands is more widespread, incidence of lymphoma is higher and the autoantibody profile is different.

Females are affected more often than males in the ratio of 10:1. Typically patients are middle-aged. The presenting complaint is usually of the underlying connective tissue disorder and only later does the patient become aware of a gritty feeling in the eyes (due to conjunctivitis in the dry eyes) or a dry mouth. In the primary disorder, the complaint will be related to reduced lachrymal or salivary flow. Occasionally there is enlargement of the parotid glands bilaterally and even more rarely the enlarged parotids are painful. Although total xerostomia causes the mucosa to become parchment-like and is obvious, lesser degrees of xerostomia may cause problems for the patient but may not be obvious on clinical examination. Superinfection with *Candida albicans* is common. Less frequently, the patient develops bacterial sialadenitis due to ascending infection from the mouth. The condition does not invariably progress to total xerostomia and for any individual patient it is not possible to predict the outcome. The characteristic feature of the condition is progressive lymphocytic infiltration, acinar destruction and proliferation of duct epithelium of all salivary and lachrymal tissue.

The diagnosis is often based on the characteristic history: no laboratory investigation is pathognomonic of either primary or secondary Sjögren's syndrome. However, the following investigations are usually undertaken:

- sialography reveals the progressive damage from punctate sialectasis to total parenchymal destruction leaving no more than a grossly dilated duct (Fig.14.12)
- labial salivary gland biopsy can be misleading, particularly if only one minor gland is harvested. The characteristic lymphocytic infiltration is focal and a single gland may not show the changes. A minimum of three glands should be submitted to the pathologist
- estimation of salivary flow may be unhelpful as the normal variation in flow rates makes interpretation of the results difficult
- vital staining of the cornea with rose Bengal and examination of the cornea with a slit-lamp is a very sensitive assessment of a dry eye
- autoantibody screen reveals salivary duct antibody, rheumatoid factor, SS-A and SS-B antibodies and rheumatoid arthritis precipitin

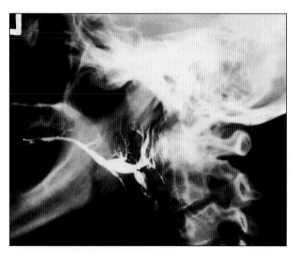

Fig. 14.12 Parotid sialogram showing gross destruction of parotid parenchyma in a patient with advanced Sjögren's syndrome.

- blood tests usually show a moderately raised erythrocyte sedimentation rate and a mild microcytic anaemia (the anaemia of chronic disease).

The management of Sjögren's syndrome must be symptomatic. No known treatment modifies or reverses the xerostomia and keratoconjunctivitis sicca. Artificial tears are essential to preserve the cornea. For the dry mouth various artificial saliva preparations are available (e.g. Saliva Orthana, Glandosane, Luborant) but often the patient prefers to use frequent drinks and learns to carry a bottle of water with them at all times. If a dentate patient is to use saliva substitutes the product should not have a low pH and should contain fluoride because rampant dental caries is a frequent complication. Other complications are recurrent infections in the mouth, ascending parotitis and those relating to any underlying connective tissue disorder. There is also increased incidence of developing MALT lymphoma (most commonly monocytoid B-cell lymphoma) in patients with Sjögren's syndrome. The risk is highest in those with primary Sjögren's syndrome. The onset of lymphoma is often heralded by immunological changes (falling immunoglobulin levels, falling titre of rheumatoid factor, rising B2-microglobulin titre, rising serum macroglobulin titre and the appearance of monoclonal light chains in the serum and urine), lymphadenopathy and weight loss.

Management of Sjögren's syndrome—symptomatic only

- Artificial tears
- Artificial saliva
- Frequent unsweetened drinks
- Fluoride mouthwash if dentate
- Antifungal therapy for candida
- Trial of pilocarpine tablets

'Benign' lymphoepithelial lesion

Use of the word 'benign' to describe this lesion is misleading because approximately 20% of patients with benign lymphoepithelial lesion or Sjögren's syndrome ultimately develop MALT lymphoma.

Histologically it is not possible to distinguish benign lymphoepithelial lesion from Sjögren's syndrome. Both are characterized by lymphocytic infiltration, acinar atrophy and ductal epithelial proliferation. Indeed, they may well be manifestations of the same condition.

Clinically benign lymphoepithelial lesion presents as diffuse swelling of the parotid gland. The swelling is firm and often painful and in 20% of cases is bilateral. Most patients are female (80%) and most are over 50 years old at presentation. Parotidectomy is mostly undertaken in order to establish the diagnosis, but if any parotid remnants are left, the swelling may recur with the risk of lymphomatous change. Prolonged follow-up is essential.

Mikulicz syndrome

In 1888 Mikulicz described benign, asymptomatic, symmetrical enlargement of the lachrymal and salivary glands. His original publication presented a series of patients who clearly had a variety of different conditions: benign lymphoepithelial lesion, Sjögren's syndrome, lymphoma, lymphocytic leukaemia, sarcoid and sialosis can all present in this way. The term Mikulicz syndrome is thus not helpful and should not be used.

Xerostomia

A complaint of dry mouth is common in oral surgery and oral medicine clinics. It seems to be particularly frequent in postmenopausal women, who also complain of a burning tongue or mouth. Normal salivary flow decreases with age in both men and women, although of course postmenopausal women are the group most likely to develop Sjögren's syndrome.

The situation is further confused as patients with Sjögren's syndrome are frequently unaware of having a dry mouth and patients who complain of dry mouth frequently have normal salivary flow rates. The most common causes of xerostomia, in order of frequency, are:

1. Chronic anxiety states and depression
2. Dehydration, which, if long term, often also leads to bacterial sialadenitis
3. Drugs—many have been implicated in causing xerostomia as an undesirable side effect
4. Salivary gland diseases—Sjögren's syndrome, benign lymphoepithelial disease, radiation damage, sarcoidosis, HIV infection.

Xerostomia can be difficult to treat. Treatment is aimed at relief of symptoms and avoidance or control of complications. Artificial salivas are not well accepted but their lubricant properties may be particularly useful at mealtimes. Cholinergic drugs such as pilocarpine can be used but their adverse effects (diarrhoea and pupillary dilatation) often outweigh any benefit. Furthermore there must be some remaining functional salivary tissue for such drugs to have any effect.

Rampant caries and destructive periodontal disease due to oral infection are major complications. Meticulous oral hygiene and the weekly use of topical fluoride is essential. There is a high incidence of oral candidosis and antifungal drugs are necessary. Conventional tablets and lozenges to be sucked are not well tolerated as the mouth is too dry to dissolve the drug: miconazole gel or ketoconazole suspension are better tolerated. Ascending parotitis is treated with antibiotics as required. Sometimes it is necessary to perform a parotidectomy and tie off the parotid duct to prevent further episodes of infection.

Sialorrhoea

Some drugs and painful lesions in the mouth increase salivary flow rates. In normal health this is rarely noticed as the excess saliva is swallowed spontaneously. 'False ptyalism' is more common and is a well-recognized delusional symptom or occurs due to faulty neuromuscular control leading to drooling despite normal saliva production. Uncontrollable drooling is usually treated surgically. As the submandibular gland contributes most resting saliva attention is directed at these glands bilaterally. The submandibular ducts can be mobilized and repositioned in the base of the anterior pillars of the fauces. Alternatively, the two glands may be excised.

FURTHER READING

Cawson R. A., Gleeson M. J., Eveson J. W. (1997) *Pathology and surgery of the salivary glands*. ISIS, Oxford, UK.

Langdon J. D. (1998) Sublingual and submandibular gland excision. In: Langdon J. D., Patel M. F. (eds) *Operative maxillofacial surgery*. Chapman & Hall, London, pp. 375–380.

Langdon J. D. (1998) Parotid surgery. In: Langdon J. D., Patel M. F. (eds) *Operative maxillofacial surgery*. Chapman & Hall, London, pp. 381–390.

Langdon J. D. (2000) Salivary gland disorders. In: Russell R. C. G., Williams N. S., Bulstrode C. J. K. (eds) *Bailey & Love's short practice of surgery*, 23rd edn. Arnold, London, Ch 42, pp. 651–668.

Norman J. E. DeB, McGurk M. (1995) *Colour atlas and text of the salivary glands*. Mosby-Wolfe, London.

SELF-ASSESSMENT

1. What features of mumps might help distinguish it from a spreading infection of dental origin?
2. A patient noted an otherwise symptomless lump under the angle of the jaw one month previously, which does not appear to have changed. Bimanual palpation reveals a rounded, smooth, firm lump 1.5 cm in diameter in the submandibular gland. What are the likely diagnoses and what investigations should be performed?

3. List two 'organic' and two 'functional' causes for the complaint of dry mouth.

4. A patient presents with a swelling on the lower labial mucosa, which intermittently swells and bursts.
   (a) What is the most likely diagnosis?
   (b) What would the treatment be?
   (c) What complications may arise?

5. A patient presents with a smooth-surfaced lesion to one side of the junction of the hard and soft palate (Fig. 14.13), which has grown slowly over about 4 years.
   (a) What is the likely diagnosis?
   (b) If confirmed at biopsy, what is the recommended treatment?

Answers on page 268.

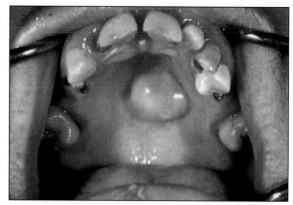

Fig. 14.13   See question 5.

15 The maxillary antrum

K. H. Taylor

- The maxillary antrum is closely related to the roots of the maxillary premolar and molar teeth and is frequently visualized on oral and facial radiographs. The signs and symptoms of antral disease may mimic those of dental disease (and vice versa).
- Dental surgery in the maxillary molar and premolar region may be complicated by the creation of an oroantral communication, the displacement of whole teeth, roots or other foreign bodies into the antrum or a fracture of the maxillary tuberosity.
- Antral disease may cause facial pain and the antral wall may be fractured during facial trauma.
- Malignant disease within the antrum often presents late but may be first diagnosed from its oral signs and symptoms.

ASSUMED KNOWLEDGE

It is assumed that at this stage you will have knowledge/competencies in the following areas:

- anatomy of the maxillary antrum and maxillary teeth, including an understanding of their innervation and normal radiographic appearance
- clinical features and diagnosis of pain of dental origin
- principles of dental extraction and the surgical removal of teeth (see Ch. 4).

If you think that you are not competent in these areas, revise them before reading this chapter or cross-check with relevant texts as you read.

INTENDED LEARNING OUTCOMES

At the end of this chapter you should be able to:

1. Distinguish signs and symptoms originating in the maxillary antrum from those of dental origin. Understand the common investigations and surgical procedures performed for antral disease and know when their use is indicated
2. Recognize situations in which dental extraction/minor oral surgery may be complicated by the creation of an oroantral communication or the displacement of a foreign body, tooth or root into the antrum
3. Know how to treat a newly created oroantral communication or a foreign body displaced into the antrum and how to minimize the risk of these complications occurring
4. Anticipate and minimize the risk of a fracture of the maxillary tuberosity occurring during tooth extraction and know how to treat this complication
5. Recognize the characteristic features of malignant disease of the maxillary antrum
6. Distinguish between those conditions of the maxillary antrum suitable for treatment in general dental practice and those requiring referral to a specialist.

THE IMPORTANCE OF THE MAXILLARY ANTRUM TO DENTAL SURGERY

The maxillary sinus is often referred to as the maxillary antrum (or more simply the 'antrum'). It is important to the dental surgeon because of its close relationship to the posterior maxillary teeth (generally from first premolar to third molar). The proximity varies between individuals (Fig. 15.1) but tends to increase with age as the antrum enlarges. The antrum can encroach into alveolar bone after tooth extraction, and periapical bone loss resulting from dental disease may further decrease the amount of bone separating it from the teeth. This close anatomical relationship can lead to diagnostic difficulties because both the antrum and the maxillary teeth are innervated by branches of the maxillary division of the trigeminal nerve. In

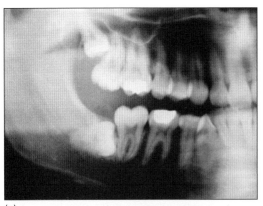

(a)

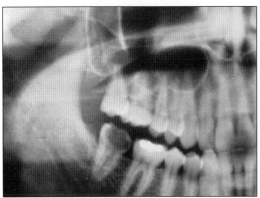

(b)

(a) A small maxillary antrum that does not reach the apex of the second premolar. (b) A large maxillary antrum that reaches to the apex of the lateral incisor.

addition, infection may spread from the periapical region of the posterior maxillary teeth to the antrum (and in the opposite direction) and the antrum is at risk of iatrogenic damage during certain dental procedures.

The ability to distinguish between dental and antral symptoms enables the dental surgeon to decide when dental treatment is indicated and when referral (e.g. to a general medical practitioner, an oral and maxillofacial surgeon or an ear, nose and throat (ENT) surgeon) is appropriate.

The antrum is visualized on oral and facial radiographs (notably periapical views of the posterior maxillary teeth, orthopantomogram (OPT) and occipitomental views) and a knowledge of its normal radiographic appearance is essential in the diagnosis of both dental and antral disease. Evidence of antral pathology may be incidentally discovered by the general dental practitioner (GDP) on these radiographs.

Although the GDP is unlikely routinely to perform elective surgery within the antrum, there will be occasions when dentoalveolar surgery with a degree of antral involvement is necessary—for example, to repair a newly created oroantral communication. It is necessary for the GDP to be able to recognize and deal with problems such as oroantral communication and foreign body in the antrum and he or she should be capable of explaining the commonly performed antral investigations and surgical procedures to a patient who requests information. The GDP may also recommend other procedures that involve antral surgery (e.g. 'sinus lift'/alveolar ridge augmentation procedures used prior to the placement of osseointegrated implants).

Summary of the importance of the maxillary antrum to dental surgery

- The roots of the upper premolars and molars and the floor of the maxillary antrum are closely related and share a common innervation. As a result dental symptoms and antral symptoms can mimic each other
- Dental procedures may be complicated by problems involving the antrum, including creation of an oroantral communication, displacement of a foreign body into the antrum and fracture of the maxillary tuberosity
- Antral pathology may be incidentally demonstrated on dental radiographs

DISTINGUISHING SIGNS AND SYMPTOMS OF DENTAL PATHOLOGY FROM THOSE OF SINUSITIS

Maxillary sinusitis is common and the dentist needs to be able to distinguish it from dental disease. It is usually an acute condition, but chronic sinusitis may also develop following an acute episode and may persist or recur if drainage from the antrum to the nasal cavity is poor or when a foreign body is retained.

Acute sinusitis may affect any of the paranasal sinuses but is usually confined at any one time to a single sinus. It is a bacterial infection and typically occurs after a viral upper respiratory tract infection (URTI)(*Haemophilus,Pneumococcus,Streptococcus, Staphylococcus* species and anaerobes are commonly found).

Maxillary sinusitis is usually related to impaired antral drainage, which may be caused by:

1. Mechanical obstruction of the ostium resulting from
   (a) inflammatory oedema of the nasal mucosa (due to a common cold)
   (b) ethmoid polyps or
   (c) deviated nasal septum
2. Impaired mucus clearance resulting from
   (a) poor ciliary action (e.g. related to the mucosal damage caused by chronic infection or surgical stripping) or the viral damage caused by a common cold (or occasionally due to rare conditions such as primary ciliary dyskinesia)
   (b) abnormally thick or sticky mucus (as found in cystic fibrosis).

Accumulated secretions become infected, allowing a collection of pus to develop in the antrum.

Dental diseases (including periapical pathology, infected odontogenic cysts and periodontal disease) may also cause sinusitis. Other possible causes include the presence of contaminated foreign bodies, trauma or infections of non-odontogenic cysts or malignant tumours.

Signs and symptoms of sinusitis

Symptoms of acute sinusitis usually appear a few days after the acute cold symptoms have resolved.

Pain, headache, nasal obstruction, a purulent nasal secretion and 'post-nasal drip' (a discharge of 'mucopus' into the pharynx) are commonly found and there may also be fever and malaise. The pain is dull, heavy, throbbing and located over the cheek and in the upper teeth. It may resemble toothache but is not related to hot, cold or sweet stimuli, although it may be increased by biting. Typically all of the posterior teeth on the affected side are painful and tender to percussion, although often no obvious dental cause can be found. Leaning the head forwards increases the pain (as it leads to an increase in venous congestion which, together with collected secretions, occludes the ostium and increases pressure within the antrum). However, leaning the head backwards reduces congestion, allowing the ostium to become patent, reducing internal antral pressure and consequently relieving pain. Although the pain usually overlies the affected sinus it may be referred from the antrum to the frontal and retro-orbital regions.

Clinical signs of sinusitis

- Signs of a recent upper respiratory tract infection, e.g. rhinorrhoea and nasal redness, dryness or crusting
- Tenderness of the cheek (especially in the infraorbital region and canine fossa)
- Tenderness of teeth in whole buccal segment to percussion or pressure
- Tenderness over the anterior antral wall, intraorally
- Swelling and inflammation of the cheek (rare in sinusitis)

THE INVESTIGATION OF ANTRAL DISEASE

A diagnosis of sinusitis can usually be made from the findings of the history and examination. The teeth and surrounding tissues should be examined for disease (although remember that sinusitis may itself have a dental cause). Transillumination, using a torch shone from inside the mouth, may demonstrate antral congestion but this is a rather crude test and may fail to detect tumours. Radiographs are not usually required to confirm the diagnosis of sinusitis as the diagnosis can be made on clinical grounds alone. Radiographs are only required to exclude the possibility of dental disease, trauma or pathology within the antrum. If pathology or trauma is suspected, occipitomental radiographic views are often taken in specialist centres. A 'fluid level' may be visible which represents a collection of pus, although following trauma it may be due to the presence of blood and suggests that there is a fracture of the wall of the antrum. Opacities due to polyps, cysts, thickened antral lining, tumours and radio-opaque foreign bodies may also be demonstrated.

Other useful radiographs include:

- the OPT (to show foreign bodies, oroantral communication (or at least a bone defect suggestive of such a communication), the size of antrum and its relationship to maxillary teeth, cysts and tumours)
- periapical views (for the relationship between roots and antrum)
- computed tomography (CT) scans (useful to demonstrate tumours or comminuted fractures involving the orbit or zygomatic complex).

Much useful information can be gathered by endoscopy of the antrum. This is better performed by someone with experience of endoscopy in the region (such as an ENT surgeon).

DENTAL EXTRACTIONS AND THE ANTRUM

The following complications may occur during the extraction of posterior maxillary teeth because of their close proximity to the maxillary antrum:

- creation of an oroantral communication
- displacement of a tooth or root into the antrum
- fracture of the maxillary tuberosity.

Maxillary premolars and permanent molars are most frequently implicated, although permanent canines may occasionally be very close to the antrum. Complications may also occur during the surgical removal of impacted partially erupted or unerupted teeth (e.g. canines, premolars and third molars). The extraction of deciduous teeth does not present a risk due to the relatively small size of the antrum in children and the presence of the developing permanent teeth.

An assessment of the size and proximity of the antrum before extraction or periapical surgery on a posterior maxillary tooth may help to anticipate and avoid these complications. When a complication does occur, it should be recognized and dealt with promptly.

The following factors should be taken into account during clinical and radiographic examination in order to anticipate and avoid complications:

- the size of the antrum and its relationship to the teeth
- the size and shape of the tooth and roots and evidence of any periapical pathology
- the patient's age
- the patient's past dental history.

If the dental history reveals the creation of an oroantral communication during a previous extraction there is likely to be an increased risk of this complication occurring during the subsequent extraction of adjacent or contralateral teeth. Similarly, if there is a history of difficult extractions, due perhaps to hypercementosis or dense bone, there may be an increased risk of tuberosity fracture.

OROANTRAL COMMUNICATION AND FISTULA

An oroantral communication (OAC) is an abnormal connection between the oral and antral cavities; an oroantral fistula (OAF) is an epithelialized OAC (although the terms OAC and OAF are often used interchangeably).

The creation of an OAC most commonly follows the extraction of a maxillary tooth closely related to the antral floor (typically the first molar (Fig. 15.2), which lies close to the lowest point of the antral floor, although any premolar or molar may be affected). An OAC may also form as a result of an alveolar fracture running through the antral floor or wall, or be due to direct trauma from a bur or chisel. Left untreated, an OAC may heal spontaneously or persist as an OAF (Fig. 15.3).

The following signs indicate OAC formation:

- a visible defect between the mouth and antrum

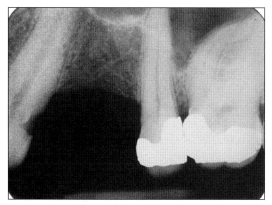

Fig. 15.2   A maxillary molar in close relation to the maxillary antrum.

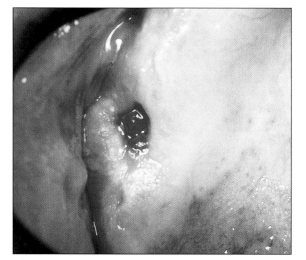

Fig. 15.3   Oroantral fistula in the first molar region with pro-liferation of soft tissue.

- bone fragments with a smooth concave upper surface (antral floor fragments) adhering to the root of the extracted tooth.

Investigation of a suspected OAC

The presence of an OAC can often be confirmed by careful examination using a mirror and a good light, although bleeding may obscure visibility. The interior of the antrum may be visible or there may be a bony defect lined by intact antral mucosa. Gentle suction applied to the socket often produces a characteristic hollow sound. The temptation to confirm the presence of a suspected OAC by probing or irrigation (to demonstrate transfer of fluid through the OAC into the antrum and nose) should be resisted. Both methods carry the risk of causing sinusitis by introducing oral flora or pushing contaminated bone fragments or other foreign bodies into the antrum. Even gentle probing may breach an intact antral floor or mucosal lining to create an OAC where one previously did not exist. It may also increase the size of an existing OAC, lessening the chances of spontaneous closure and complicating future surgical repair.

To test for a suspected OAC, a patient may be asked to attempt to blow the nose whilst pinching the nostrils. Air, which is unable to escape through the closed nostrils, is forced into the mouth through any OAC, producing bubbles of blood or saliva. Established OAFs often have small slit-like or pinhole oral openings concealing much wider underlying bony defects. They can also be detected using the above test and if sinusitis is present pus may be expressed or may discharge spontaneously into the mouth.

A patient with an untreated OAC or established OAF will typically give a history of an upper molar or premolar extraction followed by the development of:

- salty-tasting discharge or the awareness of an unpleasant smell
- reflux of fluids and food (and smoke in smokers) into the nose from the mouth
- escape of air into mouth during nose blowing
- recurrent or chronic sinusitis on the affected side
- difficulty in smoking a cigarette or playing a wind instrument
- proliferation of soft tissue around the fistula.

Radiographs (e.g. periapical views or OPT) are useful to confirm the diagnosis of OAC/OAF and to assess the size of the bone defect, although small defects may not be demonstrated.

Prevention of OAC formation

Where the risk of OAC formation is anticipated, the patient should be warned preoperatively and steps should be taken to avoid this complication. Surgical exodontia is preferable to forceps extraction because it allows more control over bone removal and, by tooth division, enables individual roots to be delivered away from the thin antral floor. If a mucoperiosteal flap is raised its design should allow it to be adapted for OAC repair if necessary.

The diagnosis and enucleation of cysts near the antrum can be problematic, as an extension of the antrum may be mistaken for an odontogenic cyst during the preoperative assessment and at operation. Both have a similar radiographic appearance, although a radio-opaque line can usually be seen to separate a cyst cavity from the antrum, whereas an extension of the antrum will appear continuous with the main antral cavity. Because the healthy antrum contains air but a cyst contains fluid, the following simple test is often useful to distinguish between the two at operation. The thin bony wall is pierced using a wide-bore needle connected to a large syringe and the cavity contents aspirated. Air is aspirated if the antrum has been pierced; fluid would be recovered from a cyst. Unfortunately, this test is not foolproof as pus may be aspirated from an infected antrum or the contents of a cyst may be too thick to enter the needle, giving the impression of an empty cavity.

Treatment of OAC and OAF

The immediate treatment of a new OAC is aimed at preventing the development of a persistent OAF and chronic sinusitis. Larger communications require surgical closure although small defects (up to 5 mm wide) may heal spontaneously (it is likely that many close without being detected). However, early surgical closure is recommended whenever possible as it is difficult to predict when spontaneous healing will occur.

Immediate treatment of new OAC

This aims to encourage the regeneration of new bone between the oral and antral cavities. Treatment is directed at protecting the blood clot within the socket whilst organization and bone formation take place and at preventing infection of the wound or antrum.

Where further surgery is delayed or contraindicated an acrylic base plate or extension of an existing denture can be used to support the clot, or a dressing such as ribbon gauze (soaked in an antimicrobial agent) may be sutured across (*not into*) the defect. In smokers this has the advantage of protecting the clot from disturbances due to the changes in intraoral pressure associated with inhalation. However, care

must be taken not to force impression material through the OAC into the antrum (the defect can be covered with sterile gauze while the impressions are taken).

If there is sufficient soft tissue, the opposing palatal and buccal mucosa may be held together with mattress sutures. A strong, preferably non-resorbable, suture material should be chosen (e.g. 3/0 black silk) and sutures retained for 10–14 days to ensure that healing is complete before they are removed. Reducing the height of the bony socket edges with a bur and slightly undermining the tissue margins helps to bring the margins together where there is a shortage of soft tissue. However, there is often insufficient mucosa for this simple technique and because the sutures are unsupported by bone there is a risk of wound dehiscence. If there is insufficient mucosa a buccal mucoperiosteal advancement flap is used to cover the defect. This is a more demanding procedure, which should be undertaken by a general dental practitioner only if he or she has adequate training, experience and facilities.

Further options for the treatment of OAC/OAF

If the immediate measures are insufficient or fail to lead to healing of an OAC (e.g. in the case of a large OAC) further treatment becomes necessary. Tissue from local flaps is most often utilized to close oroantral defects, although distant flaps (e.g. from the tongue) and grafting are also possible. The choice of method depends on the size and position of the communication. Of the variety of local flaps which have been described the most common is the buccal advancement flap.

Buccal advancement (Rehmann's) flap (Fig. 15.4)

This technique is suitable for the closure of new OACs and chronic OAFs.

1. A sharp probe is used to locate the edges of the bony defect (which may be considerably larger than the soft-tissue defect—especially in a long-standing OAF).
2. The epithelium lining the fistula tract (if present) and soft-tissue margins is excised with a No. 11 scalpel blade, leaving a 2- to 3-mm rim of exposed bone, which enables the

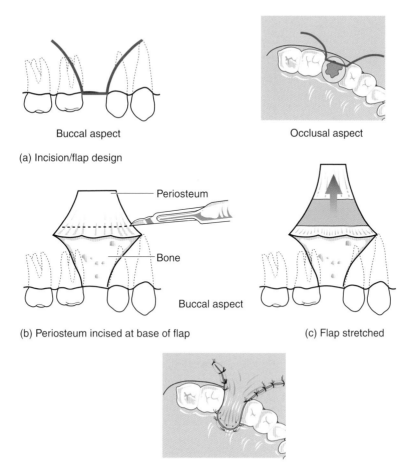

Buccal aspect

Occlusal aspect

(a) Incision/flap design

Periosteum

Bone

Buccal aspect

(b) Periosteum incised at base of flap

(c) Flap stretched

(d) Flap advanced across defect and sutured

Fig. 15.4   Closure of an oroantral fistula with a buccal advancement flap.
(**a**) The incisions outlined from the buccal and occlusal aspects.
(**b**) Incision of periosteum only, high up in the reflection of the sulcus.
(**c**) Extension of the flap following 'release'.
(**d**) Closure with vertical mattress sutures, seen from the occlusal aspect.

suture line to rest on sound bone. Alternatively, the fistula may be turned in on itself, up into the antrum. This presents, in the place of an empty tract, a connective tissue surface for the underside of the buccal flap to lie against.

3. A broad-based three-sided buccal mucoperiosteal flap, which extends to the full depth of the sulcus, is cut and reflected.

4. The periosteum lining the inner surface of the flap is cut parallel to and close to its base, allowing the flap to be stretched ('advanced') without tension to meet the palatal mucosa. Although the full width of the periosteum must be divided in order to mobilize the flap, care

must be taken not to compromise the blood supply by creating a 'button-hole' in the thin buccal tissue. To prevent this the back of a scalpel blade may be used with repeated light strokes until the periosteum is cut through.

5. The palatal margin is slightly undermined and the wound closed with mattress sutures. This author recommends 3/0 non-resorbable (or a long-lasting resorbable) suture material and that sutures should be retained for 10–14 days.

This is a simple, well-tolerated procedure with a good success rate. It can be performed under local anaesthesia in a cooperative patient and may be performed in general dental practice if adequate skill and facilities are available. Although this technique initially reduces sulcus depth, this is usually temporary.

In OAFs with large bony defects or where previous surgical closure has been unsuccessful, more complicated surgery may be required to close the defect. An adaptation of the buccal advancement flap utilizing a buccal fat pad (BFP) graft is often used. This is performed under GA in order to achieve adequate analgesia and as surgery is more prolonged. A broad-based three-sided mucoperiosteal flap is raised and periosteum incised (Fig. 15.4). The BFP is then located using a vestibular incision in the region of the upper first permanent molar and mobilized using blunt dissection with artery forceps. This tissue is then advanced to cover the bony defect and the mucoperiosteal flap is sutured using a non-resorbable material. A high success rate using the BFP graft has been reported.

Palatal rotation flap (Fig. 15.5)

This is used less commonly than the buccal advancement flap.

1. The epithelial lining (if present) is excised with a No. 11 scalpel blade (Fig. 15.5a).
2. An elongated full-thickness mucoperiosteal palatal flap, which follows the course of the greater palatine artery and which extends for a short distance anterior to the oroantral defect is designed, cut and raised. It should be long enough for its free end to be rotated to cover the defect. As the flap relies upon the greater palatine artery for its blood supply, care must be taken not to cut or damage this vessel or to reduce flow through it by bending the flap too acutely.
3. The flap is sutured across the defect (Fig. 15.5b) using mattress sutures (as for the buccal advancement flap). The resultant area of exposed bone is covered with a dressing such as ribbon gauze (soaked in an antimicrobial agent) held in place with sutures, or a periodontal dressing (secured with sutures or an acrylic base-plate), which should be retained for 10–14 days.

This technique provides a thick, strong repair, which heals readily due to its good blood supply and does not adversely affect the buccal sulcus. However,

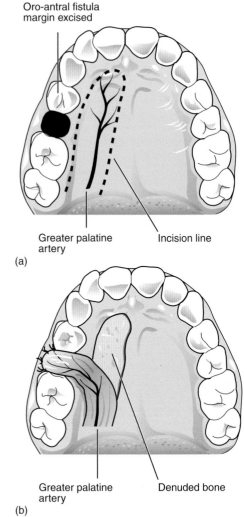

(a)

(b)

Fig. 15.5 Closure of an oroantral fistula with a palatal rotation flap.
(a) The incision outlined.
(b) The flap mobilized, rotated into the defect and sutured.

palatal flaps are relatively inelastic and can be difficult to raise and mobilize. In addition, it can be difficult to judge the precise length of tissue required. Under local anaesthesia, this procedure is more unpleasant for the patient than the buccal advancement flap is and a raw area of exposed palatal bone is produced. Although, it could be tackled in general dental practice under local anaes-thesia it is more commonly performed in a specialist setting under GA.

For all methods of OAC/OAF closure, the patient should be warned not to blow the nose during the first 10 postoperative days, as this raises pressure within the antrum and may disrupt the healing tissue. Compliance with this instruction may be greater if a patient is given a simple explanation for it. Prophylactic antibiotics and nasal decongestant drops are prescribed by some surgeons to prevent infection and encourage antral drainage.

FOREIGN BODIES IN THE ANTRUM

This complication occurs when teeth or roots are closely related to the antrum. Roots of maxillary premolars and molars are the most common foreign bodies although whole teeth may also be displaced into the antrum. Their entry into the antrum occurs during attempts at removal and is associated with OAC formation. Other foreign bodies include materials introduced during root-filling procedures, via an OAF (food, impression material, cotton buds) and during trauma.

The displacement of a root into the antrum occurs because of:

- failure to detect a large antrum or a close relationship between a root and a thin or perforated antral floor
- use of an inappropriate technique or insufficient care during removal of the root.

As a root can be pushed through a very thin antral floor using the lightest touch it is essential to avoid applying any upward pressure. The risk is particularly high when an elevator is used blindly within a socket. Root removal should therefore be performed under direct vision using a transalveolar approach. Elevators are used to apply gentle pressure towards the mouth (never towards the antrum) and forceps should not be applied without a clear view of both the palatal and buccal root surfaces. Consideration may be given to leaving a small (less than 3 mm) vital root fragment rather than risk displacing it into the antrum. If this decision is taken the patient should be informed and the reasons explained, relevant radiographs should be taken to confirm the size and position of the retained root and an entry should be made in the patient's notes. The root should be reviewed periodically and removed if symptoms develop. Whole teeth may be pushed into the antrum, with partially erupted and unerupted teeth, especially

those with a single conical root, being at the greatest risk (e.g. upper third molars, impacted canines and premolars).

A root may be displaced:

- into the antrum
- under the buccal or palatal mucosa
- out of the socket into the mouth
- out of the mouth—e.g. into suction tubing, onto patient's clothing, onto floor.

A root not removed with the tooth must be accounted for, due to the dangers of inhalation and infection. First look in the oral cavity, socket and adjacent tissues, next search extraorally and then take radiographs if necessary. Radiographs that are suitable for demonstrating a root in the antrum include periapical (Fig. 15.6) and oblique occlusal views or an OPT. The presence of a root canal confirms that a radio-opaque image represents a root.

Roots should be removed from the antrum as soon as possible to prevent an OAF and chronic sinusitis from developing. If left they may become embedded in granulation tissue, polyps or fibrous tissue or an antrolith (antral 'stone') may form around them. They are occasionally expelled through an OAF into the mouth or through the ostium into the nose from where they may be inhaled or expelled by sneezing. In general dental practice, the recommended immediate treatment for a root in the antrum is to provide simple treatment for the OAC (see above), inform the patient and arrange prompt referral to an oral and maxillofacial surgeon.

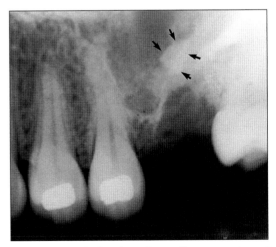

Fig. 15.6   A root displaced into the maxillary antrum (arrows).

Roots can sometimes be removed through the extraction socket, although often access is better via a window in the anterior antral wall, made using the Caldwell-Luc operation. As an alternative, consideration should be given to possible removal of small roots by endoscopy.

Surgical removal via an extraction socket

If a root in the antrum is near its socket, it can sometimes be removed by raising a buccal flap and removing the buccal wall of the socket to create an enlarged opening into the antrum. Suction and irrigation are used to locate the root, which is then recovered. The defect is closed by advancing a buccal flap across it.

Caldwell-Luc operation (Fig. 15.7)

This gives surgical access to the interior of the antrum though the mouth and is usually performed in hospital under GA. It can be used to remove roots, teeth and other foreign bodies from the antrum.

1. A horizontal incision is made in the buccal sulcus from the upper lateral incisor to the upper first molar and a mucoperiosteal flap is raised (in the edentulous ridge a two-sided buccal flap with an anterior relieving incision is used). A chisel or bur is used to create an opening in the antral wall in the canine fossa.
2. The root is located using suction and good lighting and removed with an artery clip or Fickling forceps.
3. If blood clot, granulation tissue or polyps are present they may be carefully removed, but

the antral lining should be disturbed as little as possible (problems with mucus clearance and subsequent chronic sinusitis may result).
4. Finally, the antrum is irrigated with normal saline and the incision is closed with interrupted non-resorbable sutures.

Summary of extractions and the maxillary antrum

- The extraction of maxillary teeth may be complicated by OAC/OAF formation, the introduction of roots, teeth or other foreign bodies into the antrum and fracture of the maxillary tuberosity
- These complications are more likely to occur where the antrum is large and closely related to the teeth
- The GDP should know how to predict, avoid, detect and treat these conditions and should understand whether treatment by a GDP or a specialist is appropriate

---

FACIAL FRACTURES INVOLVING THE ANTRUM

Fractures of the antral walls occur in several common types of facial fracture including zygomatic complex, mid-third (Le Fort I, II and III), orbital blow-out and alveolar fractures (see Ch. 13). The presence of a fracture through the antral wall does not preclude the extraction of a maxillary molar or premolar, although forceps should be avoided in favour of a surgical approach in the initial 6 weeks following trauma.

ANTRAL CYSTS AND TUMOURS

Antral mucosal cysts are frequently discovered as incidental findings on dental radiographs (Fig. 15.8). They are generally symptomless and have no long-term significance, but care should be taken to differentiate between truly antral lesions and cysts of odontogenic origin (apical cysts, dentigerous cysts and odontogenic keratocysts), which do require treatment.

Benign tumours arising in the antrum include papillomas and osteomas. Although they rarely cause symptoms, they may interfere with antral drainage or cause nasal obstruction by growing through the

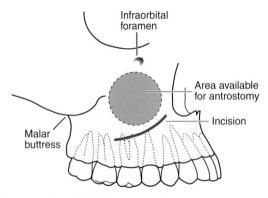

Fig. 15.7 The Caldwell-Luc operation.

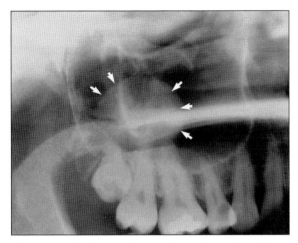

Fig. 15.8 A benign antral mucosal cyst (arrows) may be an incidental finding on a dental radiograph.

ostium, and they occasionally herniate through an OAC. More often, however, they are discovered incidentally on radiographs.

Malignant tumours arising in the antrum are less common, but often have a poor prognosis as they tend to present at an advanced stage. This is because they develop in a concealed location and early symptoms may be absent, or mistaken for sinusitis. When symptoms of antral malignancy do develop, a patient may consult a dentist believing he or she has a dental problem. This makes it especially important that dentists are able to recognize the typical presenting signs and symptoms (see also Ch. 10, p. 136). These vary according to the direction in which the tumour is spreading (see box).

Radiographs of early malignant antral tumours appear normal or may show cloudiness or an irregular soft-tissue outline. Erosion of the antral wall is seen in later stages. Whenever antral malignancy is suspected referral should be made without delay to an oral and maxillofacial surgeon, initially by telephone or fax.

THE ANTRUM AND FACIAL PAIN

Sinusitis and antral malignancy both produce facial pain, which may not have an immediately obvious cause. These conditions should be included in the differential diagnosis of facial pain (their typical signs and symptoms are described above and facial pain is discussed in detail in Ch. 16).

Signs and symptoms of antral malignancy (dependent on direction of spread)

- All directions:
  symptoms of sinusitis which are unresponsive to treatment, i.e. pain in the maxilla, unilateral nasal obstruction and purulent nasal discharge
- Towards mouth:
  unaccountable mobility of a maxillary tooth
  excessive bleeding or herniation of tumour through socket following dental extraction
  swelling in the buccal sulcus or palate (may affect the fit of an upper denture)
  oral ulceration
- Towards nose:
  epistaxis (worrying in older patient (40+ years) if no other possible explanation)
  nasal obstruction
  nasal discharge
- Towards cheek:
  extraoral swelling
  redness over the maxilla
  paraesthesia in the distribution of the infraorbital nerve (very suggestive of malignancy)
- Towards orbit:
  diplopia
  raised pupil and proptosis on affected side
- Infratemporal spread:
  trismus (due to invasion of the muscles of mastication)

PHARMACOLOGICAL TREATMENT OF ANTRAL DISEASE

Antibiotics, decongestant nasal drops and steam inhalations are prescribed for the prevention of sinus infection following the creation of an OAC. Broad-spectrum antibiotics are useful in the treatment of acute sinusitis (although they are not a substitute for the drainage of pus) and decongestant nasal drops and steam inhalations can be used to encourage drainage. An analgesic such as paracetamol or ibuprofen may be recommended for relief of pain in acute sinusitis.

Antibiotics

Amoxicillin or erythromycin is a suitable choice.

Decongestants

Sympathomimetic drops, such as ephedrine 0.5%, encourage antral drainage by causing vasoconstriction, which reduces vascular engorgement within the nasal mucosa. This decreases mucosal swelling and thus increases the patency of the ostium. Ephedrine drops should not be used for more than 7 consecutive days as rebound vasodilatation occurs with long-term use, leading to further mucosal congestion (also note that ephedrine should not be prescribed for a patient taking monoamine oxidase inhibitors). Pseudoephedrine tablets may be taken as an alternative.

Steam inhalations

Steam inhalations help to decrease the viscosity of mucus, allowing it to drain more easily (use hot rather than boiling water to avoid the risk of scalding). Menthol and eucalyptus may be added to the water to make this treatment more pleasant and, although this has no proven medical benefit, it increases patient compliance.

FURTHER READING

Awang M. N. (1988) Closure of oroantral fistula. *International Journal of Oral and Maxillofacial Surgery* 17: 110–115.

McGowan D. A., Baxter P. W., James J. (1993) *The maxillary sinus and its dental implications*. Wright, Bristol, UK.

SELF-ASSESSMENT

1. During the extraction of an upper first molar you notice a fragment of bone with a smooth, concave superior surface adhering to the palatal root. The preoperative radiograph shows a close relationship between this tooth and the maxillary antrum.
   (a) What has happened, and how can you confirm this?
   (b) What should you do immediately?
   (c) What postoperative instructions and follow-up treatment should you provide the patient?
   (d) Which other teeth may be affected by this complication?
2. During the attempted extraction of a maxillary left third molar (Fig. 15.9) you become aware of an unusual amount of movement of a large section of alveolar bone surrounding this tooth.
   (a) What has happened?
   (b) How should you proceed?
   (c) What radiographic signs warn of this possible complication?
3. During an attempt to remove the palatal root of an upper first molar, using an elevator, it suddenly disappears from view.
   (a) List the possible locations in which the root may now lie.
   (b) How would you go about locating it and how might the order in which you search the possible locations be important?

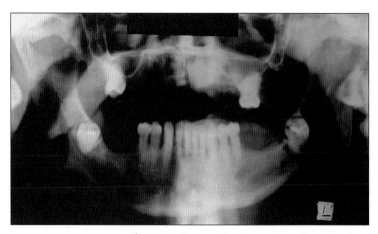

Fig. 15.9   See question 2.

c) What precautions should have been taken before and during the removal of this root?

4. List the typical symptoms, signs and radiographic features of acute sinusitis. How do these differ from those of chronic sinusitis?

5. List the signs and symptoms that would lead you to suspect that a patient may have a malignant antral tumour. What would you do on discovering such signs or symptoms?

Answers on page 269.

16 | Facial pain and temporomandibular disorders

J. Pedlar

- Most pain experienced in the teeth and jaws arises from common diseases of the teeth and periodontium.
- Differentiation of pain arising in the muscles of mastication and the temporomandibular joints from pain of non-dental origin can be difficult if the clinician is not aware of the possibilities.
- 'Temporomandibular disorders' is a term that encompasses both muscular and joint-centred conditions of the masticatory apparatus of a variety of aetiologies.
- Many such conditions do not require a surgical solution, but they must be distinguished from the few which may.
- Some clinicians have a particular interest in these disorders but treatment is not specifically in the remit of any dental (or medical) specialty.

ASSUMED KNOWLEDGE

It is assumed that at this stage you will have knowledge/competencies in the following areas:

- anatomy and physiology of pain experience in the face, head and neck
- structure and movements of the masticatory apparatus.

If you think that you are not well equipped in these areas, revise them before reading this chapter or cross-check with texts on those subjects as you read.

INTENDED LEARNING OUTCOMES

At the end of this chapter you should be able to:

1. Identify key clinical features of temporomandibular disorders
2. Distinguish disorders of the masticatory muscles from those centred within the temporomandibular joint and from disorders of dental origin
3. Distinguish those cases which may require surgical treatment
4. List possible conservative treatments and select a scheme of management for a patient with a temporomandibular disorder
5. Determine the success or otherwise of treatment of such a patient
6. Identify key clinical features of atypical facial pain[1]
7. Distinguish atypical facial pain from other facial pain of central neurological or vascular origin
8. Delimit the role of dental management for those with atypical facial pain and other non-dental chronic pain.

---

[1] 'Atypical facial pain' is a widely used term that nonetheless is not universally accepted. The International Headache Society prefers the term 'persistent idiopathic facial pain'. The author feels that such a change in terminology gains little and may tend to confuse.

PAIN OF DENTAL ORIGIN

Whilst it is not the purpose of this book to reiterate the diagnosis of common dental disorders, it is worth restating some features of these conditions to aid in the distinction from pain not caused by disease of the teeth (see Table 16.1).

In general, pain of dental origin is of relatively rapid onset (hours to days) and very well localized to the causative quadrant of the mouth or even to the tooth itself. Pulpal pain is typically worsened by thermal stimulation. Periodontal pain (apical or lateral) is associated with tenderness of (usually) one tooth to biting or to finger pressure. There are other specific features that may be sought, such as caries, loss of vitality and radiographic signs of periodontal bone loss. Even in the case of more difficult diagnoses such as cracked teeth, local signs may be elicited.

Soft-tissue disorders such as aphthous ulceration, pericoronal infection and acute ulcerative gingivitis can occasionally be confusing, but nonetheless tend to have a short natural history, or at least rapidly make themselves obvious.

It is also worth noting that studies that have attempted to distinguish dental disorders from each other on the basis of the nature of the pain have shown little success.

Table 16.1 Distinguishing pain of temporomandibular disorders from that of dental origin

	Dental pain	Pain associated with temporomandibular disorders
Site	Teeth or alveolus. Almost always unilateral	Preauricular, temple, angle of mandible. May be bilateral
Duration	Hours to days	Weeks to months
Aggravated by	Thermal stimulation or pressure on a specific tooth	Jaw movement, chewing, yawning, cold windy weather
Relation to time of day	No	Often yes

CLINICAL FEATURES OF TEMPOROMANDIBULAR DISORDERS

The term 'temporomandibular disorders' encompasses a group of conditions which can be the source of great controversy. As far as possible, this chapter will deal in fact, accepting that almost anything written may be challenged. It is the intention of the author to give enough information to allow the reader a basic understanding, sufficient to deal with those patients attending a general dental practice and to read further on the subject.

The group is recognized by one or more of three principal clinical features:

1. Pain associated with the temporomandibular joint (TMJ) and/or the masticatory muscles
2. Noises associated with the TMJ
3. Limitation of jaw movement.

Unfortunately, each of these characteristics may take a variety of forms. This not only causes confusion for the learner but is partly responsible for the controversies concerning terminology and classification so common amongst the 'experts' in the field. Patients too may have considerable difficulty putting into words the experiences associated with their suffering.

Pain

Pain of muscular origin is often described as aching, but may also be throbbing or sharp, or described as 'burning', 'stiffness', 'tightness', 'pressure', 'fullness' or even 'numbness'. It may be unilateral, but is the only common pain of the head and neck experienced bilaterally (Table 16.1). That may aid distinction from pain derived from third molar infection, which is rarely bilateral (at any one time). Muscular pain may be clearly localized to a 'trigger point' centred in one muscle (e.g. masseter), or may be less well defined in distribution in, for example, the preauricular or temporal areas.

The time scale of the pain is also important as it rarely develops to a point which causes a patient to seek help over less than a few weeks, in contrast to pain of pulpal or periodontal origin, which tends to develop over hours to days. Activities involving stretching or use of the masticatory muscles, such as chewing, yawning, laughing or singing, usually worsen the pain. Variation over time is common, with pain often being worse in the mornings, but this is by no means always so.

Pain may also derive from the TMJ itself, in which case it tends to be more localized to the joint (but is not always), may be sharp, aching or throbbing, tends to vary less during the day and is usually worsened by joint movement.

Tenderness of the muscles or joints

Sites of origin of pain are often tender to gentle palpation. Masseter and temporalis muscles are accessible to palpation over most of their surfaces. Medial pterygoid can only readily be felt on the midpoint of its anterior border (a finger can be run back along the occlusal surfaces of the teeth until it meets the muscle) or possibly where it joins the pterygo-masseteric sling beneath the mandible. Access to the lateral pterygoid, however, is very restricted, it being found by passing a small finger between the maxillary tuberosity and the coronoid process of the mandible. Caution is needed in interpreting apparent tenderness of the masticatory muscles, as normal muscles may be quite sensitive to firm palpation; a major difference between the sides of the face is usually of diagnostic value.

Noises

The most common noise associated with the TMJ is clicking (or snapping, cracking, bumping or popping). The noise may be experienced by the sufferer only or may be audible to others, but is always associated with joint movement. The clinician may detect inaudible sounds by palpation or auscultation over the joints during joint movement. Often clicking is worse during eating and occasionally it is audible to others over the sound of conversation at a considerable distance.

A number of surveys have demonstrated that clicking of the TMJ is common, possibly affecting one-third of the adult population. Most people with a clicking TMJ do not 'suffer' from their joint noise to the point that they seek help, and that brings us to one of our difficulties. If a majority of people who have a clicking TMJ do not seek help about them, can clicking per se be regarded as an abnormality? The resolution of that question is probably beyond the scope of this book, but it is right to caution against the *automatic* treatment of all people with a clicking TMJ.

Other noises encountered come under the general term 'crepitus' and may be described by the patient as 'grating', 'grinding', 'crackling', 'rubbing' and other terms. Such noises are rarely audible to others, but again may be detected by palpation or auscultation. These noises should be clearly distinguished from clicking-type noises as they almost certainly represent different aspects of disease.

Limitation of jaw movement

This may take the form of 'stiffness' or pain on attempted mouth opening, thus restricting mobility. Where this is associated with muscular problems, it is often slow in onset (and recovery) and variable in severity.

Muscular stiffness should be distinguished from 'locking', which is very sudden in onset (and, if relieved, recovery is also instantaneous).

To determine the degree of restriction some measure of the normal, which is itself very variable, is required. A reasonable measure of the lower limit of interincisal opening for an adult with a class 1 occlusion is 40 mm, measured between the upper and lower incisal edges. The upper limit of the range is about 65 mm. However, these values should be used with caution as some normal people have measures outside this range. Lateral excursive and pro-trusive movements give some degree of measure of translatory movement within the joints and may be less affected than interincisal opening by muscular influences. Lower limits for these measures are approximately 7 mm. Some allowance should be made for variation in incisor relationship and for bodily size (the larger the body, the greater the opening).

A CLASSIFICATION OF TEMPOROMANDIBULAR DISORDERS

Classification of temporomandibular disorders is one area in which controversy is rife. It is worth taking a little time to consider the value of classification before suggesting a pragmatic approach to these disorders.

The setting of a variety of entities into more or less coherent groups enables rules to be drawn concerning the behaviour of these groups. As far as disease is concerned, this should allow a prognosis to be offered, specific treatments to be selected and research to be conducted, particularly to determine whether treatments are *predictably* successful. If a group of very different disorders is considered as if they are one condition, prognosis, treatment and research results are likely to be very confused. It is the case with temporomandibular disorders that disease is defined in terms of a wide range of overlapping and ill-defined symptoms and physical signs, and both causes and predisposing factors are poorly understood. It should not be surprising that there remains uncertainty as to whether one, three or many conditions are being dealt with.

It is clear, however, that some distinctions can be made. Young adult patients do present with pain, muscle tenderness, variable stiffness, but no clicking or locking; similarly there are young patients with clicking and/or locking of the TMJ with no history of muscle-associated pain or stiffness; a third group is also seen with onset in middle life of joint-associated pain, joint tenderness, crepitus and radiological signs of bone loss within the joints. It is difficult to see these three 'pure' forms as parts of the same disorder, although 'pure' forms are relatively uncommon. There is also evidence that these disorders do interact with each other in some patients and some practitioners believe that there is a strong element of progression from one type to another.

At the other extreme there is a temptation to continue to subdivide and subdivide each category, which, without a clear understanding of the nature of the disorders, runs the risk of creating an unwieldy and confusing hierarchy of conditions when it cannot be certain they are all different.

The classification used in this chapter is pragmatic and based on that recommended by the American Academy for Orofacial Pain (McNeil 1993).

Temporomandibular disorders

- Myofascial pain dysfunction
- Disc displacement with/without reduction
- Degenerative joint disease
- Systemic arthropathies

MYOFASCIAL PAIN DYSFUNCTION

Diagnosis

In its pure form this is a condition affecting only the muscles, though it may affect neck and scalp musculature as well as masticatory ones and is probably analogous to 'fibromyalgia' affecting more distant muscle groups. It is predominantly a young patient's condition and (at least as far as hospital practice is concerned) affects women far more commonly than men. Muscles are painful, particularly during use, often particularly so in the mornings. Specific tender spots (trigger points) may be found in individual muscles, or many muscles may be tender. The condition often develops over weeks to months but with some degree of variation in severity over that time.

Mouth opening is often, but not always restricted, but interincisal opening is rarely less than 15 mm. There is usually some capacity to extend opening with passive stretching by finger pressure; this is also often accompanied by a hesitant or jerky jaw movement. Occasionally the condition appears in a severe form of rapid onset. In this case mouth opening may be restricted to a few millimetres.

The condition appears to be almost always self-limiting over a period of a few weeks to a few years, although for some patients the condition can be remarkably persistent. The cause(s) is unknown. However, several factors have been linked to it:

- parafunctional activity such as clenching or grinding of the teeth, finger nail, pencil or cheek chewing
- stress, psychological disturbance or psychiatric illness
- occlusal disturbance
- physical injury
- true joint disease in the TMJ or cervical spine
- other local inflammatory conditions.

Almost certainly each of these factors is of some importance in individual cases, but no one factor has been shown to be consistently present in all cases, nor are all those who exhibit these features affected by myofascial pain dysfunction. This inconsistency must shed some doubt on either the causative role of these factors or the coherence of the diagnostic category, and probably implies some form of 'susceptibility' which as yet is not understood.

Principal clinical features of myofascial pain dysfunction

- Muscle-associated pain
- Limited mouth opening (variable)
- Possible normal translatory movement of joint
- Association with time of day
- Possible association with stress, anxiety, parafunction
- Often bilateral

Treatment

Apparently successful treatment may take many forms. It is usual to recommend a range of conservative measures: keeping the muscles warm, minimizing chewing, analgesics (NSAIDs if the patient can tolerate them) as well as asking the patient to watch for and control daytime parafunctional activity.

A common second line is the soft vinyl mouthguard (Fig. 16.1), which, although claimed by some to worsen bruxism, does appear to work for many patients and is both inexpensive and simple to construct, requiring only one lower impression. The author recommends this appliance for night use only, for about 6 weeks: as it cannot be adjusted precisely to the occlusion, wearing the appliance 24 hours per day does result in uneven tooth movement. If it has not brought any improvement in 6 weeks, the likelihood of success is small and its use should be discontinued. Many other designs of appliance are used for this condition and it is beyond the scope of this book to review them all. The occlusally balanced or stabilization appliance is a rigid acrylic device made to fit closely into the occlusal surfaces of both upper and lower teeth when the jaw is held in a retruded position with the teeth marginally apart. It may be retained with clasps or ball cleats attached to the teeth. It can be worn all day, but there is little evidence that results are better than that achieved by night use only.

Physiotherapy of various forms has been shown to be effective in reducing pain and increasing mobility. It is, however, expensive to provide and often inconvenient for the patient because repeated visits are needed.

Antidepressant medications such as amitriptyline, dothiepin, fluoxetine or paroxetine have been used with considerable success for some patients and it has been argued that some such drugs may act more by altering the pain experience centrally than by having a direct antidepressant effect in this condition.

It is certainly worthwhile treating any obvious local causes, such as pericoronal infection affecting a third molar close to the affected muscle, or a high restoration. However, the practitioner should not undertake irreversible treatments, particularly if the factor being treated does not seem related in time to the onset of the condition.

If there are considerable signs of associated anxiety, depression or psychiatric disturbance, help should be sought from a psychologist or psychiatrist; this may generally be better done through the general medical practitioner.

DISC DISPLACEMENT WITH REDUCTION

Diagnosis

Most clicking of the TMJ has been shown to be associated with disc displacement.

Many anatomy texts show the disc within the TMJ to be superior and slightly anterior to the condylar head when the teeth are in occlusion, with the two main ridges of the disc placed one behind and one in front of the condyle (Fig. 16.2). During mouth opening the condyle rotates against the disc and the disc slides forwards and downwards along the articular eminence, but the ridges on the disc remain on either side of the condylar head (Fig. 16.3). This forward slide in the upper joint space is called *translation*. In general, much of the early part of mouth opening occurs as a hinge movement in the lower joint space and later in opening a greater part of the movement is translatory.

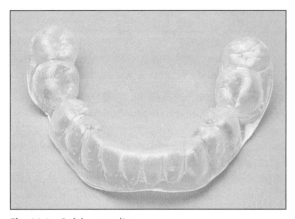

Fig. 16.1 Soft lower splint.

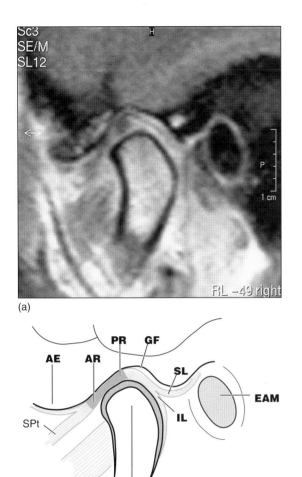

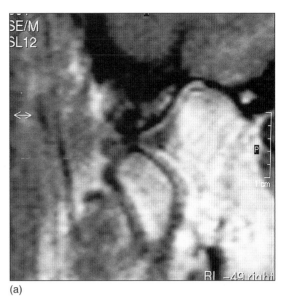

(a)

(a)

(b)

(b)

Fig. 16.2 (a) MRI of the normal disc/condyle relation, mouth closed. (b) Diagram of the same. AE = articular eminence; AR = anterior ridge of disc; PR = posterior ridge of disc; GF = glenoid fossa; SL = upper lamina of posterior attachment; EAM = external auditory meatus; IL = lower lamina of posterior attachment; CH = condylar head; SPt = superior pterygoid muscle.

Fig. 16.3 (a) MRI of the normal disc/condyle relation, mouth open. (b) Diagram of the same. Abbreviations as defined in the legend to Fig. 16.2.

For most people with a clicking TMJ the disc is not in the position described above when the teeth are together. In these people the disc is *anteriorly displaced* (or anteromedially displaced). This means that the posterior ridge of the disc is actually just in front of the condyle when the teeth are in occlusion (Fig. 16.4). On mouth opening the disc displacement reduces (Fig. 16.5): the disc moves back and the condyle forward relative to each other, in a sudden movement, resulting in the click and a 'normal' relationship between the condyle and the disc. This anterior disc displacement with reduction has been demonstrated by cadaveric dissection, arthrography and MRI scanning as the major event associated with

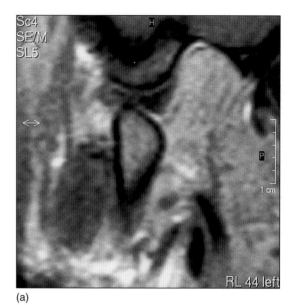

(a)

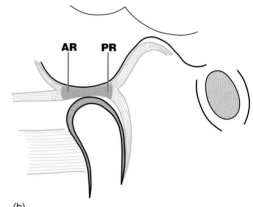

(b)

Fig. 16.5 (a) MRI showing reduction of disc displacement on mouth opening in the patient in Fig. 16.4. (b) Diagram of the same.

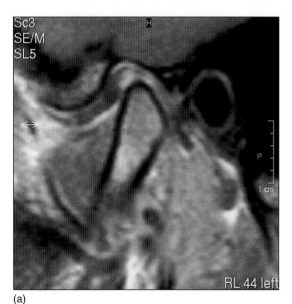

(a)

Anteriorly displaced disc

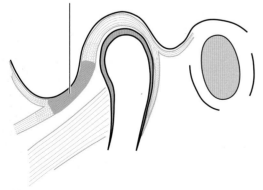

(b)

Fig. 16.4 (a) MRI of disc displacement, mouth closed. (b) Diagram of the same.

clicking of the TMJ. However, it is quite possible for joints without discs (such as finger joints) to click and therefore some clicks of the TMJ are probably due to other joint surface inconsistencies. When the individual with a reducing disc displacement closes their teeth together the disc is again displaced anteriorly.

Often the click heard on closing is much softer than that on opening and may be imperceptible to both subject and examiner, but on occasion it may be equally loud. Clicks that occur at the same time, on both opening and closing, may be described as *reciprocal*.

Causes of the condition are unclear. Associations have been made with occlusal factors, parafunction and peripheral joint hypermobility, but it is not known whether any of these is strictly causative.

There is immense variation in clicking of the TMJ. At one extreme a click may be barely perceptible to the subject and cause no distress whatever. It may on occasion, however, become much louder, be heard and remarked upon by others, become uncomfortable or frankly painful, be difficult for the subject to open past, or actually lock. There is also variation in the pattern of disturbance the problem causes over time. The age of onset may be in childhood (even in those patients who seek help in their thirties or forties), but it can appear at almost any age.

Plain radiographs are of no value in determining the position of the disc. This may be done by arthrography, arthroscopy or MRI, but for almost all cases diagnosis on clinical grounds alone is quite satisfactory.

Principal clinical features of disc displacement with reduction

- Click in the temporomandibular joint on opening, closing or both
- Possible association with myofascial pain dysfunction
- Possibly pain free
- Possible normal opening
- Often deviation on opening to side of click before clicking, with straightening afterwards

---

Treatment

Treatment of disc displacement disorders can be controversial. Whereas few would argue that the patient with a persistently painful joint should be offered what reasonable treatment is available, there are big differences of opinion as to the approach that should be taken to the symptomless click.

Where disc displacement with reduction appears to be the cause of suffering, it can be treated with relatively conservative methods, some of which achieve success. The anterior repositioning appliance (Fig. 16.6) is an acrylic device similar to the stabilization splint described earlier, but constructed to fit the occlusion with the mandible protruded and the teeth *just* not in contact. The mandible must be protruded beyond the click, so this appliance is not of value for very late opening clicks. The appliance is worn 24 hours

a day for a period of 2 months. However, this results in difficulty with talking and eating and a high risk of caries beneath the appliance. It is essential that the device is removed for cleaning of itself and the teeth after any food intake. The problem appears to be what is done at the end of the 2-month period. It is common to wean the patient off the device over a period of weeks to months. Temptation to rebuild the occlusion orthodontically or with exotic restorative procedures should be resisted, as there is evidence that teeth move and bone remodels back towards the original positions after this treatment.

For many patients who present with painful clicking, however, the problem is a complex one in which a myofascial pain dysfunction and a disc displacement disorder coexist. Where muscle tone is increased, any clicking will be both louder and more difficult to get past, making the disc displacement disorder more obvious and perhaps more painful. In such cases it is worth treating the condition as if it were entirely muscular in the first instance and reassessing after a reasonable period. It is probably equally true that inflammation within the joint secondary to a damaging disc displacement disorder is likely to aggravate the local musculature.

For a few patients clicking remains a major source of distress—whether by pain, noise or sheer difficulty in getting past the click during normal activities. These will include some patients with intra-articular adhesions. For patients with resistant physical problems a surgical solution may be sought (see Ch. 17). In these cases further imaging of the disc position before irreversible treatment may be reassuring to both patient and surgeon.

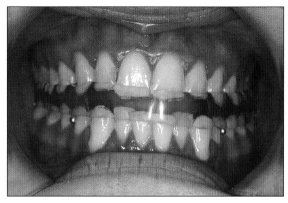

Fig. 16.6 Anterior repositioning splint in place, retained with ball cleats to the lower premolars.

DISC DISPLACEMENT WITHOUT REDUCTION (CLOSED LOCK)

Diagnosis

For those with a click, there may be no substantial change over decades (this is probably the vast majority of people with clicks) or there may be progression along one of two main paths. Intermittent painless locking may develop over months to years, with locks becoming longer and more frequent until eventually it becomes impossible to open past the click. Alternatively, joint pain is associated with the clicking, which worsens over weeks to years and leads to locking, often as a sudden event.

In these situations, the disc remains anteriorly displaced despite the patient's best effort at opening; in other words, there is *no reduction* (Fig. 16.7).

If this is considered a likely diagnosis, great care should be taken to exclude restriction of mouth opening simply due to muscular activity. In general, when locked, mouth opening will be in the range 20–30 mm (hinge movement in the lower joint space permits opening of about 20 mm). Clinical tests might include determining whether opening could be increased by passive stretching (increased opening, particularly with 'hesitation', suggests muscular restriction) and looking for signs that translatory movement in the joint is reduced (lateral and protrusive movement, rather than opening). Imaging of the disc position by MRI is valuable.

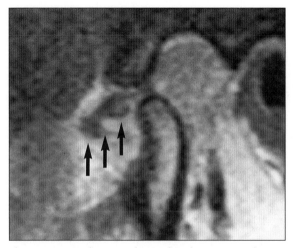

Fig. 16.7   MRI of a non-reducing disc shown in mouth open position. Black arrows point towards disc.

> **Principal clinical features of disc displacement without reduction**
>
> - Limited mouth opening
> - History of a click which has ceased
> - Possibly painful
> - Limited translatory movement

Treatment

Conservative treatment of a true closed lock is not effective in repositioning the disc or increasing mobility. However, there are people whose TMJ discs are anteriorly displaced, non-reducing, but non-painful and associated with apparently normal mobility! Up to 50% of those who develop a closed lock eventually do return to normal, comfortable mobility, without clicking, and many more will see their symptoms improve over a few years. Unfortunately predicting which ones will improve and over what time scale is an inaccurate science.

For those with severe and persistent symptoms surgical options should be considered (see Ch. 17).

DEGENERATIVE JOINT DISEASE

Diagnosis

This condition has close parallels with osteoarthritis as seen elsewhere in the body. In general onset is in middle age. The joint(s) is generally very painful, especially on movement and is often quite tender on palpation of the lateral pole or endaurally. Limitation of movement, particularly translational movement, is often severe with interincisal opening often around 20 mm and sometimes less than that. There is often (but not always) a grating or crackling crepitus on joint movement and the patient will often describe a 'grinding' or 'grating' noise in the joint. Onset is over a few weeks and there is rarely a discrete history of symptomatic temporomandibular disorder before this event.

There is evidence that large-scale molar tooth loss may be associated with this condition, although tooth loss is so common and this condition so uncommon that tooth loss alone cannot be the cause; it is assumed that there must be some form of susceptibility.

This is a temporomandibular disorder in which radiography helps to confirm the diagnosis. There may be erosion, osteophytes or traction spurs in active disease (Fig. 16.8) and marked irregularity of the condylar surface in the resolving phase.

It is now recognized that the disorder has a natural history. A painful inflammatory, erosive, phase lasting up to 3 years is followed by a phase of resolution in which the bone surfaces recover and to some degree smooth out again.

Principal clinical features of degenerative joint disease

- Pain centred in the joint
- Tender joint
- Crepitus
- Limitation of mouth opening
- Limited translatory movement
- Radiological signs (erosion, traction spurs, remodelling)

Treatment

The principle of treatment is to maintain comfort with analgesics (NSAIDs if tolerated) and taking load off the joint by ensuring maximum occlusal support, while awaiting natural resolution. Note that this is likely to take many months. For a few patients it is not possible to achieve satisfactory pain relief in this way and consideration may be given to irrigation of and injection into the joint of steroids, or more invasive surgery. In general, these actions are better taken by those with experience of intra-articular procedures.

SYSTEMIC ARTHROPATHIES

The TMJ may be affected by a wide variety of systemic arthropathies. The juvenile form of rheumatoid arthritis can be very destructive, but fortunately the adult form is rarely so. Ankylosing spondylitis, reactive arthritis, gout, systemic lupus erythematosus and psoriatic arthritis are all seen in the TMJ periodically and all have the capacity to cause permanent damage to joint surfaces with loss of condylar height (Fig. 16.9). Reactive arthritis seems particularly prone to causing adhesions in the joint.

Treatment of the TMJ problem is best taken as part of the overall management of the arthropathy and is therefore usually left in the hands of the rheumatologist. It can, however, be beneficial to reduce loading on the affected joint if that is possible. Sometimes surgical treatment local to the TMJ is appropriate.

ATYPICAL FACIAL PAIN AND OTHER NON-DENTAL CAUSES OF PAIN

The remaining disorders mentioned in this chapter are included primarily for purposes of differential

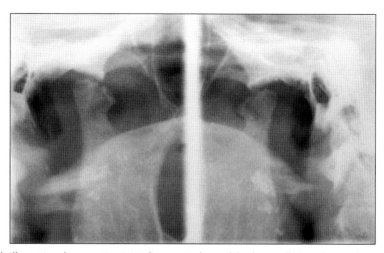

Fig. 16.8 Radiograph illustrating degenerative joint disease. Both condyles have a flattened, irregular superior surface; there is an active erosion centrally in the right condyle.

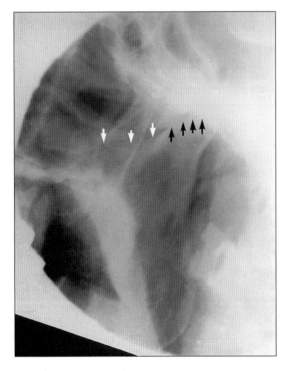

Fig. 16.9 Radiograph showing destruction of the condyle due to ankylosing spondylitis. White arrows show the sigmoid notch, the black arrows show the margin of what remains of the condyle.

diagnosis and to clarify what the dentist is, or is not, fitted to assist with.

Atypical facial pain

Atypical facial pain was originally a 'dustbin' diagnosis; that is, when all other possible causes of pain had been carefully considered and excluded, the pain was considered to be 'atypical'. It is now recognized that the group of patients who describe this painful condition often describe a similar pattern of events and there are sufficient common features to consider this as one disorder.

The origin of the pain is often associated with an item of dental treatment, although sometimes careful questioning reveals a significant period of pain that caused the patient to seek treatment. The pain persists, despite the best efforts of the dentist, who may restore the tooth, root fill it or extract it, all to no benefit. The author's experience is that dry socket is commonly diagnosed after extraction and that this too seems uncommonly delayed in resolution.

It is not unusual for such wounds to be surgically explored without abnormal findings. There may be some brief respite in the pain but soon it is back at the same site or nearby, prompting the patient's response that the wrong tooth has been removed and that something more must be done to put the condition right. Further local dental treatment does not bring that relief.

It is not surprising that the patient becomes frustrated by the apparent ineffectiveness of the dentist, often then migrating from dentist to dentist, and doctor to doctor in a vain search for relief.

The pain itself is variable in nature and in severity but remarkably chronic in duration, lasting for years. Indeed it is often more than a year before the diagnosis is made. In general the pain is continuous. It may be sharp, aching, throbbing, burning, with some variation in intensity over time and responds poorly to common analgesics. It is often associated with allodynia (pain experienced as a result of stimuli not normally capable of causing pain), but there are no local signs such as inflammation or discharge. The pain may also migrate from one site to another although generally it remains within the same quadrant.

There is a strong predilection for women and the more common age for diagnosis is the late forties or fifties. There is a strong association between this condition and anxiety and depression, although there has never been any proof that the psychological disturbances are causative. There is also a strong element in these patients of 'somatization', suggesting a mechanism by which pain *might* result from psychological sources. It is probable that the process of neuronal plasticity plays a role in the development and maintenance of the condition, though why these particular people are afflicted is not known.

No investigations are of great value in diagnosis, except where they actively exclude other local causes of pain. For that reason the practitioner must be on the lookout for pain that does not correspond to local disease and the pattern of poor response to treatment described above.

Treatment of atypical facial pain

Treatment of atypical facial pain may take the form of general analgesics, antidepressant therapy, referral to a psychologist or psychiatrist, transcutaneous electrical nerve stimulation (TENS) or other pain

---

Principal clinical features of atypical facial pain

- Pain not evidently associated with current dental disease
- Pain persistent and not responsive to dental treatments
- Pain not consistent with common neurological causes (neuralgias and migraine)
- Common history of demands for treatment, leading to conservative, then extraction treatment
- Common history of dry socket
- Tendency for pain to migrate from original site over a period of months to years

---

management strategies. Beware, though! Great care should be taken in treatment planning not to give the impression that the pain is in any way 'imagined' or not real, or that the dentist is washing their hands of a troublesome patient. These patients suffer very real pain, are deserving of proper attention and require thorough evaluation. However, also beware the opposite extreme. It is possible, by repeatedly attempting dental solutions where none will bring relief, to reinforce the patient's belief that this is a dental condition and that the practitioner is patently incompetent, failing to cure the condition.

A sound policy is:

- recognize the condition as early as possible
- remedy any obvious local causes of pain
- avoid irreversible treatments
- advise the patient on the diagnosis and prognosis
- be supportive
- ensure real dental disease is managed on its own merits
- refer to a specialist early.

Three statistical rules or guidelines on chronic facial pain may be of help:

1. Pain present for more than one year, despite reasonable efforts at diagnosis and treatment, is unlikely to respond to local treatment now
2. The greater the number of hospital specialists the patient has seen concerning the pain, the lower the chance of success with dental treatment
3. There is often a buried tooth on the side of the face afflicted by the pain, *but its removal almost never brings relief.*

These guidelines may appear fatuous, but they can help to prevent the unwary practitioner from being pushed into unhelpful treatments and hence delaying treatments offering the best chance of benefit.

Atypical facial pain should be clearly distinguished from well-defined neurological and central causes of facial pain.

Trigeminal neuralgia

The pain of trigeminal neuralgia is experienced within the distribution of the trigeminal nerve, usually either the maxillary or mandibular division and usually unilaterally. Classically it is severe, sharp, electrical or needle-like in quality, coming in multiple short bursts, usually on light touch or gentle stimulation of a skin or mucosal surface (a trigger zone). There may be after-pain, but usually there is relief between episodes. Sometimes firm palpation of the trigger zone fails to elicit the pain.

The condition is treated with anticonvulsants, the first line being carbamazepine, but phenytoin and sodium valproate are also used successfully. The author's view is that this condition is better managed in the longer term by a neurologist, although it is acknowledged that, provided thorough monitoring is carried out, it may be managed by a dental specialist. There has been a vogue for surgical resection or cryotherapy of the peripheral nerves in the distribution of the pain, but the pain relief these treatments bring is of relatively short duration (1–2 years). They also cause numbness which the patient sometimes finds almost as bad as the pain. Radiofrequency lesions of the trigeminal ganglion or, in extreme cases, dissection of the trigeminal nerve roots in the posterior cranial fossa appears more valuable in cases resistant to medical management.

Trigeminal neuralgia is almost exclusively a condition of the older person. Therefore, when the diagnosis is made in someone under 50 years of age, early referral to a neurologist is wise to exclude disorders such as multiple sclerosis or intracranial neoplasms.

Migraine and cluster headache

Migraine is a very common condition, but is generally a cause of headache rather than facial pain. Classic migraine associated with nausea, visual disturbance and photophobia is relatively uncommon, most migraines being what is called 'common migraine' which is a periodic headache without these additional features. Common migraine is thought to be of vascular origin and usually responds to prophylactic treatment with triptans ($5HT_1$ antagonists). It is also treated with simple analgesics in many sufferers. The chief distinction to be made for the dentist is that from myofascial pain, particularly where the latter affects the temporalis muscle (or occipitofrontalis) and thus causes headache. There is evidence that some migraine responds to treatment with occlusal appliances; this is a controversial area for dental involvement.

Cluster headache is a very similar pain that may be experienced in the head and face, sometimes associated with flushing of the skin, congestion and running of the nose.

Giant-cell arteritis

This is one of very few painful conditions of the face for which early diagnosis can make a major difference to the outcome. The condition, which affects only elderly people is recognized by pain that is severe, inflammatory in type and centred over the worst affected arteries. There is a severe vasculitis, which, although it may present primarily in the head and neck region, is a systemic disorder. This is confirmed by biopsy. The superficial temporal artery, if affected, is enlarged, hardened and tender. If untreated, the risk of occlusion of the retinal arteries is high, with resultant permanent blindness: early treatment with systemic steroids is very effective in preventing this.

The dentist's role is in recognition and *early* referral.

Referred pain

Occasionally pain in the face may be referred from more distant sites. The typical example cited in textbooks is of pain due to angina pectoris being felt in the left mandible, in addition to the more classical sites for anginal pain (centrally in the chest, at the left shoulder and down the inner aspect of the left upper arm). The author has also witnessed a patient requesting extraction of a lower left molar tooth, when the cause of pain was a left-sided spontaneous pneumothorax. Pain in the jaws may also derive from the pharynx, ear and neck.

It is beyond the scope of this book to deal in detail with all possible non-dental causes of facial pain, but dentists should be aware of the possibility that pain felt in the jaws may not be caused within their area. Great care should therefore be exercised if difficulty is being experienced in diagnosis.

FURTHER READING

Feinmann C., Harris M. (1984a) Psychogenic facial pain. Part 1: the clinical presentation. *British Dental Journal* 156: 165–168.

Feinmann C., Harris M. (1984b) Psychogenic facial pain. Part 2: management and prognosis. *British Dental Journal* 156: 205–208.

Gray R. J. M., Davies S. J., Quayle A. A. (1995) *Temporomandibular disorders: a clinical approach*. British Dental Journal, London.

Hall E. H., Terezhalmy G. T., Pelleu G. B. (1986) A set of descriptors for the diagnosis of dental pain syndromes. *Oral Surgery* 61: 153–157.

Harrison S. D. (2002) Atypical facial pain and atypical odontalgia. In: Zakrewska J. M., Harrison S. D. (eds.) *Assessment and management of orofacial pain*. Pain Research and Clinical Management, Vol 14. Elsevier, Amsterdam, Netherlands, pp. 255–266.

Helkimo M. (1976) Epidemiological surveys of the masticatory system. In: Melcher A. H., Zarb G. A. (eds.) *Oral Sciences Reviews No 7 Temporomandibular joint function and dysfunction III*. Munksgaard, Copenhagen, Denmark, 7: 54–69.

Kurita K., Westesson P-L., Yuasa H., Toyama M., Machida J., Ogi N. (1998) Natural course of untreated symptomatic temporomandibular joint disk displacement without reduction. *Journal of Dental Research* 77: 361–365.

McNeill C. (ed.) (1993) *Temporomandibular Disorders. Guidelines for classification, assessment and management.* Quintessence, Chicago, IL.

Morris S., Benjamin S., Gray R. J. M., Bennett D. (1997) Physical, psychiatric and social characteristics of the temporomandibular disorder pain dysfunction syndrome: the relationship of mental disorders to presentation. *British Dental Journal* 182: 255–260.

Nitzan D. W., Samson B., Better H. (1997) Long-term outcome of arthrocentesis for sudden onset, persistent, severe closed lock of the temporomandibular joint. *Journal of Oral and Maxillofacial Surgery* 55: 151–157.

Okeson J. P. (1989) *Management of temporomandibular disorders and occlusion*, 4th edn. Mosby, St Louis, MO.

Okeson J. P., Bell W. E. (eds.) (1995) *Bell's orofacial pain*, 5th edn. Quintessence, Chicago, IL.

Sarnat B. G., Laskin D. M. (1992) *The temporomandibular joint. A biological basis for clinical practice*, 4th edn. Saunders, Philadelphia, PA.

Schnurr R. F., Brooke R. I. (1992) Atypical odontalgia: update and comment on long-term follow-up. *Oral Surgery* 73: 445–448.

Seligman D. A., Pullinger A. G. (1991) The role of functional occlusal relationships in temporomandibular disorders: a review. *Journal of Craniomandibular Disorders* 5: 265–279.

Westling L. (1992) Temporomandibular joint dysfunction and systemic joint laxity. *Swedish Dental Journal* Supplement 81: 1–79.

SELF-ASSESSMENT

1. List four features of muscular pain that help to distinguish it from pain of purely dental origin.
2. Name two features that distinguish pain arising from inflammation in the TMJ from muscular pain.
3. By what means can limitation of mouth opening due to myofascial pain dysfunction be distinguished from that due to disc displacement without reduction?
4. In what circumstances should a surgical solution be considered for a disc displacement disorder?
5. What is the significance of a grating noise in the TMJ associated with a tender joint and severe limitation of joint movement?
6. A patient attends with a 2-month history of worsening bilateral preauricular pain and tenderness of the masseter and lateral pterygoid muscles associated with interincisal opening of 28 mm. There is no evident local dental disease. She suggests that recently she has been clenching her teeth quite a lot because of difficulties at work and wakes with severe pain every morning. What advice should you give, and what treatments are available?
7. What features noted in the history or on examination would alert you to the possible diagnosis of atypical facial pain?
8. How does the pain of trigeminal neuralgia differ from that of atypical facial pain?
9. How should the diagnosis of atypical facial pain modify general dental treatment planning?

Answers on page 270.

17 Surgery of the temporomandibular joint

J. Pedlar

- Most disorders of the masticatory apparatus do *not* require surgical treatment.
- Those disorders which benefit from a surgical approach often present first to the general dental or medical practitioner.
- Some such disorders prevent normal dental treatment because of limited mouth opening.
- Surgery can range from closed manipulation to major reconstruction of the joint.

ASSUMED KNOWLEDGE

It is assumed that at this stage you will have knowledge/competencies in the following areas:

- structure (including radiology) and movements of the masticatory apparatus
- variation within the population at large in position of the intra-articular disc and its function
- clinical features and non-surgical management techniques of temporomandibular disorders (as described in Ch. 16).

If you think that you are not well equipped in these areas, revise them before reading this chapter or cross-check with texts on those subjects as you read.

INTENDED LEARNING OUTCOMES

At the end of this chapter you should be able to:

1. Distinguish temporomandibular disorders that may require surgical treatment from those which do not and evaluate the degree of urgency for such treatment
2. Describe investigations that would help to clarify the nature of a particular disorder
3. Describe surgical approaches to the temporomandibular joint and anticipate anatomical sources of surgical complication
4. Evaluate, with a patient, the advantages and disadvantages of the more common surgical treatments of the temporomandibular joint
5. Describe a method for successful reduction of a dislocation of the temporomandibular joint.

MINIMALLY INVASIVE TECHNIQUES

Injection into the joint

Entry into the joint with a needle, from the skin surface, may be necessary for the instillation of steroid or local anaesthetic solution and is a prerequisite for insertion of an arthroscope as the joint needs to be distended with fluid from within.

The upper joint space is most easily approached from below and behind, starting from a point 10 mm in front of the point of the tragus, just below a line that joins that point to the outer canthus (Fig. 17.1). With the mouth open, or the mandible protruded, the needle is inserted upwards, forwards and medially, until it penetrates the capsule just above and behind the condyle; this may be as deep as 2 cm from the surface. To check that the needle is in the joint, a small quantity of saline is injected then drawn back. It should be readily possible to flush fluid in and out of the joint. If no fluid can be withdrawn, the tip of the needle is unlikely to be in the joint and the position should be reassessed and adjusted. The average joint may be distended with about 2 mL of fluid.

Closed manipulation for adhesions: method and results

In cases of disc displacement without reduction, it is common that adhesions prevent the normal movement of the disc in the upper joint space. It is sometimes possible to release the lock and increase mobility by closed manipulation.

In general, pain during the procedure would be considerable if no form of anaesthesia were provided: muscle guarding in such circumstances is too powerful to permit the necessary manipulation. Local anaesthesia is often sufficient and is achieved by placing the local anaesthetic (lidocaine with epinephrine) posterior to the joint, close to the auriculotemporal nerve or in the joint itself. Patients

should be warned in advance that occasionally local anaesthetic might diffuse from the site of injection to the facial nerve, giving rise to a temporary facial palsy. Should there be any weakness of the eyelids, the affected eye should be taped shut for the duration of the local anaesthetic.

It is important, after the local anaesthetic has been placed, to measure the mouth opening, in order later to be able to determine the change that has taken place. The operator stands beside the patient, who is seated and leaning slightly backwards. The operator holds the mandible, with the thumb from the opposite hand inside the patient's mouth, resting on the posterior teeth and the fingers placed beneath the body of the mandible (Fig. 17.2). The patient's head is held fast against the operator's body with the other hand, the fingers of which are placed over the TMJ to feel any movement within it. The thumb is used to push down on the posterior teeth and distract the joint, then slowly the mandible is drawn forwards with increasing force until increased mobility is achieved. This often happens as one or two sudden releases. When maximum movement is achieved, mouth opening should be measured again.

It is often possible to gain considerable mobility in closed lock by this technique. Unfortunately it can result in considerable pain over the following few days, leading to the patient moving their jaw little

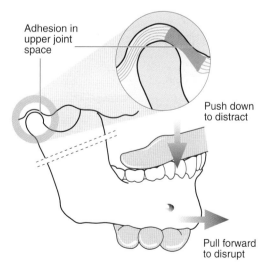

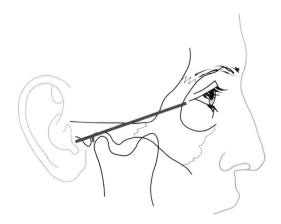

Fig. 17.1 Anatomical landmarks for needle entry into the TMJ. An imaginary line may be drawn from the tip of the tragus to the outer canthus; injection point is noted approximately 10 mm forward along this line and 2 mm below it.

Fig. 17.2 Closed manipulation for anterior disc displacement with reduction. The thumb is placed on the posterior teeth and the fingers beneath the jaw. The joint is distracted downwards then the jaw is pulled forwards to disrupt the adhesions.

and the consequent reforming of adhesions. This effect can be reduced by giving NSAIDs before and after the treatment, but a considerable inflammatory exudate still remains within the joint. The pain and immobility can be eased further by irrigating the joint with saline and instilling a small quantity of steroid (see pp. 242, 245).

Arthroscopy

An arthroscope is an endoscope designed specifically for use within a joint (Fig. 17.3). TMJ arthroscopes are up to 2.8 mm in diameter and rigid. With these devices it is possible to inspect the whole of the upper joint space without formally dissecting the joint, all through a skin puncture a few millimetres in diameter.

The joint is distended by injection of about 2 mL saline (see above). Initially the sheath is inserted through a skin puncture with a pointed but round-ended trocar inside it. This is pushed upwards, inwards and forwards until it reaches the joint capsule. At this stage the trocar may be replaced with a more round-ended one to enter the upper joint space itself. Entry into the joint is far easier if the capsule has been distended with saline and is taut. Once into the joint, the trocar is removed, leaving the sheath in place, and is replaced with the arthroscope, which is attached to the fibreoptic light source and saline for irrigation. Because there tends to be some bleeding into the joint at the point of entry, vision would rapidly deteriorate if the joint were not washed through, but at this stage there is only one portal for both entry and exit. So, now a needle (or a second arthroscope port) is placed about a centimetre further forwards and parallel to the arthroscope itself; this can act as the exit (or egress) cannula. Saline is now slowly flushed through the joint as it is examined.

The joint can be examined by direct vision, but it is more common to attach a video camera to the scope and to display what is seen on a television monitor (Fig. 17.4).

With the simplest of equipment the joint can be inspected, usually starting with the posterior recess, looking at the position of the disc, the condition of the posterior attachment tissues and the synovium on the medial aspect of the joint. The scope is then swept anteriorly over the top of the disc to look at the anterior parts of the joint. By inspection alone it is possible to detect disc displacement, adhesions, degenerative changes in the disc and cartilage over the glenoid fossa and articular eminence and synovial inflammation. It is possible, if adhesions are

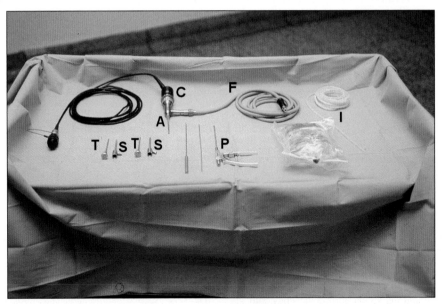

Fig. 17.3 Arthroscopy equipment. A = arthroscope; C = camera; F = fibreoptic cable; I = irrigation tubing and saline to run through; T = trocars; S = sheaths through which trocars and scope are passed; P = biopsy punch and other tools for use with arthroscope.

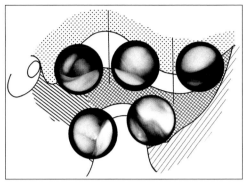

Fig. 17.4 Views of the TMJ obtained through the arthroscope (courtesy of Dr K.-I. Murakami and Harcourt Brace Publishers). Top left = upper posterior synovial pouch; top middle = intermediate space showing disc below; top right = upper anterior synovial recess; bottom left = lower posterior synovial pouch; bottom right = lower anterior synovial pouch.

detected, to replace the blunt-ended trocar and sweep around within the joint to break them down. The joint must be thoroughly irrigated at the end of the procedure and many surgeons will finally instil a steroid before leaving the joint. It is often necessary to place one suture in the skin wound.

If two arthroscope ports are used it is possible to perform surgery within the joint under direct vision. Procedures including disrupting adhesions, biopsy and smoothing roughened areas may be relatively straightforward for the expert arthroscopist, but attempts are also being made to shorten the posterior attachment tissues and reposition the disc by laser surgery. In time such procedures may become more routine.

Selection of patients is very much a matter of personal judgement. Great reliance has been placed on a failure to respond to conservative measures, with persistent pain being a central criterion. Nonetheless, if arthroscopy is intended to be therapeutic and not just a diagnostic procedure there must be some real expectation of a mechanical problem within the joint. Therefore disc displacement disorders and degenerative joint disease resistant to conservative treatments may be indications for arthroscopy, whereas painful muscular conditions are not.

Studies of the effectiveness of arthroscopy have been very encouraging, with a success rate of approximately 90%, but there have been few randomized controlled trials against conservative or more aggressive surgical treatments to allow thorough scientific evaluation. Success rates must depend upon which patients are entered into the studies, and details of patient selection in reported trials have been scanty.

Arthroscopy is a procedure associated with few serious complications. The most common problem is failure to enter the joint cleanly, or at all, although the incidence of this decreases with experience. For this reason, considerable training is recommended before independent use of arthroscopes. Poor entry into the joint results not only in physical injury to the joint capsule and/or the joint surfaces but also in greater leakage of irrigant into the surrounding tissues leading to massive swelling. Bleeding along the entry tract or into the joint is an occasional problem, but is usually readily controlled with pressure. The scope may be misdirected towards the external ear canal or upward towards the middle cranial fossa (the bone of the glenoid fossa is paper thin) or may be placed deep to the joint in the pharyngeal wall. These are serious complications and great effort must be taken with technique to avoid them.

Summary of arthroscopy technique

- Insert a sheath with a trocar into the joint
- Replace the trocar with the scope
- Illuminate the joint fibreoptically
- Irrigate the joint via the sheath and an egress cannula
- View the joint via a camera attached to the scope
- Sometimes instrument the joint via a second port

Advantages of arthroscopy

- Minimally invasive
- Diagnostic information obtained

Disadvantages of arthroscopy

- Limited scope for reconstructive surgery
- Requires high level of operator skill

Arthrocentesis

In view of the success of simple arthroscopy, attempts have been made to achieve the benefits without the use of extremely expensive equipment. There are several reports of great benefit from simply irrigating the joint with a considerable flow of saline.

Irrigation is best performed with two needles in the joint, placed as for arthroscopy, and can be used either alone to flush out inflammatory mediators from an inflamed joint or combined with a closed manipulation for closed lock. It is of course a 'blind' procedure and therefore offers little diagnostic information, and there is some risk that sharp needles within the joint over a period of an hour or more will damage joint surfaces, but it appears from clinical results that this is not a major problem.

Success rates with arthrocentesis appear comparable with those for arthroscopy for both painful non-reducing disc displacement and for degenerative joint disease, although studies of direct comparison are few and involve small numbers of subjects.

SURGICAL APPROACHES TO THE TMJ (FIG. 17.5)

Preauricular approach

The most common surgical approach by which the TMJ is entered is via a vertical incision about 3 cm in length immediately in front of the ear, extending to just below the tragus. This relatively less vascular plane gives access at its upper end to the temporalis fascia and through that to the root of the zygomatic arch. The dissection remains above the main trunk

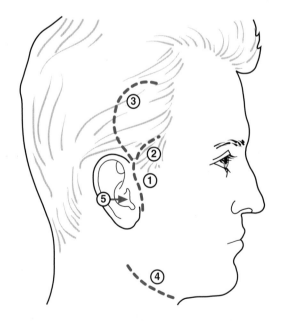

Fig. 17.5 Surgical access to the TMJ. 1. Preauricular incision; 2. temporal extension; 3. 'question mark' extension; 4. submandibular incision for access to the condylar neck; 5. endaural approach.

of the facial nerve and allows dissection along the zygomatic arch at a subperiosteal level, beneath the zygomatic and temporal branches of the seventh cranial nerve. The joint capsule is exposed from a posterosuperior aspect.

The approach is relatively simple and, provided one resists the temptation to dissect too close to the external auditory meatus (which is directed forwards as it extends inward), the risks are small. Some degree of temporary injury to the auriculo-temporal nerve and the zygomatic and temporal branches of the facial nerve due to traction occasionally occurs. The incision leaves a scar on an exposed facial surface (although this is rarely unsightly).

The incision can be extended upwards and forward to give better access, or into a question mark shape to additionally minimize damage to the auriculo-temporal nerve. However, most surgeons feel that the additional access gained by these extensions is of little advantage.

Submandibular approach

The preauricular approach gives good access to the joint itself, but access to the condylar neck is poor. Where such access is necessary, a submandibular approach may be made. The skin incision is usually about 5 cm in length and two finger breadths below the angle of the mandible, in a skin crease. Dissection is carried through in layers to the deep investing layer of fascia to minimize inadvertent risk to the marginal mandibular branch of the seventh nerve. Once bone is reached at the lower border of the mandible, dissection is continued at a subperiosteal plane upwards to the condylar neck. However, access is still not good.

Endaural and other approaches

Other approaches that attempt to overcome the problems of the two previously mentioned have been described. These have included entering the joint posteriorly, through the external ear canal, or by a skin incision behind the ear, folding the whole ear forwards. These may improve the visible scarring, but do relatively little for access, unless it is essential to focus on the posterior aspect of the joint and they do increase the potential for ear damage. Access to the condylar neck may be gained by an incision posterior to and nearly parallel with the posterior border of the ascending mandibular ramus, with dissection taken through parotid to masseter muscle and thence to the mandible. Access to the condylar neck is extremely good but there is an increased risk of facial nerve damage.

DISC DISPLACEMENT DISORDERS

Meniscectomy (discectomy), disc replacement or disc repositioning

For patients with persistent mechanical problems of the joint such as painful reducing or non-reducing disc displacement, or restricted mouth opening due to such disc problems it may be appropriate to open the joint surgically to reposition or remove the disc. Sometimes the disc is perforated, fragmented or so tightly tethered that it cannot be satisfactorily repositioned. Consequently it must be removed.

It has often been believed that if the disc is removed and not replaced there is an increased risk of degenerative joint disease. However, several reports of long-term follow-up of discectomy have shown few clinical signs of that. Various strategies have been employed in relation to that supposed risk. The simplest has been to accept the risk and deal with the problem if and when it arises. Alternatively, an alloplastic material such as Silastic may be placed instead of the disc. If left in the longer term this material fragments, causing multiple granulomas in the joint and a worsening problem. However, if a thin sheet is left for a period of months, a layer of fibrous tissue forms around it; this has been considered as a reasonable replacement for the disc. There is inadequate information to judge this view.

It is also possible to replace the disc with tissue, in the form of either a free graft of tissue such as dermis (from the abdomen or buttock) or local viable tissue such as temporalis fascia or muscle. The fascia tends to be rather thin and if a substantial muscle flap is brought down into the joint there tends to remain an aesthetic defect at the temple. Consideration should certainly be given to replacement of the disc if discs are to be removed from both joints, as the likelihood of developing anterior open bite is high in this situation.

Surgical access is by a preauricular approach, opening the joint capsule horizontally to gain access to both joint spaces, leaving enough capsule attached to the zygomatic arch to permit closure. The disc is mobilized and either pulled back into position, and tethered by ligating it laterally to fascia behind and lateral to the joint or is removed with or without replacement.

Disc repositioning surgery was regarded as the treatment of choice through much of the later part of the twentieth century, but it became apparent that although success in relief of pain was fairly good, the disc frequently remained malpositioned, suggesting our understanding of how such operations work was limited. All surgery to the disc within the joint carries a significant chance of failure to control symptoms.

TOTAL REPLACEMENT OF THE TMJ

With the success of replacement hip, knee and other prostheses, it is inevitable that consideration should be given to total replacement of the TMJ. Early experiences with Proplast-Teflon prostheses, however, set a very bad precedent. The surfaces of the alloplast were subject to wear, leading to loose fragments in the tissue and some very severe inflammatory reactions.

More recently, prostheses which appear to be better tolerated have been developed and the track record of the currently available prostheses is well documented. Nonetheless, total joint replacement is expensive and leaves no easy escape if the surgery is unsuccessful and symptoms continue. It should be regarded as a last resort for the few cases of true joint disease where other approaches are just not viable (such as where significant height has been lost in the condyle due to bone erosion) or where simpler surgery has been unsuccessful.

DEGENERATIVE AND INFLAMMATORY JOINT DISEASE

The recommended mainstream treatment of degenerative joint disease is conservative, as it frequently resolves spontaneously over a few years. However, in some cases pain is severe and not readily controlled by restorative and pharmaceutical approaches. In such circumstances, as a short-term measure, it may be valuable to irrigate the joint and instil a short-acting steroid (such as aqueous hydrocortisone) to reduce inflammation. Repeated use of depot steroid preparations can cause significant bone resorption and therefore is best avoided.

Now that there is good evidence that degenerative joint disease affecting the TMJ tends to have a limited period of activity, after which it tends to resolve, the role of surgery in the disorder needs to be considered carefully. If, however, there is severe bone change with roughened irregular surfaces preventing simple joint movement, operation to smooth surfaces or to interpose a soft-tissue flap between bone ends can be justified.

Where a systemic or local arthropathy has caused significant bone loss and a reduction in condylar height, an anterior open bite can result. In this situation, provided that the inflammatory process has ceased (this may be determined on repeat radiographs or by an isotope bone scan), it may be appropriate to carry out an osteotomy to lengthen the ramus or to place a prosthetic joint.

DISLOCATION OF THE TMJ

Diagnosis

Dislocation of a joint is a displacement of one component of the joint beyond its normal limits, without spontaneous return to its normal position.

Dislocation of the TMJ is a diagnosis that is simple to make and generally requires no further investigation. The history is of an event following wide mouth opening (such as yawning, vomiting, laughing, dental treatment or trauma), after which the patient can no longer close their mouth. If both joints are dislocated and the patient is dentate the mouth remains wide open, although sometimes the patient may be able to close *towards a protruded position*. If only one joint is dislocated there is a marked deviation to the opposite side and the teeth may be brought closer together but still nowhere near back into occlusion. For a few hours after the event there remains a depression just in front of the ear where the condyle would normally be found, but in time that fills with oedema and, although palpable, it ceases to be clearly visible. The condition is painful, may become increasingly so with time and is associated with considerable muscle guarding.

The condyle of the dislocated joint is in front of the articular eminence and the mandible is rotated downwards, leaving the posterior face of the condyle resting against the anterior aspect of the eminence (Fig. 17.6).

Treatment

The short-term treatment is manual reduction. This may be helped by local anaesthesia or sedation, but these are rarely necessary.

The author's technique is to stand behind the patient, who is lying down on a trolley or in the dental chair, with their head at the operator's waist level. Both thumbs are placed inside the mouth, resting on the molar teeth, with fingers of both hands beneath the patient's chin. The operator presses down on the posterior teeth at the same time as lifting the chin occlusally. Pressure is increased steadily until the joints 'pop' back into place. Sometimes, if there is considerable resistance, it helps to press more on one side than the other and reduce the joints separately.

The next stage is almost as important. There is a natural tendency when the joints are reduced for the patient to immediately open their mouth wide again, reproducing the dislocation. Therefore the patient should be warned about it in advance and should keep the mouth firmly shut for about 30 seconds to a minute after reduction, only slowly easing the upward chin pressure. Redislocation is common within the first 24 hours, so patients should

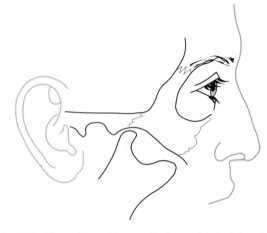

Fig. 17.6 The position of the mandibular condyle in dislocation, forwards of the articular eminence and rotated.

be warned not to open their mouth wide during this time.

Some dislocations are not repeated, but for many patients, repeated episodes of dislocation occur, despite great care. This very distressing condition may be managed entirely conservatively, either by the patient learning to avoid situations in which dislocation is likely or by training friends or family members to reduce the dislocations as they occur. For some the frequency of the events or the difficulty of reduction may warrant more active attempts to prevent further dislocation.

Some success has been reported with the injection of *Botulinus* toxin into the lateral pterygoid muscle. This causes prolonged muscle weakness, aimed at preventing the forward displacement associated with dislocation. It is not yet widely accepted and long-term study of its effects must be awaited. Operative surgery is the alternative.

Reduction of dislocation of the TMJ

- Have the patient supine
- Stand behind the head
- Place the thumbs on the posterior teeth and the fingers under the chin
- Press increasingly firmly on the posterior teeth while pulling gently up anteriorly
- If there is great resistance concentrate on one side at a time
- When reduced hold the mouth shut for 30 seconds or so
- Advise restricted mouth opening for at least 24 hours

Surgery for recurrent dislocation

Many operations have been described (this is usually a testament to a poor success rate) and it is not appropriate to deal in detail with all of them here.

The principles of their action are, however, relatively simple. Techniques fall into several categories:

- prevention of forward condylar movement by placing a block (bone, cartilage, alloplast) on the articular eminence, in front of the condyle
- prevention of condylar movement by tightening the constraints of the capsule
- limitation of the forward pull of lateral pterygoid (by section)

- permitting easier reduction of the dislocation by reduction of the height of the eminence.

All procedures have their advocates, all can be successful, all can fail and comparative success rates are not available. Selection of procedure therefore tends to be a matter of personal preference.

ANKYLOSIS OF THE TMJ

Diagnosis

The pathology of this condition is described in pathology texts, but it is worth reminding readers that ankylosis is the physical union of two bones that normally are partners in a movable joint. The union may be partial or total and either fibrous or bony (Fig. 17.7). In the TMJ the cause may be trauma (especially intracapsular fractures), infection or a systemic arthropathy such as juvenile rheumatoid or reactive arthritis.

The principal clinical feature is severe restriction of mouth opening (no more than a few millimetres). The onset may be traced to a particular event (infective or traumatic) or it may be slowly progressive. In either event there is no relief. Investigation should include CT and/or MR imaging as well as conventional radiographs to determine the bone relationships (not only in the joint but also between the coronoid process and the zygomatic arch, maxilla and squamous temporal). Care should be taken to

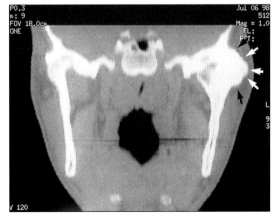

Fig. 17.7 CT scan showing ankylosis of the TMJ. An extensive mass of bone (arrows) extends around the lateral aspect of the left joint and the joint space is not visible. There is also loss of joint space in the right joint.

exclude muscular causes of limited opening and the rare hysterical reactions which do not derive from the joint at all.

Treatment

Treatment is directed either at mobilizing the existing joint, if there remains a satisfactory one, and attempting to prevent reformation of the ankylosis or at forming a false joint lower down in the mandible. Provided that the bony masses around the joint are not too extensive, particularly on the medial side (where they may encroach on the middle meningeal artery and other structures), mobilization of the joint is the preferred option.

To dissect the joint and restore its mobility may require access from both preauricular and submandibular approaches and is a time-consuming process. It is likely that both right and left joints will need to be dissected to achieve mobility and sometimes it is also necessary to section the coronoid processes to get the mouth open. Whether it is then felt necessary to interpose something (such as temporalis muscle or fascia) between the bone ends to prevent reformation of the ankylosis depends upon what is found at operation.

The construction of a false joint may be attempted at the condylar neck or lower in the ascending ramus and requires that the mandible be sectioned, the area of contact between the bone ends reduced and something interposed between the bone ends to prevent new bone formation. The construction of a false joint has the advantage of being somewhat easier to perform and with a more predictable short-term result. Its disadvantage is that hinge movement is all that can be achieved.

With surgical management of ankylosis the main problem is postoperative loss of the opening gained by surgery. Intensive physiotherapy in the form of opening exercises, which can be performed by the patient, reduces the loss but must be maintained for weeks to months. Pain relief is very important to permit therapy.

FRACTURE DISLOCATION OF THE NECK OF THE MANDIBULAR CONDYLE

Most fractures of the condylar neck of the mandible do not strictly involve the joint itself. They are of interest here because the surgical approaches to such fractures are the approaches to the TMJ and any active surgical treatment is undertaken because of effects of the fracture on the functioning of the joint (see p. 195).

In the event of bilateral fracture dislocations of the mandibular condylar neck, the elevator muscles pull the mandible up posteriorly and create an anterior open bite. If poorly treated, as many as 50% of patients with this condition are left with marked occlusal problems or persistent problems with their TMJ. Open reduction and internal fixation with plates or screws reduces the morbidity considerably.

Fractures within the capsule of the joint are more likely to result in ankylosis, but are not as amenable to open reduction and fixation.

TUMOURS

Tumours in or around the TMJ may be benign or malignant, local or secondary but are all relatively rare. Biopsy may be necessary on occasion, in which case generally the area will need to be formally dissected. Tumours here, as elsewhere, are dealt with according to their expected behaviour and extent. If resection is proposed it may be necessary to replace resected tissue with a graft, such as a costochondral free graft.

POST-SURGICAL MANAGEMENT

Mobility

Following any TMJ surgery there is a tendency for the patient to avoid opening the mouth because of pain. However, early mobilization is desirable to reduce the tendency for scar tissue formation to limit mobility in the longer term. This need for mobilization must be weighed against any likelihood that excessive movement in the early postoperative stages would place the wounds under too much strain and cause separation at suture lines.

The rate and extent of mobilization is therefore dependent upon the nature of the surgery performed. For example, following a meniscal repositioning procedure where a section of disc has been removed, mobilization should be treated with caution for a few weeks.

Active physiotherapy provided by therapists may be very helpful.

Feeding

It is also important to anticipate the patient's inability to chew and reluctance to move their jaw by planning for a very soft or liquid diet in advance. The capacity to take in adequate food and drink should be confirmed before discharge from hospital.

Time scale of recovery

Scar tissue in the wounds develops from about 2–3 weeks onwards, gradually increasing in strength over many months. It is expected that the jaw movement will have recovered to its best level by about 2 months after surgery. If it is necessary to apply intermaxillary fixation for a period, retrieving full mobility may be much more difficult.

Complications

Surgery to the TMJ is subject to the same range of adverse events as other surgery: bleeding, wound infection, unsightly scars, etc. However, a few addi-tional problems are specific to the site. The major complications of TMJ surgery can be anticipated from the anatomy.

Stretch injury of the branches of the facial nerve can cause weakness of orbicularis oculi, or frontalis or at the corner of the mouth. Numbness in the distribution of the auriculotemporal nerve is common.

Some occlusal disturbance is common with any intra-articular procedure, but is usually short-lived.

Injury to nearby structures such as the external auditory meatus and middle meningeal artery should be avoided but have been reported.

Probably the most irritating complication, from the patient's point of view, is Frey's syndrome (see also Ch. 14). This comprises flushing of the cheek or preauricular area with itching and sweating at times of gustatory stimulation (mealtimes). It is due to abnormal recovery following injury to the auriculotemporal nerve and is long lasting. Few treatments offer much relief.

FURTHER READING

Dimitroulis G. (2005) The role of surgery in the management of disorders of the temporomnadibular joint: a critical review of the literature. Parts 1 and 2. *International Journal of Oral and Maxillofacial Surgery* 34: 107–113, 231–237.

Dolwick M. F., Sanders B. (1985) *TMJ internal derangement and arthrosis: surgical atlas.* Mosby, St Louis, MO.

Keith D. A. (1988) *Surgery of the temporomandibular joint.* Blackwell, Oxford, UK.

McCain J. P., Sanders B., Koslin M. G., et al. (1992) Temporomandibular joint arthroscopy: a 6-year multicenter retrospective study of 4,831 joints. *Journal of Oral and Maxillofacial Surgery* 50: 926–930.

Murakami K.-I., Segami N., Moriya Y., Iizuka T. (1992) Correlation between pain and dysfunction and intra-articular adhesions in patients with internal derangement of the temporomandibular joint. *Journal of Oral and Maxillofacial Surgery* 50: 705–708.

Nitzan D. W., Samson B., Better H. (1997) Long-term outcome of arthrocentesis for sudden onset, persistent, severe closed lock of the temporomandibular joint. *Journal of Oral and Maxillofacial Surgery* 55: 151–157.

Rasmussen O. C. (1981) Description of population and progress of symptoms in a longitudinal study of temporomandibular arthropathy. *Scandinavian Journal of Dental Research* 89: 196–203.

Sanders B., Murakami K.-I., Clark G. T. (1989) *Diagnostic and surgical arthroscopy of the temporomandibular joint.* Saunders, Philadelphia, PA.

Spruijt R. J., Hoogstraten J. (1991) The research on temporomandibular joint clicking: a methodological review. *Journal of Craniomandibular Disorders and Facial Pain* 5: 45–50.

Takaku S., Toyoda T. (1994) Long-term evaluation of discectomy of the temporomandibular joint. *Journal of Oral and Maxcillofacial Surgery* 52: 722–726.

Zamburlini I., Austin D. (1991) Long-term results of appliance therapies in anterior disc displacement with reduction: a review of the literature. *Cranio* 9: 361–368.

SELF-ASSESSMENT

1. A patient attends with a 10-year history of painless clicking of both TMJs. She is not concerned but has been told by a neighbour that she should 'get something done about it'. Her interincisal opening is 55 mm. A click can be felt in both TMJs at early to mid-opening

with inconsistent late closing clicks. What is the most likely diagnosis? Should a surgical approach be considered?

2. A patient attends with pain in the preauricular area on both sides and limitation of mouth opening of several months duration. The condition is worsening but varies somewhat during the day. Her interincisal opening is 29 mm but that can be increased, with some discomfort, to 37 mm by finger pressure on the lower teeth. Masseter and lateral pterygoid muscles are markedly tender to palpation. What is the most likely diagnosis? Should a surgical approach be considered?

3. A patient attends with pain in the preauricular area on both sides and limitation of mouth opening of 4 weeks duration. He used to have clicking of both TMJs but that has stopped. His interincisal opening is 23 mm and cannot be increased by finger pressure on the lower teeth. Opening does not seem limited by pain. Lateral excursive movement is limited to about 4 mm to each side. What is the most likely diagnosis? Should a surgical approach be considered?

4. If disc displacement without reduction were considered as a diagnosis what investigations might clarify the condition?

5. What landmarks may be used to guide instruments into the TMJ for arthroscopy?

6. What nerves are potentially at risk during a preauricular surgical approach to the TMJ?

7. For a patient undergoing manual reduction of dislocation of the TMJ, what advice should be given to reduce the risk of redislocation?

Answers on page 270.

18 Surgery for the compromised patient

J. P. Rood

- With compromised patients, the history is extremely important, and *must* include information about their social circumstances, psychological state (as far as it can be assessed) and their past and present health (including medications).
- Dentoalveolar surgery is stressful for most patients. Compromised patients may not be able to tolerate even a minor procedure unless management is adapted.
- When planning care for a vulnerable patient, the benefits of surgery and the extent of the treatment recommended must be judged carefully.
- Consideration must be given to the appropriate location (whether in the practice surgery or in hospital), taking into account the need for adequate measures to control pain and anxiety.

ASSUMED KNOWLEDGE

It is assumed that at this stage you will have knowledge/competencies in the following areas:

- basic knowledge of human disease and understanding of how common disorders affect patients' abilities to respond to treatment
- the basics of pharmacology and therapeutics.

If you think that you are not competent in these areas, revise them before reading this chapter or cross-check with relevant texts as you read.

INTENDED LEARNING OUTCOMES

At the end of this chapter you should be able to:

1. Plan surgical treatment, taking into account a patient's social, psychological and medical status
2. Assess whether the patient's medications will affect the proposed treatment, including the prescription of drugs required for the surgical procedure and recovery period
3. Distinguish those patients who are suitable for treatment in practice from those requiring hospital care.

INTRODUCTION

This chapter offers guidance and general principles for dealing with patients who are suffering from a disorder that might affect their treatment. It is not possible to deal with every situation or disease state. Drug interactions and adverse effects are not described in detail.

Identifying compromised patients

Patients presenting for treatment may be compromised in a variety of ways—financially, socially, psychologically or medically. An ability to identify patients who are disadvantaged is an important clinical skill. Observation of the patient when they are first seen, and an ability to ask appropriate questions during the interview, will provide most of the information required.

Important factors include the patient's general appearance and demeanour, and whether they are accompanied when they attend the surgery. These factors become increasingly important when the patient is elderly.

During the history-taking procedure, in addition to the standard medical enquiries (see Ch. 2) it is important to explore the patient's attitude to previous treatment, and their probable responses to planned treatment. It is also advisable to assess whether the patient is unusually anxious or shows evidence of any other departures from normal behaviour. Discussions regarding the patient's social background should identify, particularly for older patients, whether they live alone or have family support.

GENERAL ASSESSMENT

When surgery is contemplated, it is in response to a patient's clinical complaint. However, it is important to ensure that the problem is given appropriate priority within the patient's general, social and health care, so that the treatment recommended is relevant and is seen by the patient to be acceptable and desirable.

For the compromised patient the likely outcome must be considered against the risks and consequences of the surgery—a treatment plan which may be routine and sensible for a healthy patient may need to be modified considerably when dealing with an elderly or sick patient.

In the general practice environment, short episodes of treatment are usually tolerated well but extensive, prolonged surgical procedures are not recommended.

Patients who are psychologically vulnerable and who may become confused when treatment is described to them should be encouraged to discuss the proposals with a family member or friend whilst in the surgery. It is often beneficial to arrange a second appointment specifically for this purpose. It is also important not to increase anxiety by emphasizing

unlikely risks, particularly if the treatment proposed is essential. If the surgery is part of a longer-term treatment plan, then the patient's ability to complete the whole course (physically and financially) must be confirmed.

A patient's aftercare must also be taken into account. The recovery period will require an adjustment for the patient in terms of daily activities and diet, and support at home (from partner, relatives or friends) is an important factor. For patients who are unwell, the effects of their illness, including their medications, on wound healing and the prescription of drugs required to aid recovery are additional important factors to take into account.

Before finalizing a surgical treatment plan which is appropriate and specific for the patient, they will have been assessed:

- socially (support, financial)
- psychologically
- medically.

ASSESSMENT OF MEDICAL STATUS

When the history is documented, a detailed medical enquiry (often obtained initially from a questionnaire completed by the patient) will have identified whether the patient has had, or is suffering from, any significant disease. It is important to remember that even if the patient has been seen at the practice for many years, the history must be checked before arranging any surgery.

Patients may be suffering from diseases of which they are unaware and the surgeon must take into account the patient's social status when interpreting the medical history; for example, an overweight, middle-aged man who consumes alcohol should be considered a possible risk for a degree of liver dysfunction. Also, with increasing age, patients may suffer from undiagnosed cardiovascular (cardiorespiratory) disorders such as hypertension and ischaemic heart disease.

Once a disease state has been identified, there must be some attempt to categorize the illness, so that planned surgery is based on a systematic approach rather than a 'one-off' judgement.

As well as identifying the disease some attempt should be made to assess its severity. For example, the length of time the patient has suffered from the problem and the effect it has on their life and mobility are helpful measures. Direct enquiries about whether the patient has been hospitalized (and when and how often) and how the patient is managed (whether by their practitioner or with regular out-patient visits to a hospital specialist unit) will also assist.

The assessment scale first introduced by the American Society of Anesthesiologists (see Ch. 3) has provided a basis for similar classifications, such as scales for the severity of congestive heart failure or for severity of cardiopulmonary disease. This type of grading may be helpful in the assessment of a patient's general medical status. A suggested system is given below.

Grade 1:

- Fit young patient—no known disease
- Fit elderly patient—assume undiagnosed mild cardiorespiratory disease
- Psychologically vulnerable patient who has adequate family or social support
- Patient apparently well, but whose social history suggests risk factors.

Grade 2:

- Patient with mild controlled disease—little or no interference with daily activities
- Disorder which may require modification of management because of the condition or drug therapy
- Patient who denies illness, but who appears to be unwell (e.g. short of breath).

Grade 3:

- Patients with more than one disease
- Complex drug regimens that will affect management
- Elderly patients with disease, particularly those without social support
- Inadequate control of disease, causing interference with daily routines.

Grade 4:

- Severe or uncontrolled disease
- Disease which requires acute, specialized management (e.g. haemophilia)
- Confused or psychologically unstable patient, without family or social support.

Grade 5:

- Seriously ill patient.

Using a grading system to assess the patient's medical and social status provides a framework for planning the best way and location to undertake the required surgery.

Grade 1

In general terms, most dentoalveolar surgery could be provided in the practice environment, under local anaesthesia, using premedication or sedation when beneficial. It would be wise to be extremely cautious with some patients in this group if general anaesthesia is contemplated, e.g. elderly people or patients with suspected risk factors.

Grade 2

Most of these patients could be managed in the practice environment, given sensible responses to the medical history and medications required (e.g. antibiotic cover for valvular disease). In some patients (e.g. epileptic patients) the positive prescription of sedation would assist in management.

Grade 3

Simple surgical procedures could be undertaken in general practice for selected patients, but it would be wise for most patients to be managed in a hospital environment—even if the surgery is to be provided under local anaesthesia.

Grade 4

These patients must be managed in hospital—and often require admission.

Grade 5

Patients in this group are almost certainly inpatients, for whom only minimal emergency treatment is provided.

COMMON CONDITIONS AND THEIR INFLUENCE ON SURGICAL TREATMENT

Respiratory diseases

Acute respiratory tract infection

It is unwise to undertake surgery when a patient has an acute upper respiratory tract infection. Emergency surgery can be provided, but treatment would have to be of limited duration, because of respiratory difficulty and the possibility of the patient coughing during the procedure. Some diagnostic problems can arise when acute maxillary sinusitis develops associated with infection of the upper respiratory tract.

An elective general anaesthetic should not be provided when a patient has an acute respiratory infection.

Lower respiratory tract infections are commonly acute exacerbations of bronchitis. These infections cause cough, fever, breathlessness and malaise, and it is highly unlikely that a patient would attend for treatment whilst in this condition: a patient with pneumonia would be too ill to consider surgical treatment. If emergency treatment is required whilst the patient has an acute infection, it should be directed at relieving pain and be of minimal duration, under local anaesthesia.

Chronic respiratory diseases

Chronic obstructive airways disease is usually due to chronic bronchitis, in which viscous mucus accumulates in the airways. A chronic cough is usually present, and the inability to clear the mucus from the lung structures results in frequent secondary infections and may be associated with emphysema. This type of lung disorder is nearly always associated with chronic hypoxia. Patients with more severe disease cannot tolerate lengthy procedures and are extremely uncomfortable if treated supine.

Surgical procedures that can be reasonably completed in about 20–30 minutes under local anaesthesia may be undertaken in the general practice environment with the patient sitting, not supine. Intravenous sedation should be used only with carefully selected patients because, once the patient is reclined, hypoxaemia and reduced respiratory function from the disease will cause

difficulties in breathing, which are exacerbated by sedation. The use of supplementary oxygen during sedation is helpful, but the patient must be monitored carefully and continuously.

Asthma is common; it is valuable to assess the severity of the disease before planning treatment. Patients who have been hospitalized with an episode of asthma or who take systemic steroids on a regular basis should be considered as severe asthmatics and unsuitable for sedation or general anaesthesia, except in hospital. Patients suffering from milder asthma, which is controlled with inhalers, are usually suitable for management in general practice. An asthma attack can be precipitated by stress, so it is important to plan treatment in a sympathetic way to avoid anxiety from undue waiting before surgery and, where necessary, to use premedication (oral benzodiazepines are useful). Treatment under local anaesthesia is usually safe; patients should have with them their usual medications and use their inhaler before treatment.

Drug sensitivities are common, and opiates are best avoided (but are rarely indicated for pain control following oral surgery). Some asthmatic patients are sensitive to the non-steroidal analgesics (NSAIDs), the use of which can initiate bronchospasm or a severe asthma attack. It is important to enquire whether the patient reacts adversely to aspirin, ibuprofen or similar drugs. Fortunately, most asthmatics can take NSAIDs safely and should not be denied these valuable analgesics.

Cardiovascular diseases

Ischaemic heart disease

This is most frequently reported in the history as angina (crushing central chest pain, associated with myocardial ischaemia), with the patient having been prescribed drugs to relieve the symptoms. Angina may be accompanied by hypertension and some degree of heart failure—the patient should be examined for evidence of either. Mild angina does not preclude surgery being carried out in general practice, but frequent severe attacks, unstable angina and angina at rest are more worrying and the patient would be better managed in hospital. The severity of ischaemic heart disease may be judged by the distance that the patient can walk on the flat without having to stop because of chest pain, their ability to climb stairs and the frequency with which they take medication such as sublingual nitrate sprays to relieve pain.

Angina is best prevented by good patient management, including adequate pain control. Premedication and sedation are extremely useful. It is useful to advise the patient to take their spray or tablet used to alleviate angina as a prophylactic measure before surgery commences.

The use of lidocaine (lignocaine) with adrenaline (epinephrine) will provide the most profound pain control and is therefore the drug of choice. It is, as usual, important to use an aspirating system and to inject slowly. Occasionally a small, transient increase in heart rate will be induced, but this is rarely of clinical significance.

When a patient has suffered a myocardial infarction, any surgery should be deferred for at least 3 months if possible, and treatment requiring general anaesthesia for at least 6 months. Emergency treatment within these periods is best provided in hospital, where local anaesthesia and sedation are likely to be selected.

Hypertension

Hypertension is associated with increasing age and increased peripheral arterial resistance. Mild degrees of hypertension are common and are often undiagnosed. Some patients are 'controlled' with diuretics (necessitating the assessment of potassium levels before significant surgery or general anaesthesia). Hypertension may be secondary to other disease states (e.g. renal or endocrine) and this should be revealed when the history is taken.

Patients who have been hypertensive for years may well have heart failure or angina; if either is known to exist, the patient must be considered more prone to complications during or after surgical treatment.

Pain and anxiety must be avoided in hypertensive patients to prevent increases in blood pressure before and during surgery. Good pain control (local anaesthesia using lidocaine (lignocaine) with adrenaline (epinephrine)), with premedication for the obviously anxious, is essential, and intravenous sedation is valuable during surgery. Lidocaine (lignocaine) 2% with adrenaline (epinephrine) 1:80 000 is the most effective local anaesthetic currently available and, although systemic effects of the adrenaline (epinephrine) can be demonstrated, there is no evidence that moderate doses have any serious harmful effect in hypertensive patients.

Intravenous sedation is valuable for most hypertensives, as it reduces the risk of increasing blood pressure from anxiety and discomfort. For obviously anxious hypertensive patients, premedication should be considered.

Heart failure

This is a consequence of other disorders, mainly valvular disease, ischaemic heart disease or hypertension. Even when heart failure appears to be controlled, it should be taken as an indication of cardiovascular 'wear and tear'.

Patients suffering from left-sided heart failure develop pulmonary oedema, with dyspnoea and a cough. Ankle oedema may be apparent. When right-sided failure is also present, further respiratory embarrassment may occur due to congestion of abdominal organs, and more obvious peripheral (ankle) oedema will be evident.

Surgery can be undertaken for a patient with heart failure, but prolonged treatment should be avoided. Stress can induce an increased sense of respiratory difficulty; if the patient is supine, dyspnoea can be exacerbated, so patients are best managed semi-reclined or sitting upright.

Patients with heart failure can be difficult to manage although those who appear to be well controlled and live a relatively active life can be treated in the practice. Local anaesthesia will be regarded as perfectly safe, but intravenous sedation might precipitate respiratory difficulties and patients requiring sedation might be more appropriately managed in hospital. Similarly patients with poorly controlled disease, with evident breathlessness and oedema, will be better managed within the hospital environment.

Heart failure can interfere with vascular perfusion of the liver and, consequently, drug metabolism. A limiting factor in planning surgery is therefore a restriction in the dose of local anaesthetic solution that can be used. This further dictates that only short procedures should be undertaken at each visit.

The 'at-risk' endocardium

If there is turbulence in flow within the heart there is a risk of bacteria from the bloodstream settling on the endocardium and causing infective endocarditis. A bacteraemia will result from most invasive surgical procedures in the mouth (such as tooth extraction). Therefore it is necessary to identify patients who are at risk of endocarditis and provide appropriate prophylactic measures at the time of surgery. Detailed guidance from the Working Party of the Society for Antimicrobial Chemotherapy is published in the *British National Formulary*.

Haemorrhagic disorders

Disorders of coagulation are the most significant in daily practice. Although the congenital coagulation defects are usually identified when the history is taken, some others may only be revealed during the examination or suspected from the history (e.g. secondary to liver disease). Interference with platelet function is a feature of the NSAIDs and aspirin. Patients commonly take 'over-the-counter' drugs of these types.

If the history reveals episodes of troublesome or serious haemorrhage following previous surgery, or if examination reveals unusual purpura or bruising, then the patient should be fully investigated before surgery is undertaken.

Patients who may be considered likely to have a mild haemorrhagic disorder (perhaps due to other disease) or who have been taking analgesics should be treated cautiously, with limited surgery being provided in the first instance. Management under local anaesthesia, preferably avoiding deep (block) injections, with sedation if required, is acceptable, but attention to haemostasis with adequate postoperative care and follow-up is essential. Inferior dental block injections rarely seem to cause bleeding at the injection site for those therapeutically anticoagulated. However, for patients with a severe clotting defect such as haemophilia there is a risk of a substantial haematoma developing.

Those patients who have identified coagulation or platelet defects will require contemporaneous assessment and replacement therapy and should, therefore, be managed in hospital. Once there has been replacement therapy there is no need to withhold block injections.

Many patients are taking anticoagulant drugs and if a patient volunteers a relevant history, then positive enquiry into anticoagulant treatment should be undertaken.

Common conditions where anticoagulation might have been prescribed include:
• Deep vein thrombosis • Myocardial infarction • Valvular disease or replacement • Atrial fibrillation

Patients on anticoagulation therapy will carry with them a record of their drug treatment and INR assessments. If minor procedures are planned (e.g. the extraction of one or two teeth or a biopsy) then it is reasonable to proceed if the INR value on the day of surgery is no greater than 3, with strict attention to postoperative haemostasis (using a resorbable material in the socket and sutured into place). The surgical removal of teeth, and greater numbers of extractions, can be carried out with an INR of up to 4, provided that, in addition to the local measures, tranexamic acid mouthwashes are prescribed.

If the INR is greater than 4, then modification of the anticoagulant regimen will be required, in collaboration with the physician controlling the patient's anticoagulation. The treatment should be undertaken in hospital. There is variation between hospitals in recommended values of INR for particular procedures.

Problems arise with postoperative care. The use of NSAIDs is undesirable in these patients and pain control must be provided using paracetamol in the outpatient setting. If surgery is likely to induce significant pain, the patient is probably best managed in hospital, where opioids can be used. The prescription of antibiotics can also interfere with anticoagulation control, necessitating frequent reassessment.

Diabetes

The general management of diabetic patients in the dental practice is acceptable, provided that the usual protocols are adopted—that patients are encouraged to take their drugs and meals at normal times before their treatment, which must be provided at sensible times (preferably in the morning). Difficulties arise when general anaesthesia is required and patients must be starved—in these circumstances management in hospital is essential.

Problems can arise postoperatively because of interference with wound healing and secondary infection. For this reason, antibiotics are usually prescribed following surgery in and around the mouth.

Patients who suffer from milder forms of diabetes (controlled by diet alone, or sometimes with oral hypoglycaemics) can usually be managed well within the practice environment, but patients who are insulin-dependent can be a greater risk.

It is unwise to provide intravenous sedation for insulin-dependent diabetics unless the practice has the ability to check blood sugar levels before treatment, and immediately if any difficulty with managing the level of consciousness arises.

Remember that patients who have suffered from diabetes for many years may have other diseases as a consequence (e.g. cardiovascular or renal).

Musculoskeletal disorders

The disorders that are relatively common are osteoarthrosis and rheumatoid arthritis. The severity of these disorders should be noted when the patient is first examined and a history is taken.

Problems with mobility might well interfere with the patient's ability to seek advice or return to the practice if problems arise after surgical treatment. These potential restrictions must be considered when surgery is planned; family support is invaluable.

When planning a surgical procedure for a patient with severe rheumatoid arthritis it is necessary to ensure that the patient can be maintained comfortably in an appropriate position, that the mouth can be opened sufficiently widely for the anticipated duration of the procedure and that care is taken to support the neck—particularly if the patient is sedated.

Outpatients with these disorders usually take NSAIDs. The possibility of anaemia and interference with postoperative haemostasis must be taken into account. In addition, patients with severe rheumatoid arthritis may well be on steroid therapy.

Neurological disease

The most common neurological problem presenting in younger patients is epilepsy. Many patients are well controlled but are taking a variety of medications, some of which (e.g. valproate) may cause haemorrhagic tendency. Provided the well-known aspects of management are adopted (preventing anxiety and irritating 'stroboscopic' lighting defects), epileptic patients can be managed well under local anaesthesia. The use of local anaesthetics is not contraindicated: there is no evidence that local anaesthetic agents provoke epilepsy. Less well-controlled patients benefit from sedation during surgery.

In older patients with neurological diseases, difficulties of management arise primarily in people with Parkinson's disease, or those who have had significant strokes.

A patient with Parkinson's disease may appear expressionless and be uncommunicative. It is important that the treatment is discussed with the carer as well as the patient—the patient may be upset and anxious if he or she is not apparently involved in the debate. There may be postural problems and rigidity, making management in the dental chair quite difficult. Problems of rigidity or tremor are frequently overcome using intravenous sedation, although it is preferable to plan the first episode of treatment to be 'minimal', to see whether sedation is helpful to the individual patient.

Patients who have suffered a cerebrovascular accident might have significant impairment with mobility and communication. This can increase difficulties with oral hygiene, particularly if there is facial paralysis, and postoperative wound care will require additional attention. Patients may well be hypertensive (this should be investigated) and have other features of cardiovascular disease; they may well also be on anticoagulants. All of these factors make their management in the general practice environment quite inconvenient although, if the patient is mobile, their families usually welcome maintenance of local, normal dental care. In more severe cases it is preferable to carry out surgery in hospital.

Drugs

Many patients are taking prescribed medications but, when the history is obtained, it is important to enquire about other drug use, in particular over-the-counter medications and recreational drugs. Information about drugs may provide an insight into the patient's health that was not revealed during the history. It is important to assess the potential difficulties that might arise during management because of drug treatments or interactions. There are some well-known problems, but new adverse reactions and interactions continue to be reported. It is important to consult up-to-date publications regarding new drugs and their effects (e.g. BNF).

The importance of the pharmacological aspects of treatment should be considered systematically:

1. Drugs that the patient is taking when first assessed:

   - What disease does this indicate?
   - Does it give an indication of severity?
   - Will the drugs affect management?

2. Drugs that will be necessary for the surgical procedure:
   - Is there a need to administer any drugs before surgery?
   - Are there any reasons for altering the usual analgesic drug regimens?
   - Could there be any problems with sedation?

3. Drugs used in the postoperative period:

   - Are there any medical or pharmacological reasons for altering postoperative analgesic regimens?
   - Is there a need for antibiotics and should this prescription differ from standard regimens?

Summary

- Be aware of a variety of compromises
- Identify compromise and respond to it
- Careful, sensitive planning is essential
- When a disease is identified, be aware of the secondary and hidden effects of that disease—and of the medications
- Surgery should be limited at first and never prolonged
- Decide when it is prudent to have the patient treated in hospital

---

FURTHER READING

American Society of Anesthesiologists (1963) New classification of physical status. *Anesthesiology* 24: 111.

Francis G. S. (1998) Congestive heart failure. In: Stein J. H. (ed.) *Internal medicine*, 5th edn. Mosby, St. Louis, MO, pp. 156–175.

Gould F. K., Elliott T. S. J., Foweraker J., et al. (2006) Guidelines for the prevention of endocarditis: report of the working party of the British Society for Antimicrobial Chemotherapy. *Journal of Antimicrobial Chemotherapy* 57: 1035–1042.

Trieger N. (1994) *Pain control*, 2nd edn. Mosby Year Book, St Louis, MO.

Webster K., Wilde J. (2000) Management of anticoagulation in patients with prosthetic heart valves undergoing oral and maxillofacial operations. *British Journal of Oral and Maxillofacial Surgery* 38: 124–126.

SELF-ASSESSMENT

1. A 56-year-old man has pain from the retained roots of a lower first molar, incompletely removed several years ago. He gives a long history of ischaemic heart disease, with 2 myocardial infarcts 2 and 5 years ago. Two weeks ago he underwent a coronary artery bypass operation which seems to have been successful, apart from a deep venous thrombosis for which he now takes warfarin. How would you grade his current medical state using the system outlined in this chapter and what impact might that have on removing those roots in the immediate future? How are things likely to change over the next 6 months?

2. A 23-year-old woman requires removal of a partially erupted lower third molar. She tells you she is epileptic. How can you assess the likelihood of problems arising with this particular patient during operative treatment? How can you prepare for them and minimize the risk of these difficulties?

Answers on page 271.

Appendix A

SUGGESTED SURGICAL KIT

A suitable surgical kit contains the following (some of these may be kept separately packed, to open only if required):

- drapes to cover the patient's clothing
- mouth mirror and dental probe
- college forceps
- Swann Morton no. 15 surgical blade on a no. 3 handle
- periosteal elevators: Howarth's, Freer's or Fickling's
- Mitchell's trimmer
- flap retractors such as the Lack's tongue depressor or Morris rake retractor
- mosquito artery forceps, straight and curved
- straight handpiece and motor (handpiece and tubing (or sleeve) must be amenable to autoclaving)
- long-shanked surgical burs (usually tungsten carbide tipped), round and flat fissure (steel burs are available in a range of sizes, but blunt easily)
- a means of irrigation with saline (either through the handpiece or via a syringe)
- a means of aspiration: the tip must be finer than conventional dental aspirators; Jankauer's or American-pattern tips are suitable

- dental elevators: Coupland's nos 1, 2, 3, a pair of Cryer's and Warwick-James right, left and straight
- tooth extraction forceps
- cheek retractor (such as the Kilner)
- toothed tissue-dissecting forceps
- suture material—3/0 polygalactin or silk on a medium-sized (approx. 22 mm, half round or three-eighths round), side-cutting needle
- suture scissors, such as McKindoe's
- needle holders: small Mayo's, Kilner's or Ward's
- swabs.

SUGGESTED ADDITIONAL INSTRUMENTS FOR APICECTOMY

- non-toothed forceps
- ribbon gauze 0.6 cm wide
- contra-angled, micro-head handpiece
- flat plastic instrument
- ball-ended burnisher
- straight excavator
- Briault probe
- (A fine, custom amalgam carrier is recommended if dental amalgam is chosen to obtain an apical seal.)

Appendix B
Answers to self-assessment

CHAPTER 2: DIAGNOSIS: THE PROCESS AND THE RESULT

1. Any possible cause, shape, size, colour, definition of periphery, consistency, tenderness, attachment to deeper structures, pulsation, associated lymph nodes. It is certain to be warm if in the mouth.
2. A list of possible diagnoses in order of probability, used when multiple diagnoses may explain the signs and symptoms. It is used to guide the choice of special tests, which eventually eliminate diagnoses from the list.

CHAPTER 3: CONTROL OF PAIN AND ANXIETY: SELECTION OF AND PREPARATION FOR ANAESTHESIA OR SEDATION

1. Before undergoing a general anaesthetic the patient must take no food for several hours. The timing of food for the insulin-dependent diabetic is critical and omitting food means omitting insulin. It is usual to convert the patient onto soluble insulin and give glucose by intravenous infusion, matching the blood glucose level to the amount of insulin by a 'sliding scale'. This is easier to monitor on an inpatient basis.
2. General anaesthesia always carries a small risk of mortality. The risk is increased for this patient because she is overweight for her height (BMI = 42). If it is possible to deal with her problem with local anaesthesia (with or without sedation) that risk can be reduced dramatically. If not, she would have to undergo the general anaesthetic as an inpatient.
3. Gauze or other material can be placed over the back of the tongue, suction can be maintained throughout, the volume of irrigant can be kept to that which is required to cool the bur, the patient is not laid absolutely flat.
4. The patient should not drive, operate machinery, cook, look after small children, make important decisions or do anything else that requires careful use of the hands or brain. The advice should be given when the appointment is booked, just before the procedure and after it, to the escort.
5. First thoughts might go to oral or inhalational sedation, but it is worth noting that for some individuals with a 'needle phobia', the concern is primarily with needles used inside the mouth rather than in the hand and I.V. sedation may still be appropriate. General anaesthesia should be later in your list.
6. An anti-inflammatory drug such as ibuprofen may be your first choice, but paracetamol is also effective, as are combination drugs.

CHAPTER 4: EXTRACTION OF TEETH

1. The buccal beak has a point (to fit in the furcation) separating two concavities (to fit around the two buccal roots). The palatal beak has a single broader concavity. The handles have curves in two directions. When seen from the side the handles curve from the vertical beaks forward out of the mouth then down again towards the handle end. Both handles curve to the right when seen from the operator's perspective. Note: many dentists use the upper premolar (root) forceps for upper molars. For these, the beaks each have a single concavity but the handles curve as for the full molar forceps.
2. Straighten the wrist, remove index finger from between handles, move the end of the handle into the palm of the hand and, possibly, place the little finger between the handles (see Fig. 4.12).
3. (a) Standing behind, generally on the right.
   (b) Tipped back by about 30°–45°.
   (c) Below the operator's elbow.
4. Buccally until it just moves, then palatally till it just moves, then a little more each way, eventually wriggling the tooth down through the socket.
5. Limited access due to reduced mouth opening, small or tight oral entrance (e.g. burn scars), large alveolus, large tooth, severe tooth surface loss, extensive caries.
6. (a) Pain at the site of recent extraction, exposed bone in the socket, inflammation of surrounding alveolus.
   (b) Prophylactic metronidazole or irrigation with chlorhexidine. (Note: just because dry socket numbers can be reduced by these treatments does not indicate their use as a routine; indeed, the prophylactic use of metronidazole after routine extractions is *not* recommended.)
   (c) Irrigation with warm saline and placement of a sedative dressing.

CHAPTER 5: REMOVAL OF UNERUPTED TEETH

1. **Diagnosis**: pain, trismus, increased temperature, red inflamed operculum overlying 8, regional lymphadenopathy.
   Treatment: extract upper 8 if traumatizing operculum of lower, antibiotics (if systemic involvement), analgesics, improve oral hygiene (e.g. chlorhexidine mouthwashes), irrigate operculum with antiseptic (e.g. chlorhexidine).
2. Recurrent infection (e.g. pericoronitis). Unrestorable caries in third molar or distal aspect of second. Periodontal disease affecting the distal aspect of 7. Cysts or tumours affecting 8. External/internal resorption.
3. Resorption of adjacent teeth, pathological change around the unerupted crown, caries or periodontal disease if this area is not cleaned properly, recurrent pericoronitis.
4. Your surgical skills and technical back-up, a patient who refuses local anaesthesia, at the patient's request or for a patient who is very anxious, if the operation would take longer than 30 minutes, complication within medical history.
5. Pain, swelling, bruising, trismus, possible para/anaesthesia of lip and tongue (including the possibility of permanent loss of sensation), interference with diet.
6. Diversion of inferior dental canal, darkening of the root where crossed by the canal, interruption of the white line of the canal.
7. The depth of impaction (i.e. the vertical distance from the occlusal surface of the second molar to that of the third molar), angulation, the distance between the second molar and ramus compared to the width of the third molar crown.
8. Sectioning the nerve by extending the distal relieving incision directly backwards, 'bruising' the nerve by trapping it between the retractor and bone, stretching the nerve during retraction (if lingual flap is raised), drilling through the lingual plate, suture passing through the nerve.
9. **For**: infection present (e.g. systemic involvement) or risk of infection significant (e.g. prolonged surgery), prevention of infective endocarditis in 'at-risk' patients, compromised host defence (i.e. significant medical history).
   Against: may encourage lax surgery, potential risk of allergy, unnecessary in the vast number of cases—good local hygiene is more important.

10. **Dry socket**: irrigate with warm saline or chlorhexidine; place a sedative dressing.
    Infected wound: if systemic involvement or regional lymphadenopathy, prescribe antibiotics.
    Trismus: usually resolves after a couple of weeks.
    Inferior dental or lingual nerve injury: review. Damage usually improves (up to 10% may have dysaesthesia at one week; this has reduced to <1% by 1 year). Prolonged loss of fungiform papillae associated with poor prognosis. If no significant sensibility at 4–6 weeks, consider nerve repair.

11. Ensure you discuss with the patient the risks and benefits of the operation, and that these are recorded in the patient's notes. Ideally, your dental nurse should act as a witness. Provide the patient with an information leaflet. Consider obtaining written consent in which the likely risks are outlined.

12. Distal relieving incision should be up the external oblique ridge, in a distobuccal direction, remaining on bone at all times. A common error by those inexperienced is to extend the incision distal to the 2nd molar in the direction of the midline of the molar teeth. This risks running off the bone, into the lingual nerve and causing troublesome bleeding. The anterior relieving incision for a triangular flap should include the papilla distal to the lower 2nd molar and then curve down gently in an anterior direction. This allows the flap to rest on bone after removal of bone and tooth, ensuring adequate blood supply to the flap with minimal disruption to the gingiva of the lower 2nd molar. Beware of extending the incision too far into the sulcus as this risks cutting an arteriolar branch of the facial artery. The incision should be through the periosteum to the bone and thus in the correct tissue plane such that on raising the flap bone rather than bleeding periosteum is visible.

CHAPTER 6: SURGICAL ENDODONTICS

1. (a) The root is narrow mesiodistally, with little space between it and the adjacent teeth, and it is broad labiolingually with usually two canals.
   (b) The apex is deeply placed in bone and largely hidden by the mental nerve.
   (c) The tooth commonly has two roots, the palatal of which is very deeply placed.

2. It generally gives good access allowing the margin to be replaced on bone and is easy to reposition. However, sometimes, particularly on very convex surfaces, access may be better with a three-sided flap. The risk of recession at the gingival margin seems to be greater than for a semilunar flap.

3. The wound may be packed to control haemorrage, specifically to keep the operative field as dry as possible. Packing also prevents filling material being spilled into the bone. Ribbon gauze, an alginate swab or bone wax may all be used.

4. Ongoing or developing pain, tenderness, swelling or discharge. Do not expect any radiographic change and so do not take a radiograph at this stage.

5. A radiograph should be taken shortly after the procedure (on the same day or within 2 weeks) as a baseline against which to measure future change and to confirm that the procedure appears to have been completed satisfactorily. There is no value in taking another radiograph until 6 months, the earliest time at which complete bone repair might be found. If that has not occurred, further radiographs at 6-month intervals for up to 2 years may help to clarify the outcome. Complete bone repair is the most reliable sign of success, but progressive reduction in the size of an apical radiolucency over 12 months may be consistent with elimination of infection. Remember that in large bone cavities some healing with scar tissue occurs; this does not show as bone on the radiograph.

CHAPTER 7: SPREADING INFECTION

1. (a) Cellulitis.
   (b) Because oedema tends to expand in lax tissues with little fascial constraint.
   (c) The buccal space/canine space.

(d) Temperature, pulse and respiration; feel intraorally for fluctuance; vitality test; intraoral radiographs of tooth 13 or orthopantomogram.

(e) The time scale is far too short and the swelling is dominated by oedema.

(f) Antibiotics to control the spread of infection, removal of the cause by opening the causative tooth to drain or extraction, possibly under general anaesthesia.

2. (a) Masticator and/or lateral pharyngeal spaces (in this case the masticator space).

(b) Is there difficulty or pain on swallowing, or breathing? (You should be concerned about possible lateral pharyngeal involvement, but cannot inspect it directly.)

(c) CT, MRI.

3. (a) The distribution of the swelling is far too localized and well away from the teeth.

(b) The parotid gland.

(c) Is there any change at meal times?

4. (a) Alveolar abscess.

(b) Incision and drainage (extraction would probably not be enough in this case because of the extent of suppuration beyond the bone).

(c) Injected local anaesthetic or general anaesthesia.

(d) Bone.

5. (a) Metronidazole, 400 mg three times daily for 5–7 days, would be satisfactory. Some people would choose a cephalosporin (despite allergic cross-reactivity between the penicillins and the cephalosporins); some would add another drug to the metronidazole and still others would use a drug such as erythromycin.

(b) Certainly no more than 2 days. The author would tend to review at 24 hours, by which time there should be some slight improvement and maybe signs of localization.

6. (a) This is osteomyelitis, but you should consider the possibility of a malignancy, particularly a secondary carcinoma.

(b) Is she taking, or has she taken, corticosteroids for her asthma?

7. (a) The duration, the history of trauma, the intermittent discharge.

(b) A chronic infection: actinomycosis or osteomyelitis.

(c) Any history of numbness of the lip; do the teeth come together properly (considering a possible fracture)? Is there anything in the medical history which indicates an increased risk of infection? What treatment has been offered so far?

(d) Sample pus for culture and sensitivity; radiographs of the mandible for possible fracture, dental disease, bone loss, periosteal new bone or sequestration.

(e) Oral penicillin for 3 months (this is actinomycosis).

CHAPTER 8: ORAL LESIONS: DIFFERENTIAL DIAGNOSIS AND BIOPSY TECHNIQUES

1. (a) Fibrous epulis or fibroepithelial polyp. You might also consider pyogenic granuloma (or pregnancy epulis) or peripheral giant-cell granuloma.

(b) Excision biopsy with a scalpel if it does not seem excessively vascular; consider electrocautery if it is particularly inflamed.

2. (a) Excisional biopsy.

(b) Under local anaesthesia avoiding distortion of the lesion, pass a suture beneath the lesion to hold it and avoid damage to it, use an elliptical incision to include a band of surrounding normal tissue; primary closure using interrupted sutures.

(c) Place in a container with 10% formal saline, complete a pathology form including full and relevant clinical observations.

(d) A histological diagnosis; evidence of epithelial dysplasia.

3. (a) Duration, change in size or shape, any symptoms including pain, ulceration, bleeding, any precipitating factors, including trauma.

(b) Site, size, consistency, whether it is raised, firmness, fluctuance, ulceration, tenderness, presence of inflammation.

(c) Normal circumvallate papilla, papilloma, polyp, median rhomboid glossitis.

4. (a) Torus palatinus.
   (b) A salivary neoplasm would be soft and to one side of the midline, where normal salivary tissue is found.
   (c) If asymptomatic, observe and reassure; if being traumatized or interfering with the fit of a denture, consider surgical removal.
5. Should be a representative sample of the mass; must include some normal tissue; should be deep enough to include a substantial zone of connective tissue; should be wide enough to permit a number of complete sections to be made after processing; should be amenable to closure.
6. Plain radiographs, aspiration, angiography. Do *not* take an incisional biopsy!

CHAPTER 9: CYSTS

1. (a) It may be asymptomatic with or without swelling in the buccal sulcus or palate, depending on size; discolouration of the tooth; if acutely infected pain, diffuse or localized swelling; tooth tender to percussion.
   (b) Vitality tests, tooth usually non-vital; a periapical radiograph: if not infected, well-defined apical radiolucency, if acute, diffuse borders.
   (c) Acute phase, drain through tooth and/or incision in the sulcus if tooth is to be restored or extract tooth; following acute phase, endodontics with or without apicectomy at the time of cyst enucleation.
2. (a) Apical periodontal cyst (or residual cyst); incisive canal cyst.
   (b) Could be asymptomatic, presenting as swellings; if they become infected they would have signs and symptoms of an acute infection; firm or fluctuant, dependent on the thickness of the overlying bone.
   (c) Vitality tests—apical periodontal cyst associated with non-vital tooth; appropriate radiography to visualize whole lesion; aspiration—to relieve pressure and gain a sample.

   (d) Apical periodontal cyst—extraction or apicectomy with cyst enucleation; incisive canal cyst—enucleation; complications—haemorrhage, wound breakdown, recurrence (rare if removal complete).
3. Slow growth over years; periodic associated infection; smooth, rounded surface, either bony hard or clearly fluctuant; normal function in adjacent tissues.
4. Displacement of teeth; mobility of teeth; pathological fracture (but this is more commonly associated with tumours and osteomyelitis); non-vital tooth (but remember that most non-vital teeth do not have associated cysts).
5. Treatment involves making a window in the cyst and keeping that open while the cyst shrinks away from the teeth and nerve. Initially the wound will be packed open, then a bung will be made to seal the opening. Treatment may take up to 2 years and there will be a number of visits in that time. It may be necessary to operate later to remove the residual tissue.

CHAPTER 10: MALIGNANT DISEASE OF THE ORAL CAVITY

1. Tobacco use (smoking or chewing) and alcohol consumption.
2. (a) Risk about 3–6%.
   (b) Risk may be greater than 50%.
   (c) Difficult to quantify for the UK, but in India one study noted one in three subjects to have a slow-growing carcinoma.
   (d) The common, reticular pattern does *not* appear to be premalignant, but there is an association between erosive or atrophic lichen and cancer (1.2%).
3. (a) Excision, with a margin and primary closure.
   (b) Lip split and mandibulotomy followed by excision, with a margin, in continuity with the lymphatic drainage on that side and reconstruction (probably by free tissue transfer). That may be supplemented by external beam radiotherapy.
   (c) Excision of abnormal areas either by laser excision or by conventional surgery, followed by skin grafting.

4. Regular 6-month monitoring for life; early attention to all new caries or periodontal disease; continuing use of fluoride mouthwash indefinitely; urgent referral of patient if any suspicion of recurrence or new cancer; absolute avoidance of dental extractions or surgery in patients who have received radiotherapy.

5. **Surgery**: destruction of complicated structures, need for reconstruction, lengthy operation and hospital stay.

   Radiotherapy: severe mucositis at the time of treatment, dry mouth if salivary glands involved, permanent damage to bone and soft tissue, not effective if bone involved.

CHAPTER 11: SURGICAL AIDS TO PROSTHODONTICS, INCLUDING OSSEOINTEGRATED IMPLANTS

1. Where a discrepancy in the height, width or regularity of the denture-bearing area, or discrepancy in arch sizes renders conventional prosthodontics unsatisfactory.

2. Reposition displaced alveolar bone, trim sharp bone edges, minimize bone loss during surgical removal of teeth, alveoplasty (particularly if there is a considerable bony undercut).

3. *Endosseous implants* (literally within the bone) are usually covered by mucosa for a period of months awaiting osseointegration and subsequent uncovering and loading. *Subperiosteal implants* consist of a metal frame inserted as an onlay directly on to the surface of cortical bone with abutments protruding through the mucosa. The frame is fabricated from impressions of the exposed surface of the jaw. Wound dehiscence and infection are common problems. *Transosseous implants* extend all the way through the bone and may be indicated for a severely atrophic mandible in which endosseous implants are contraindicated.

4. Biocompatibility of the implant material, design of the implant, surface characteristics, physical health of the patient, anatomical conditions, patient's cooperation, oral

hygiene status and smoking habits; operator experience; loading of the implants after osseointegration.

5. Use only sharp drill bits; run the drill slowly, with little pressure, applied intermittently and with thorough cooling using saline; increase the drill size progressively; insert the implant slowly.

CHAPTER 12: SURGICAL AIDS TO ORTHODONTICS AND SURGERY FOR DENTOFACIAL DEFORMITY

1. (a) Between the ages of 11 and 12.
   (b) No problems, dentigerous cyst formation, resorption of the roots of the adjacent teeth.
   (c) By: (i) the use of parallax radiographic technique, (ii) direct clinical examination to determine the position of swellings and the angulation of adjacent teeth.

2. (a) Typically at age 6–7. Local causes include early loss of deciduous predecessor, dilaceration, impaction with a supernumerary tooth. Systemic causes include cleidocranial dysostosis, Down's syndrome, hypothyroidism, achondroplasia.
   (b) Complications include trauma to the roots of adjacent teeth, postoperative resorption or mobility of adjacent teeth and loss of attached gingivae.
   (c) This is an unerupted midline supernumerary tooth (mesiodens).

3. (a) This is an apically repositioned flap.
   (b) To preserve the keratinized attached gingivae around the tooth.
   (c) Packing the exposure using an antiseptic material on ribbon gauze and securing it with sutures (e.g. Whitehead's varnish or BIPP).
   (d) In this case a bracket could be bonded to the external buccal surface of the tooth and a gold chain used to apply traction in conjunction with the existing fixed appliance.

4. (a) Direct traction and observation of blanching of the incisive papilla or using an intraoral periapical radiograph.

(b) Indications for lingual fraenectomy include severe impairment of normal speech development (although this is debatable) and high fraenal attachments, which interfere with oral hygiene and periodontal health.

5. (a) Class II skeletal relationship (retrognathism).
   (b) Treacher-Collins syndrome or Apert's syndrome.
   (c) Reversed overbite, reversed overjet, class 3 malocclusion, proclination of upper incisors and retroclination of the lower incisors.
   (d) Analysis of OPT, cephalometric and PA radiographs; articulated study models; photography.
   (e) Pain, swelling, nerve damage (inferior dental and lingual nerves), malocclusion and relapse. The risk of the last two complications arising is minimized by careful planning.

6. (a, b) Repair of the lip at 4–6 months; repair of the palate by the first birthday; alveolar bone grafting as needed aged 8–9; orthognathic surgery aged 16–18 as needed.
   (c) To allow normal development of the premaxilla and the eruption of the canines.
   (d) It allows a functional repair giving a better cosmetic result as the child grows; it is safer from an anaesthetic viewpoint; it enables the child to grow and therefore have more tissue available.

CHAPTER 13: MAXILLOFACIAL TRAUMA

1. Assess the airway, bleeding problems and the level of consciousness. Manage bleeding with pressure (such as with gauze or by bringing fracture ends together with a ligature around the adjacent teeth). Clean and suture soft tissue injuries. Seek any further injuries, take radiographs and refer if appropriate.

2. Abrasions, lacerations, haemorrhage, haematoma, swelling may all overlie sites of fracture. Reluctance to use muscles that move the jaw (guarding), deviation on jaw movement, bone deformity, displacement of the eye or abnormality of eye movement may be signs of fractures.

3. Fixation is the process in which the bone ends on either side of a fracture are prevented from moving relative to each other, after they have been repositioned (reduced). Often fixation is achieved with 'mini-plates'.

4. Assess. If the injury needs to be treated under general anaesthesia, refer to hospital. If not, give local anaesthetic, examine, thoroughly clean, remove necrotic tissue only, close in layers: vermilion, then muscle, mucosa and skin.

5. Enquire about sleep disturbance, jumpiness and flashbacks. If you suspect PTSD, refer the patient to her family practitioner or, with the patient's consent, consult a clinical psychologist or a voluntary organization such as Victim Support or Women's Aid.

CHAPTER 14: SALIVARY GLAND DISEASE

1. Recent contact with mumps; swelling anatomically in the parotid(s); pain worsens on eating and drinking; lack of suppuration; reduced salivary flow usually bilateral.

2. Such a symptomless lump is most likely to be a stone. Plain radiographs (OPT and lower occlusal) should demonstrate it. If no stone is demonstrated, consider a neoplasm (benign or malignant) and arrange a CT or MRI.

3. **Organic**: Sjögren's syndrome, benign lymphoepithelial lesion; radiation damage; sarcoidosis; HIV infection.
   Functional: depression; dehydration; drugs (such as antidepressants).

4. (a) Mucocele is by far the most likely, but consider traumatized fibroepithelial polyp or papilloma.
   (b) Enucleation of mucocele (usually with an ellipse of mucosa) and the minor gland beneath.
   (c) Scarring, but mucosa usually heals well; mucoceles can recur, probably due to traumatizing adjacent glands during surgery.

5. (a) Pleomorphic adenoma in the minor salivary glands.

(b) Wide excision down to periosteum; pack the cavity and await secondary epithelialization; if the defect is large consider a flap to close.

CHAPTER 15: THE MAXILLARY ANTRUM

1. (a) An OAC has been created. Ask the patient to pinch the nostrils and gently attempt to blow their nose. The appearance of bubbles at the socket confirms the presence of an OAC.

   (b) Explain the situation to the patient. Close the defect immediately if possible (the buccal advancement flap is usually most appropriate). If closure is not possible (e.g. due to inadequate facilities or experience, patient unfit for further surgery) place mattress sutures across socket to encourage spontaneous closure (for small OAC) or cover with an acrylic base plate or ribbon gauze/Whitehead's varnish and refer promptly to an oral and maxillofacial surgeon.

   (c) Advise against nose blowing and smoking (the pressure changes disturb healing). Prescribe antibiotics and possibly a decongestant to encourage drainage and prevent infection. Smaller OACs may resolve spontaneously but if they persist after 2 weeks arrange surgical closure. Defects over 5 mm in diameter require surgical closure (refer to oral and maxillofacial surgeon as necessary— depending on size and position of defect, available facilities and your experience).

   (d) Upper premolars and molars, which are closely related to the antrum.

2. (a) The maxillary tuberosity has fractured.

   (b) Stop at once, consider splinting the tooth and removing it surgically when the bone has healed, or proceed to surgical removal if the fragment is small.

   (c) Large antrum encroaching into the tuberosity and around the roots; lone standing tooth; hypercementosis.

3. (a) Still in socket, near socket (e.g. pushed into cyst or abscess cavity or adjacent socket), beneath palatal or buccal mucosa, in antrum either within antral cavity or between antral lining and bone, elsewhere in oral cavity (e.g. floor of mouth, dorsum of tongue, oropharynx), swallowed or inhaled, outside patient (on clothing, chair, floor, suction equipment, sink).

   (b) Ask patient to sit up and spit out, search the mouth and pharynx to minimize the subsequent risk of inhaling the root if it has dropped to back of mouth; then search other possible locations (as above) using good light and suction—don't forget to consider possibility of the root being on clothes, chair, sink or floor and search suction if necessary. Take radiographs if necessary—a periapical will demonstrate a root in the socket or periapical tissues and may also show a root in the antrum (a root under the palatal mucosa may appear to be in the socket); an oblique occlusal view can show the antral floor better and gives a second angle with which to locate the root; an occipitomental may show a root in the antrum (look for a root canal to indicate a root). If the root cannot be found despite these careful searches, consider referral for chest/abdominal films.

   (c) Examine the radiograph, note the proximity of the root to the antrum; do not use elevators blindly, but remove the root by a transalveolar approach, raise a buccal mucoperiosteal flap, remove bone carefully with bur, coax root towards mouth with elevator, without any upwards pressure with any instrument.

4. Signs and symptoms of acute sinusitis: history of recent URTI (or extraction with OAC formation, recent introduction of foreign body into antrum or other trauma to antrum); headache and pain over affected antrum and in premolars and molars of affected side, tenderness in buccal sulcus over anterior antral wall. The pain is typically throbbing, dull and heavy in character and worse when head is inclined forwards, but is not affected by temperature or sweet stimuli. Purulent nasal discharge and/or postnasal drip may

be present. A radiograph will show mucosal thickening and, perhaps, a fluid level due to a collection of pus, but radiography is not usually necessary. Chronic sinusitis usually follows acute sinusitis, may persist or recur over a prolonged period of time, but is largely asymptomatic between acute attacks.

5. **Signs and symptoms** of a malignant antral tumour depend on the direction of tumour spread. They include pain in maxilla; nasal obstruction; nasal discharge; swelling and/or ulceration in buccal sulcus, palate or extraorally over the maxilla; redness of skin over the maxilla; mobility of teeth adjacent to the antrum; herniation of tumour through an extraction socket; excessive postextraction bleeding; epistaxis; paraesthesia in the distribution of the infraorbital nerve; diplopia; raised pupillary level; proptosis; trismus.

   Action: Refer immediately to ENT or oral and maxillofacial surgeon. Stress that an urgent appointment is required.

CHAPTER 16: FACIAL PAIN AND TEMPOROMANDIBULAR DISORDERS

1. Any four of: location to masticatory muscles or preauricular region, duration of onset and persistence of the pain, association with jaw movement rather than chewing, often bilateral, relation to time of day, lack of a 'dental' cause, tenderness of muscles.

2. Any two of: specific location of pain to preauricular area, tenderness of TMJ itself, limitation of lateral excursive movement.

3. Disc displacement without reduction usually results in restriction of mouth opening that is of sudden onset; if eased it also releases suddenly; there is no significant variation in opening with time; there is a history of clicking; it is not possible to extend opening with finger pressure; on imaging the disc with MRI or arthrography the disc is seen to remain forwards of the condyle throughout the range of movement.

4. Surgery should be considered if the patient is *suffering* from the disorder, if conservative treatments have been unsuccessful, if it

is unlikely that symptoms will subside spontaneously in a reasonable time.

5. They are common clinical features of degenerative joint disease, but on their own they do not exclude the rarer systemic inflammatory arthropathies.

6. **Advice** should include the benign nature of the condition, local heat, resting the jaw muscles as much as possible, avoiding daytime clenching, the use of regular analgesics (NSAIDs if tolerable).

   Treatment is likely to include an appliance, such as a soft bite guard, but physiotherapy should be considered and antidepressants can be used.

7. Features include prolonged pain (months to years), limited (or no) response to treatment, few features typical of dental pains (e.g. thermal stimuli), allodynia or hyperalgesia, history of repeated dry socket and poor healing after extraction, tendency of the pain to migrate, decreasing confidence of the patient in dental (and medical) advice.

8. Trigeminal neuralgia should exhibit sudden onset of short periods of intense pain with pain-free periods (or much reduced pain), a trigger zone, precise location within a division of the trigeminal nerve, responsiveness to carbamazepine, patient not woken by pain.

9. General dental treatment planning for those with atypical facial pain should include irreversible treatments only when they are justified for demonstrable dental disease. Patients should be counselled in advance that that line will be taken, but that justified treatment will be offered as normal.

CHAPTER 17: SURGERY OF THE TEMPOROMANDIBULAR JOINT

1. Disc displacement with reduction. If the patient is not concerned she should merely be reassured. Conservative treatments may be tried, but surgery is hard to justify in the absence of symptoms.

2. Myofascial pain dysfunction. There is no place for surgery in this condition.

3. Disc displacement without reduction. Surgery may be considered, although it is

not essential. Note that as many as 50% of patients may become symptom-free within 2 years, and many of the remainder will see an improvement in symptoms, without surgical treatment. Closed manipulation with or without arthrocentesis may work well, or an open procedure might be considered. In either event, many surgeons would investigate further to confirm (or otherwise) the diagnosis.

4. MRI or arthrography to determine disc position and mobility.
5. Often an imaginary line is drawn from the point of the tragus to the outer canthus of the eye. A point is marked 10 mm forwards along that line and 2 mm below it. With the mouth open, the line of approach to the joint from there is upwards, forwards and inwards.
6. Auriculotemporal and both zygomatic and temporal branches of the facial nerve.
7. The mouth will be held closed for about a minute after the dislocation. Patient should be careful to restrict mouth opening for at least 24 hours and great care taken in activities such as yawning, laughing and biting not to open the mouth more than absolutely essential.

CHAPTER 18: SURGERY FOR THE COMPROMISED PATIENT

1. He would be grade 3 because of multiple diseases and a complex drug regimen which would affect management. He is still not out of the period where further infarcts are likely. The vein grafts to his coronary system will not have healed and his myocardium will still not yet be well perfused. There is little capacity for his heart to respond to a demand for extra work. In addition the warfarin does increase the likelihood of bleeding following extraction. If the grafting is successful, his exercise tolerance will improve and provided he has no other risk factors for venous thrombosis, he will be taken off warfarin (although he is likely to remain on aspirin). If everything goes well he will be much better able to tolerate stressful surgery in 6 months time.

2. Firstly ask what type of epilepsy the patient suffers, the frequency of seizures, whether hospital admission has ever been required for persistent seizures, whether there are any precipitating factors such as stress and whether they get any warning or 'aura'. Ensure that you and your team are aware of how to manage epileptic fits and that oxygen and suction are always available. Make sure the patient knows they are to take their normal medication prior to the visit. There is no requirement to change your choice of local anesthetic drugs, but sedation can reduce the likelihood of fitting in less well-controlled individuals.

Index

ABC, life support, 185, 186
abscess, 84, 85
   alveolar, 87-8
   cervicofacial space, 88, 91
   discharge, 85
   drainage, 90-1
      drain insertion, 91, 92
      dressings, 92
   fluctuance detection, 84-5
   pus microbiology, 89, 90-1
   salivary gland, 202
   systemic clinical features, 87
   use of antibiotics, 92
access
   extraction of teeth, 26
   implant surgery, 157
   surgical endodontics, 70
   third molar surgery, 46, 61-2
   torus removal, 153
acinic cell carcinoma, 209
acromegaly, 174
actinomycosis, 60, 96
activated partial thromboplastin time (APTT), 43
adenocarcinoma, salivary gland, 209
adenoid cystic carcinoma, 116, 209
adenoma, salivary gland, 208
adenomatoid odontogenic tumour, 106
aftercare, compromised patient, 254
airway protection
   general anaesthesia, 19, 21
   maxillofacial trauma, 185
   sedation, 17
alcohol consumption
   implant surgery contraindication, 157
   leukoplakia association, 131
   maxillofacial trauma association, 185, 186, 197
   oral cancer risk, 128, 143
   sialosis, 210
alendronate, 42
allergic sialadenitis, 203
alveolar abscess, 87-8
alveolar bone loss, 147
alveolus cancer of, 135, 136, 141, 142
alveolus cysts of, 125
alveolus fracture of, 43
alveoplasty, 152-3
amalgam tattoo, 102
ameloblastoma, 50, 104, 105-6, 116, 122, 124

American Society of Anesthesiologists (ASA) grading scale,
   19, 20, 255
amethocaine gel, 14
aminoglycosides, 93
amitriptyline, 232
amoxicillin, 47, 92, 225
ampicillin, 93, 202
anaemia, 20
analgesics, 22
   asthmatic patients, 256
aneurysmal bone cyst, 126
angina, 256, 257
angled elevators, 35
anterior open bite, 173, 174
   maxillofacial trauma-related, 189, 250
anterior repositioning appliance, 235
antibioma, 92
antibiotics
   ascending bacterial sialadenitis, 202
   cancrum oris (noma), 97
   cyst enucleation, 121
   diabetic patients, 259
   facial laceration repair, 196
   implant surgery, 162
   infection of dental origin, 92-3
   infective endocarditis prophylaxis, 258
   maxillary antral disease, 225
   maxillofacial trauma, 195, 196
   oroantral communication closure, 223
   osteomyelitis, 95-6
   pericoronitis, 47, 49
   recurrent parotitis of childhood, 202
   surgical endodontics, 78, 80
   third molar surgery, 59, 60, 63
   tooth extraction, 41
      transalveolar, 40
anticoagulant therapy, 25, 43, 258, 259
antidepressants, 232, 238
antiplatelet drugs, 43
anxiety, 14, 15
   compromised patient, 254
   control, 12-23, 72
      epileptic patients, 259
      general anaesthesia, 18
      hypertensive patients, 257
      non-pharmacological, 15-16
      sedation, 16-17
   definitions, 13-14

recognition, 14
Apert's syndrome, 174, 175, 179
apicectomy, 68, 75-6, 80
    instruments, 261
    recurrent infection, 78-9
    repeat, 80
apicectomy retractors, 74
arthrocentesis, 245-6
arthroscope, 244
arthroscopy, 244-5
artificial saliva, 212, 213
aspirin, 43, 59, 93, 258
asthma, 256
atypical facial pain, 237-9
auriculotemporal nerve damage, 246, 251
autotransplantation of unerupted teeth, 167, 168, 170-1

bacterial sialadenitis
    acute, 201-2
    chronic, 202
basal bone, 147
benign lymphoepithelial lesion, 211, 212
benign naevus, 102
benzocaine, topical, 14
benzodiazepines, 72, 256
betel (arecha nut) use, 128, 131, 132
bimaxillary anomalies, 173
    assessment of need for surgery, 175
biopsy, 109-12
    acute necrotising sialometaplasia, 204
    care of specimens, 112
    consent, 113
    cysts, 119
    cytological techniques, 111-12
    excisional, 109-10, 113, 119
    fine needle aspiration, 119, 137, 143, 208
    in general dental practice, 113
    giant-cell arteritis, 240
    incisional, 110-11, 113, 119, 137
    leukoplakia (white plaques), 102, 130, 131
    oral cancer, 134, 137
    oral lesions, 101, 109-13
    pigmented lesions, 102
    punch, 111
    referral criteria, 113
    salivary gland tumours, 208
    soft-tissue lesions, 102, 103, 104
    submucosal solid lesions, 104
    trephine, 111
bismuth iodoform paraffin paste (BIPP), 41, 122
bisphosphonates
    implant surgery contraindication, 157
    osteonecrosis association, 42, 69, 108, 109
bleeding control
    cyst enucleation, 121
    impacted maxillary canine extraction, 63
    incisional biopsy, 111
    maxillofacial trauma, 185
    surgical endodontics, 75, 79, 80

third molar surgery, 58, 62
bleeding, postextraction, 33, 34, 42-3
bleeding tendency, 43, 69, 258, 259
blood clotting function tests, 42-3
body temperature measurement, 87
Bohn's nodule (gingival cyst of childhood), 125
bone augmentation, 154-5
    implant surgery, 158
bone removal
    apicectomy, 68
    cyst enucleation, 120
    impacted lower third molar surgery, 54, 56
        lingual split technique, 59
    impacted maxillary canine surgery, 63
    surgical endodontics, 74-5
    unerupted teeth exposure, 169
bone wax, 42, 77, 121
botryoid cyst, 125
Botulinus toxin, 249
Bowdler-Henry retractor, 74
branchial cyst, 126, 211
Briault probe, 77
bronchitis, 256
bruising (ecchymosis), complicating third molar removal, 60
buccal advancement (Rehmann's) flap, 220-2
buccal fat pad graft, 222
buccal mucosal cancer, 130
    clinical presentation, 136
    treatment, 141
buccal mucosal lesions, 101
buccal space
    abscess drainage, 91
    spread of infection, 86
buccal sulci, 7
bupivacaine, 22

calcifying epithelial odontogenic tumour, 106
Caldwell-Luc operation, 224
cancrum oris (noma), 96-7
candidiasis
    chronic hyperplastic, 132
        malignant potential, 130, 132
    xerostomia-related, 213
canines
    extraction, 32
    impacted maxillary, 62-4
        radiographic localization, 62-3
        surgical removal, 63-4, 218
    maxillary, spread of infection, 87
carbamazepine, 239
carcinoma in-situ, 131
cardiovascular disease, 256-8, 259
    severity grading, 255
cefradine, 92, 93
cellulitis, 85
    clinical features, 88
    spreading in floor of mouth (Ludwig's angina), 93-4
cemento-osseous dysplasia, 104, 106
cementoblastoma, 104, 106

cephalosporins, 92, 96
cerebrovascular accident, 259
cervicofacial space abscess, 88
    drainage, 91-2
chaperone, 5
chemotherapy, 129
cherubism, 107
children
    general anaesthesia, 19
    intravenous sedation, 17
chloramphenicol, 203
chlorhexidine, 41, 47, 49, 72
chrondrosarcoma, 108
cisplatinum, 129
clarithromycin, 93
cleft lip and palate, 46, 174, 175, 180
    principles of repair, 180
cleidocranial dysostosis, 46
clindamycin, 202
clopidogrel, 43
cluster headache, 239-40
compromised patient, 253-60
    aftercare, 254
    general assessment, 254
    identification, 253-4
    medical status assessment, 254-5
    treatment planning, 254
computerised tomography (CT)
    cysts, 118
    implant treatment planning, 159
    maxillary antral disease, 218
    odontogenic keratocysts, 124, 125
    oral cancer, 137-8
    salivary gland tumours, 207
    temporomandibular joint ankylosis, 249
condylar hyperplasia, 174
connective tissue grafts, 158
conscious sedation see sedation
consent, 8-9
    biopsy, 113
    disclosure of confidential information, 197
    extraction of teeth, 25
    general anaesthesia, 21
    implant surgery, 160
    sedation, 17, 21
    surgical endodontics, 72, 80
    third molar removal, 52, 60
Coupland's elevator, 35, 36, 37, 39, 56, 58, 63
cowhorn extraction forceps, 29
craniofacial anomalies, 173
    assessment of need for surgery, 175
Crohn's disease, 102
Crouzon's syndrome, 175, 179
Cryer's elevator, 35, 36, 58, 61
Cumine Scaler, 120
cyst-like lesions, 126
cysts, 115-26
    alveolar, 125
    biopsy, 119

definition, 116
dentigerous (follicular), 124
enucleation, 119, 120-1, 124, 125
    adjunctive care, 121
    wound repair, 121
eruption, 125
follow-up care, 123
imaging investigations, 118-19
inflammatory, 124
keratocyst (odontogenic keratocyst), 124
    multiple, 125
marsupialisation, 119, 121-3, 124, 125
    healing period, 122-3
    indications, 121-2
maxillary antrum, 123, 224
patterns of growth, 117-18
presenting symptoms/signs, 116-18
radicular (dental), 116, 117, 118, 124
site, 117
soft-tissue, 126
treatment principles, 119
cytological smears, 112

day stay general anaesthesia, 21
decisional support systems, 10
decongestant nasal drops, 225-6
demographic details, 5
dental trauma, 196-7
dentigerous (follicular) cyst, 50, 116, 118, 124, 224
dentoalveolar preprosthetic surgery, 151-2
dentofacial deformity, 166, 173-80
    assessment of need for surgery, 173-5
denture-induced hyperplasia, 103
dermoid, 117, 126, 211
dexamethasone, 22, 59
diabetes mellitus, 19, 157, 170, 210, 258-9
diagnosis, 4-11
    definitive, 8
    expert practice, 9
    guidelines, 9-10
    process, 5
    record keeping, 5-6
diagnostic wax-up, implant surgery, 160
diathermy, bleeding control, 42, 121
differential diagnosis, 7-8
discectomy (meniscectomy), 247
discoid lupus erythematosus, 130, 133
distraction anxiety control, 15
diuretics, 257
dothiepin, 232
drain insertion, 91, 92
dressings
    abscess drainage, 92
    dry socket, 41
drug history, 259-60
dry socket, 40-1, 237
dyskeratosis congenita, 130, 134

eagle beak extraction forceps, 29

ectopic teeth, 46
  dentigerous cysts association, 124
edentulous alveolar ridge
  alveoplasty, 152-3
  assessment for preprosthetic surgery, 149
  bone augmentation, 154-5
  hyperplastic oral mucosa excision, 149-50
  mapping for implant surgery, 159
  radiography, 149
edentulous jaw
  alveolar bone loss, 147
  atrophic ridge, 148
  classification, 148
  effects on facial aesthetics, 148
  ideal ridge, 148
  surgical aids to prosthodontics see preprosthetic surgery
  tooth loss-related anatomical changes, 147-8
elderly people, 254
  general anaesthesia, 19
  oral cancer, 134, 140
  oral tissue changes, 146-7
  treatment planning, 254
elevators tooth removal, 34-5
  applications, 35-7
  principles of use, 35
  retained root removal, 35-6, 223
  third molar surgery, 54
elevators periosteal, 38
EMLA cream, 14
endodontics
  conventional treatment failure, 67-8, 69
  surgical see surgical endodontics
endotracheal intubation, 21, 185
enostoses (solitary bone islands), 106
enucleation, cyst, 119, 120-1, 124, 125
  adjunctive care, 121
  wound repair, 121
envelope flap, 55-46
ephedrine, 225-6
epidermoid cyst, 126
epilepsy, 259
epithelial dysplasia, 131
Epstein's pearls (gingival cysts of childhood), 125
epulis, 101
  treatment, 103
eruption cyst, 125
erythromycin, 93, 225
erythroplakia (red plaques), 102, 130, 131
  definition, 131
  malignant potential, 130, 131
  management, 131
escort requirement
  general anaesthesia, 21
  sedation, 17
ethyl chloride, 90, 91
etidronate, 42
eugenol dressings, 41
examination, 5, 6-7, 9
  extraction of teeth, 25

extraoral, 7
  implant treatment, 156
  intraoral, 7
  maxillofacial trauma, 186-9
  oral cancer, 137
  orthognathic surgery, 176
  preprosthetic surgery, 149
  soft-tissue lesions, 101-2
  surgical endodontics, 70
examination setting, 5
excisional biopsy, 109-10, 113
  cysts, 119
  submucosal lesions, 110
  superficial lesions, 109-10
exfoliative cytology, 111
exostoses, 104, 106, 107
exposure plus orthodontics, unerupted teeth, 167, 168
  mechanical traction application, 170
  technique, 168-70
extraction forceps, 26-9
  design variants, 29
  for left-handed operators, 27
  for lower teeth, 28
  position in hand, 29-30
  for upper teeth, 26-8
extraction of teeth, 24-44, 90
  anticoagulated patients, 43
  with blood-clotting disorders, 43
  clinical examination, 25
  complications, 40, 40-3, 218, 223-4
  consent, 25
  extraction socket care, 33
  fracture, 34
    of alveolus, 43
  history-taking, 25
  indications, 25-6
  mandibular
    canines, 32
    incisors, 32
    molars, 33
    premolars, 32
  maxillary
    canines, 32
    incisors, 32
    molars, 33
    premolars, 32-3
  movements, 31-3
    modifying techniques, 33
  operator/patient position, 30, 32
    for lower teeth, 30, 32
    supporting hand, 30-1
    for upper teeth, 30, 32
  postoperative bleeding, 33, 34, 42-3
  postoperative instruction for patients, 33-4
  preprosthetic surgery, 151-2
  radiographic assessment, 25
  record keeping, 34
  transalveolar approach, 37-40, 223
    surgical procedure, 38-9

extraction of teeth, *continued*
  suturing, 39-40
  unerupted *see* unerupted teeth
extraoral examination, 7

facial laceration repair, 195-6
facial lymph nodes, 87
facial nerve, 200, 202, 210, 246, 247, 251
  salivary gland tumour involvement, 207, 209
facial pain
  atypical facial pain, 237-9
  dental pain, 229
  maxillary antral disorders, 225
  non-dental causes, 237-40
  temporomandibular disorders, 229-30
facial trauma
  medicolegal issues, 197
  scar revision, 197
  see also maxillofacial trauma
fever, 87
fibroepithelial polyp, 101, 102, 103
  excisional biopsy, 109
  treatment, 103
fibrous dysplasia, 104, 107-8, 174
Fickling's forceps, 58
fine needle aspiration cytology, 111, 112
  cysts, 119
  oral cancer, 137
   lymph node involvement, 143
  salivary gland tumours, 208
floor of mouth, 7
  cancer, 130, 131
   clinical presentation, 135
   treatment, 141
  spreading cellulitis (Ludwig's angina), 93-4
flucloxacillin, 202
flumazenil, 17
5-fluorouracil, 129
fluoxetine, 232
foreign bodies, maxillary antrum, 223-4
fracture fixation, 192
  historical aspects, 194-5
  Le Fort pattern fractures, 193
  mandibular condylar neck fracture dislocation, 250
  mandibular fracture, 194, 195
  mini-plates, 192, 193, 194, 195
fraenectomy, 150, 172-3
  labial, 172
  lingual, 172-3
Frey's syndrome (gustatory sweating), 210, 251

gag reflex, 17, 69, 153
Gardner's syndrome, 104, 107
gastric contents aspiration, 17, 20
general anaesthesia, 17-22
  advantages, 17-18
  airway management, 21
  anaesthetist competency, 19
  Caldwell-Luc operation, 224

contraindications, 256
cysts treatment, 119
diabetic patients, 258
equipment, 19
facial laceration repair, 196
fitness measures, 19, *20*
indications/referral criteria, 19
  difficult cases, 21-2
inpatient versus outpatient treatment, 21
intraoral abscess drainage, 90, 91
investigations, 20
maxillary/mandibular torus removal, 153
oroantral communication closure, 222
patient instructions, 18
preparatory starvation, 20-1
problems, 18-19
recovery/discharge, 21
giant-cell arteritis, 240
giant-cell epulis, 101
giant-cell granuloma, 102, 107
  central, 107
  treatment, 103
giant-cell tumour of bone, 107
Gillies' procedure, 192, 193
gingival cancer, 135
gingival cyst, 117, 125
  of childhood, 125
glandular odontogenic cyst, 117, 125
Glasgow Coma Scale, 186
Gorlin Goltz (basal cell naevus) syndrome, 123, 125
granulomatous sialadenitis, 202-3
gustatory sweating (Frey's syndrome), 210, 251

haemangioma, 101, 104
  intrabony lesions, 108
  salivary gland, 210
haematomas
  complicating impacted maxillary canine extraction, 63
  complicating lower third molar removal, 60
  haemorrhagic disorders association, 258
  maxillofacial trauma, 187, 189, 190
   nasal bones, 193
haemostatic agents, resorbable, 42, 43
hamartomas, 104, 105, 106
hard-tissue lesions, 104-9
  odontogenic, 104-6
  osseous, 106-9
hard-tissue preprosthetic surgery, 151-4
hearing loss/tests, maxillofacial trauma, 188, 190
heart failure, 257
hemifacial atrophy, 174
hemifacial microsomia, 174
hemisection, 81
history of presenting complaint, 5-6
history-taking, 5, 9
  compromised patient, 254
  drug history, 259-60
  extraction of teeth, 25
  impacted lower third molars, 46

implant treatment, 156
  maxillofacial trauma, 185-6
  medical status, 254-5
  oral cancer, 137
  orthognathic surgery, 176
  preprosthetic surgery, 149
  surgical endodontics, 70
  unerupted teeth, 46
HIV infection, 102
  cystic lymphoid hyperplasia, 211
  salivary gland lymphomas, 210
  sialadenitis, 203-4
Howarth's periosteal elevator, 38, 54, 61, 63
hyperparathyroidism, 107
hyperplastic oral mucosa excision, 149-50
hypertension, 20, 257, 259
hypnosis, 15
hypoglossal nerve, 202

ibuprofen, 22, 40, 47, 59, 225
impacted teeth see unerupted/impacted teeth
implant burs, 161
implants, endosseous, 146, 155-64
  bone grafting, 158
  complications, 163-4
  consent, 160
  contraindications, 157
  diagnostic wax-up, 160
  exposure (second-stage surgery), 162-3
  factors affecting success, 156
  flap design, 160-1
  insertion, 161-2
    bone preparation, 161-2
    cover screw placement, 162
    immediately after extraction, 161
  investigations, 157-9
  optimum length determination, 159
  osseointegration, 156
  position, 159
  postoperative care, 162
  prior extraction of teeth, 151
  prosthodontic rehabilitation, 163
  record keeping, 159
  ridge mapping, 159
  soft-tissue grafting, 158
  systems, 156
  treatment planning, 156-7
  wound closure, 162
implants, subperiosteal, 155
implants, transosseous, 156
incisional biopsy, 110-11, 113
  cysts, 119
  oral cancer, 137
  soft-tissue repair, 111
  submucosal lesions, 110
incisors extraction, mandibular/maxillary, 32
infection, 83-99
  antibacterial chemotherapy, 92-3
  inpatient management, 93

investigations, 89
local features, 84-5
localisation, 85
methicillin-resistant Staphylococcus aureus (MRSA), 97
microbiology, 89
necrotising, 96-7
neoplastic disorders differentiation, 88-9
normal response, 89
presentation, 87-8
spread, 85-7
supportive care, 93
surgical treatment (drainage), 90-2
systemic features, 87
infective endocarditis, 59, 258
inferior alveolar nerve damage, 60, 72, 163
inflammation, 84, 85
inflammatory cysts, 124
infraorbital nerve damage, 72
inhalational sedation, 16
injection
  into temporomandibular joint, 242-3
  pain reduction, 14-15
instructions for patients
  extraction of teeth, 33-4
  general anaesthesia, 18
  sedation, 17, 18
international normalised ratio (INR), 43, 258
interrupted sutures, 39
  facial laceration repair, 196
  implant surgery, 162
  incisional biopsy repair, 111
  labial fraenectomy, 172
  surgical endodontics, 77
intraoral examination, 7
intravenous sedation, 16-17, 157
investigations, 8
  before general anaesthesia, 20
ischaemic heart disease, 10, 25, 69, 240, 256-7

jugulodigastric lymph node, 87
juvenile rheumatoid arthritis, 174, 249
  temporomandibular joint involvement, 237

keratocyst, 50
ketoconazole, 213
Kuttner tumour, 202, 211

labial fraenum
  denture displacement, 147
  prominent tissue excision (fraenectomy), 150, 172
Lack's tongue retractor, 38
Langerhans cell histiocytosis, 107, 108
laryngeal mask, 21
Laster's retractor, 61
lateral periodontal cyst, 117, 125
lateral pharyngeal space infection, 86, 88
Le Fort I fracture, 187, 188, 224
Le Fort I osteotomy, 179
Le Fort II fracture, 187, 188, 224

Le Fort II osteotomy, 179
Le Fort III fracture, 187, 188, 224
Le Fort III osteotomy, 179
Le Fort pattern fractures, 187-8, 189
    antral wall involvement, 224
    infection risk, 195
    surgical intervention, 193
leukaemia, 25
leukoplakia (white plaques), 102, 130-1, 135
    aetiology, 131
    biopsy, 110, 130, 131
    definition, 130
    malignant potential, 130, 131
    management, 131
lichen planus, 102, 130, 133
lidocaine, 41
    with adrenaline, 22, 243, 257
    topical, 14
ligation, postextraction haemorrhage control, 42
lincosamides, 93, 96
lingual fraenectomy, 172-3
lingual nerve, 200, 202
    injury during third molar removal, 54-5, 60
lingual retractor, 54-5
lip
    carcinoma, 140
    soft-tissue lesions, 101
lipoma, 210
lobulation, cysts diagnosis, 118
local anaesthesia, 14-15
    compromised patients, 257
    cysts treatment, 119, 122
    epileptic patients, 259
    excisional biopsy, 109, 110
    exposure plus orthodontics of unerupted teeth, 168, 170
    extent required, 15
    failure, 15
    fraenectomy, 172
    implant surgery, 157
    injection pain reduction, 14-15
    intraoral abscess drainage, 90, 91
    postsurgical pain relief, 22
    surgical endodontics, 72-3, 79
    temporomandibular joint closed manipulation for
        adhesions, 243
local anaesthetic with vasoconstrictor, 22, 73, 79
loupes, 72, 80
Ludwig's angina, 93-4
Luebke-Ochsenbein flap, 74
lumps, 5
    examination, 7
    soft-tissue lesions, 101
luxators, 37
lymph nodes
    examination, 7
    infection, 87
        differentiation from neoplastic disorders, 89
    oral cancer involvement, 135, 136
        aspiration biopsy, 137

management, 142-3
    treatment, 141
submucosal lesions, 102
lymphangioma, salivary gland, 210
lymphoma, 130
    salivary gland, 210

McCune-Albright syndrome, 107, 108
macrogenia, 174
macrolides, 93
magnetic resonance imaging (MRI)
    cysts, 118
    oral cancer, 137-8
    salivary gland tumours, 207
    temporomandibular disc displacement, 236
    temporomandibular joint ankylosis, 249
malaise, 87
malignant melanoma, 130
    treatment, 142
malignant osseous lesions, 108-9
mandibular anomalies, 173
    assessment of need for surgery, 173-4
mandibular condyle fracture, 190, 192, 195
    condylar neck fracture dislocation, 250
mandibular fracture, 188, 189
    complicating implant surgery, 164
    complicating lower third molar removal, 60
    infection risk, 195
    rehabilitation, 197
    surgical intervention, 193-5
mandibular osteotomy, 177-8
mandibular teeth extraction
    canines, 32
    incisors, 32
    molars, 33
    operator/patient position, 30, 32
    premolars, 32
mandibular torus, 104
    preprosthetic removal, 153-4
marsupialisation, cyst, 119, 121-3, 124, 125
    healing period, 122-3
    indications, 121-2
masseter muscle tenderness, 230
masticator space infection, 86, 88
maxillary alveolar bone loss, 147
maxillary anomalies, 173
    assessment of need for surgery, 174, 175
    bimaxillary, 175
maxillary antrum, 215-27
    anatomical relationship to posterior maxillary teeth, 216
    cysts, 123, 224
    dental extraction-related disorders, 218
    facial pain, 225
    foreign bodies, 223-4
    fracture, 218, 224
    investigations, 217-18
    radiography, 216, 218
    sinusitis, 219, 220
        dental pathology differentiation, 217

pharmacological treatments, 225-6
tumours, 136-7, 142, 224-5
see also oroantral communication; oroantral fistula
maxillary Le Fort pattern fractures *see* Le Fort pattern
        fractures
maxillary osteotomies, 179
maxillary teeth extraction
    canines, 32
    incisors, 32
    molars, 33
    operator/patient position, 30, 32
    premolars, 32-3
    see also canines, impacted maxillary; third molars
        removal, maxillary
maxillary torus removal, 153-4
maxillary tuberosity
    fracture complicating third molar removal, 63
    hyperplastic, reduction, 150-1
maxillofacial trauma, 183-98
    acute management, 185, 186
        assessment of brain injury, 186
    causes, 184-5
    dental injuries, 196-7
    examination, 186-9
    facial laceration repair, 195-6
    history-taking, 185-6
    infection risk, 195
    investigations, 189-90
    medicolegal issues, 197
    prevention, 185
    psychological injury, 196
    radiography, 186, 189-90
    rehabilitation, 197
    surgical intervention, 190, 192-7
        principles, 192
mediastinal infections, 87
meniscectomy (discectomy), 247
menopausal changes, 146
mental nerve damage, 72, 73
methicillin-resistant *Staphylococcus aureus* (MRSA), 97
methylene blue dye, root fracture identification, 76
metronidazole, 40, 41, 47, 92, 93, 97
miconazole, 213
microbiology, 89
microgenia, 174
micrognathism, 174
midazolam, 16, 17
migraine, 239-40
Mikulicz syndrome, 212
mini-plate fracture fixation, 192, 193, 194, 195
    osteogenesis promotion, 195
minor salivary glands
    mucoceles, 206
    sialadenitis, 204
    stone formation, 204
    tumours, 101, 102, 110, 130, 136, 142, 153, 208
        treatment, 209
Mitchell's trimmer, 75, 120
molars

extraction, 33
    maxillary third, 61-2
    retained root removal, 35-6, 37
    see also third molars, impacted mandibular
morbid obesity, 19
mucocele, 101, 126, 206
mucoepidermoid carcinoma, 209
mucoperiosteal flaps, 37-8
    apicectomy, 68
    canine removal, impacted maxillary, 63
    cyst marsupialisation, 122
    envelope, 55-46, 62
    gingival margins recession, 72, 73-4, 80
    implant surgery, 160
    local anaesthesia, 15
    Luebke-Ochsenbein, 74
    oroantral communication closure, 211, 222
    palatal, 63, 222
    semilunar, 74
    surgical endodontics, 72, 73-4
    suturing, 39-40
    third molar removal
        impacted mandibular, 54-6
        maxillary, 61
    three-sided, 37, 54-5, 73-4, 211, 222
    transalveolar tooth extraction, 37, 38
    two-sided, 37, 73
mucosal grafts, 158
mucous cyst, 101, 103-4
    excisional biopsy, 110
multiple myeloma, 108
mumps, 200-1
musculoskeletal disorders, 259
myocardial infarction, 257
myofascial pain dysfunction, 231-2, 235
    clinical features, 231-2
    treatment, 232

nasal bone fracture, 193
nasal examination, maxillofacial trauma, 188
nasoethmoid fracture, 193
nasolabial cyst, 117
nasopharyngeal tube airway, 185
nasopharyngeal tumours, 109
nasopalatine duct cyst, 117, 125
necrotising infections, 96-7
necrotising sialometaplasia, 204, 211
necrotising ulcerative gingivitis, acute, 96
neurilemmoma, 102
    salivary gland, 210
neurofibroma, 174
    salivary gland, 210
neurological diseases, 259
nitrous oxide/oxygen, 16
noma (cancrum oris), 96-7
non-steroidal anti-inflammatory drugs, 258, 259

obstructive airway disease, chronic, 20, 256
odontogenic cysts, 115-26

odontogenic cysts, *continued*
  maxillary antrum, 123, 220
  see also cysts
odontogenic fibroma, 106
odontogenic keratocyst, 116, 117, 118, 124-5, 224
  follow-up care, 123
  management, 124-5
  multiple, 125
odontogenic myxoma, 106
odontogenic tumours, 104-6
  adenomatoid, 106
  calcifying epithelial, 106
  cementifying, 106
odontomes, 104, 105, 171-2
opioids, 22
oral cancer, 11, 127-44, 225
  biopsy, 134, 137
  chemotherapy, 129
  classification, 138-9
  clinical presentation, 134-7
  diagnosis, 137
  epidemiology, 128
  follow-up, 143
  imaging investigations, 137-8
  infection differentiation, 88-9
  management, 139-42
    age considerations, 140
    general dental practitioner's role, 139
    neck, 142-3
  multiple primary tumours (field change), 128, 140, 143
  premalignant lesions, 130-4
  radiotherapy, 129
  reconstruction, 128-9, 141, 142
  referral, 101, 137
  resection, 128
  risk factors, 128
  sites, 129-30
  staging, 138-9, 142-3
oral lesions, 100-14
  biopsy, 101, 109-13
  hard-tissue *see* hard-tissue lesions
  referral, 101
  soft-tissue *see* soft-tissue lesions
oral sedation, 16
oral submucous fibrosis, 130, 132
orbit
  examination, maxillofacial trauma, 188
  infection, 87
oroantral communication, 216, 218-23
  closure, 220-3
    buccal advancement (Rehmann's) flap, 220-2
    palatal rotation flap, 222-3
  complicating dental extractions, 63, 218, 223
  formation prevention, 219-20, 223
  immediate management of new communication, 220
  investigations, 219
  pharmacological prevention of infection, 225-6
  signs, 218-19
oroantral fistula, 218, 219

treatment, 220-3
orofacial granulomatosis, 102
oropharyngeal cancer *see* oral cancer
oropharyngeal tube airway, 185
oropharynx, 7
orotracheal intubation, 21
orthodontic procedures, 166, 167
  cleft lip and palate, 180
  unerupted/impacted teeth, 167-71
    radiographic assessment, 168
orthognathic surgery
  assessment of need
    bimaxillary anomalies, 175
    craniofacial anomalies, 175
    mandibular anomalies, 173-4
    maxillary anomalies, 174
  cleft lip and palate, 180
  edentulous jaw augmentation, 164
  instruments, 179
  investigations, 177
  osteotomies
    planning, 176-7
    procedures, 177-9
osseointegrated implants *see* implants, endosseous
osseous lesions, 106-9
  benign tumours, 107
  giant-cell, 107
  malignant, 108-9
  referral, 109
ossifying fibroma, 104, 106, 107
osteoarthritis, 259
osteoblastoma, 107
osteogenesis imperfecta, 25
osteogenic sarcoma, 107
osteoma, 104, 107
  maxillary antrum, 224
osteomyelitis, 41, 60, 94-6, 107, 109
  treatment, 95-6
osteonecrosis, bisphosphonates-related, 42, 69, 108, 109
osteoporosis, 146
osteoradionecrosis, 109
osteosarcoma, 104, 108
osteotomies
  instruments, 179
  planning, 176-7
  procedures, 177-9
    mandible, 177-8
    maxilla, 179

Paget's disease, 104, 107, 108
pain, 5, 10-11, 14
  definitions, 13
  history-taking, 6
  of injection, 14-15
  recognition, 13
  referred, 240
pain control, 12-23
  general anaesthesia, 17-22
  hypertensive patients, 257

local anaesthesia, 14-15
postoperative *see* postoperative analgesia
sedation, 16-17
sinusitis, 225
temporomandibular degenerative joint disease, 237
palatal cancer, 130
clinical presentation, 136-7
premalignant lesions, 131
treatment, 142
palatal rotation flap, oroantral communication closure, 222-3
palatal torus, 104
preprosthetic removal, 153-4
palate, 7
soft-tissue lesions, 101, 104
submucosal lesions, 110
palor, 87
papilloma, 103, 109
maxillary antrum, 224
see also viral papilloma (wart)
paracetamol, 22, 59, 93, 201, 225, 258
paradental cyst, 117
Parkinson's disease, 259
parotid gland, 199-200
obstruction, 204
sialosis, 210
stone formation, 204, 205
trauma to papilla, 204
tumours, 207, 208, 209, 210
parotidectomy, 209, 210
parotitis
recurrent of childhood, 202
see also sialadenitis
paroxetine, 232
past dental/medical history, 6, 254-5
Paterson-Kelly syndrome (sideropenic dysphagia), 130, 133
pathological fracture, 118
pathology request form, 112
penicillin, 96, 97
penicillin V, 92, 93, 95
pericoronitis
acute, 46
chronic, 46
impacted lower third molars, 46-7, 49, 50
periodontal disease, surgical endodontics patients, 70
periotome, 151
personal information (demographic details), 5
phenytoin, 239
phobia, 14
pigmented soft-tissue lesions, 102
platelet count, 43
pleomorphic adenoma, 208, 209
Plummer-Vinson syndrome (sideropenic dysphagia), 130, 133
polyglycolic acid sutures, 39, 42, 59
positron emission tomography (PET), oral cancer, 138
postoperative analgesia, 22
anticoagulated patients, 258
cyst enucleation, 121

impacted lower third molar removal, 59
implant surgery, 162
temporomandibular joint closed manipulation for adhesions, 243-4
transalveolar tooth extraction, 40
postoperative pain, 13
post-traumatic stress disorder, 196, 197
pregnancy epulis, 102
treatment, 103
pregnant patients
general anaesthesia, 19
sialosis, 210
premalignant lesions, 130-4
premolars
extraction, 32-3
maxillary spread of infection, 87
retained mandibular root removal, 36
unerupted/impacted
maxillary antrum complications, 218
surgical removal, 64
preoperative analgesia, lower third molar removal, 59
preprosthetic surgery, 145-65
aims/objectives, 146
deficient denture-bearing areas restoration, 154-5
hard-tissue procedures, 151-4
major procedures, 164
radiography, 149
soft-tissue procedures, 149-51
treatment planning, 149
see also implants, endosseous
presenting complaint, 5
progenia, 174
prognathism, 173, 174, 176, 177
osteotomy procedures, 178
prosthodontic surgical aids *see* preprosthetic surgery
pseudoephedrine, 226
psychological injury, maxillofacial trauma association, 196, 197
pterygoid muscle tenderness, 230
punch biopsy, 111
pus microbiology, 89
sample collection, 90-1
pyogenic granuloma, 101, 102, 103

racial deposits, 102
radiation sialadenitis, 203
radicular (dental) cyst, 116, 117, 118, 124
radiography, 8
cysts, 118-19
extraction of teeth, 25
impacted lower third molars, 47-9, 53, 54
impacted maxillary canines, 62-3
implant treatment planning, 157, 159
jaw radiolucencies differential diagnosis, 119
maxillary antrum, 216, 218
maxillary torus removal, 153
maxillofacial trauma, 186, 189-90
oral cancer, 137
oroantral communication/fistula, 219

radiography, *continued*
    orthognathic surgery planning, 177
    osteomyelitis, 95
    preprosthetic surgery, 149
    sialolithiasis, 205
    surgical endodontics, 71
        follow-up, 78
        postoperative, 77, 80
    temporomandibular degenerative joint disease, 237
    unerupted teeth, 168
radiotherapy, 59, 69
    oral cancer, 129, 139, 140, 142, 143
    salivary gland tumours, 209, 210
rake retractor, 38, 56, 74
ranula, 206
record-keeping, 5-6
    consent, 9, 25, 72
    extraction of teeth, 34
        lower third molar retained fragments, 58
    implant surgery, 159, 160
    maxillofacial trauma, 185
    preprosthetic surgery, 149
    sedation, 17
recurrent symptoms, 6
red patches *see* erythroplakia
referred pain, 240
regional block failure, 15
replantation, 82
    traumatic dental injuries, 197
    see also autotransplantation of unerupted teeth
residual cysts, 124
residual ridge, 147
    mapping for implant surgery, 159
respiratory tract infection, acute, 256
resuscitation, maxillofacial trauma patients, 185, 186
retrogenia, 174
retrognathism, 173, 174
retrograde (root end) filling, 68-9
retromolar trigone cancer, 130
    treatment, 141-2
retropharyngeal space infection, 87
rheumatoid arthritis, 259
    secondary Sjögren's syndrome, 211
rima oris examination, 7
root amputation, 81
root displacement into antrum, 223-4
    removal procedures, 224
root end (retrograde) filling, 68-9, 77, 80
root fracture, maxillofacial trauma, 197

sagittal split osteotomy, 178
salivary duct cyst, 211
salivary duct obstruction, 205-6
salivary gland disorders, 199-214
    degenerative, 211-13
    developmental, 200
    inflammatory, 200-4
    neoplasms *see* salivary gland tumours
    obstructive, 204-6

salivary gland tumours, 207-10
    biopsy, 208
    clinical presentation, 207
    epithelial, 208-10
        management, 209
    investigation, 207-8
    lymphomas, 210
    non-epithelial, 210
    salivary duct obstruction, 206
sarcomas, 104, 107, 108, 116, 130
scope of oral surgery, 3
secondary malignancy, 107, 108, 109, 128, 130
sedation, 16-17
    advantages/risks, 17
    airway protection, 17
    with chronic respiratory disease, 256
    compromised patients, 256, 257, 259
    definition, 16
    diabetic patients, 259
    epileptic patients, 259
    inhalational, 16
    instructions for patients, 17, 18
    intravenous, 16-17, 259
        implant surgery, 157
    oral, 16
    with Parkinson's disease, 259
    patient preparation/discharge requirements, 17
sequestrum, 95
sialadenitis
    acute ascending bacterial, 201-2
    allergic, 203
    chronic bacterial, 202
    chronic sclerosing, 202
    granulomatous, 202-3
    HIV-associated, 203-4
    minor salivary glands, 204
    radiation, 203
sialography, 205, 207
    Sjögren's syndrome, 211
Sialolithiasis (salivary stones), 204-5
sialorrhoea, 213
sialosis, 210
sickle cell disease, 20
sideropenic dysphagia (Plummer-Vinson/Paterson-Kelly syndrome), 130, 133
silk sutures, 39, 42, 59, 92
sinus, 85
sinusitis, maxillary, 23, 217
    diagnosis, 217-18
    oroantral communication, 219, 220
    pharmacological treatment, 225-6
    signs/symptoms, 217
Sjögren's syndrome, 203, 204, 211-12
    lymphoma, 210, 211, 212
skin examination, maxillofacial trauma, 189
social history, 6
    compromised patient, 254
sodium valproate, 239
soft vinyl mouthguard, myofascial pain dysfunction

treatment, 232
soft-tissue cysts, 117, 126
soft-tissue grafting, implant surgery, 158
soft-tissue lesions, 101-4
    anatomical relationships, 101-2
    biopsy, 102, 104
        indications, 103
    colour, 101
    consistency, 101-2
    diagnosis, 101, 103
    modifying influences, 102
    multiple, 102
    pigmented, 102
    red patches, 102
    referral, 103, 104
    site, 101
    treatment, 103-4
    vascular, 104
    white patches, 102
soft-tissue preprosthetic surgery, 149-51
specimens, pathological, 112
squamous cell carcinoma, 130, 136, 142
    salivary gland, 209
steam inhalations, maxillary antral disease, 226
steroids
    degenerative joint disease, 248
    giant-cell arteritis, 240
    lower third molar removal, 59, 61
    Ludwig's angina, 94
    postsurgical pain relief, 22, 61
    temporomandibular degenerative joint disease, 237
    temporomandibular joint postoperative care, 244, 245
Still's disease see juvenile rheumatoid arthritis
stomatitis nicotina, 204
straight elevators, 35
study casts, implant treatment planning, 157
sublingual gland, 200
    ranula, 206
    stone formation, 204
    tumours, 208
sublingual keratosis, 131
sublingual space infection, 88
submandibular abscess drainage, 91
submandibular gland, 200
    chronic bacterial sialadenitis, 202
    stone formation, 204, 205
    tumours, 207, 208, 209
submandibular lymph nodes, 87
submandibular space infection, 87
submucosal lesions, 102, 104
    excisional biopsy, 110, 113
    incisional biopsy, 110
supernumerary teeth, 64, 171
supplemental teeth, 64, 171
surgical emphysema, 72, 79-80
surgical endodontics, 67-82
    advanced procedures, 81-2
    aims/objective, 68
    apical tissue curettage, 75

apicectomy, 68, 75-6, 80
    repeat, 80
bleeding control, 75, 79, 80
bone removal, 74-5
case selection, 71
clinical examination, 70
closure, 77
complications, 71-2, 78-80
consent, 72, 80
contraindications, 69-70
debridement, 77
hemisection, 81
history-taking, 70
indications, 67-8, 69
instrumentation, 72
intentional replantation, 82
lateral perforation closure, 81
local anaesthesia, 72-3, 79
maxillary antrum lining perforation, 72, 79
mucoperiosteal flaps, 72
    design, 73-4
    reflection, 74
outcome assessment, 78
perioperative medication, 72
postoperative care, 78
preoperative advice for patients, 71
principles, 68-9
radiographic assessment, 71
    follow-up, 78
    postoperative, 77, 80
referral criteria, 71
retrograde (root end) cavity
    preparation, 76
    temporary obturation bone cavity, 77
root amputation, 81
root end (retrograde) filling, 68-9, 77, 80
surgical procedure, 72-8
treatment planning, 70-2
surgical kit, 261
surgical sieve, 10
suturing, 39
    facial laceration repair, 196
    fraenectomy, 172
    impacted maxillary canines removal, 63
    implant surgery, 162
    incisional biopsy repair, 111
    lower third molar surgery, 59
    oroantral communication immediate management, 220
    postextraction bleeding control, 42, 43
    surgical endodontics, 77
    transalveolar tooth extraction, 39-40
swelling, 5, 7
    acute apical abscess, 70
    complicating lower third molar removal, 61
    cysts presentation, 117
    fluctuant, 84-5, 117
    indurated, 84
    infection, 84, 85
        spread to neck, 87

swelling, *continued*
    malignant osseous lesions, 108
    maxillofacial trauma, 187
    salivary stones, 205
synergistic gangrene, 97
syphilitic glossitis, 130, 132-3
systemic arthropathies, temporomandibular joint
        involvement, 237

temazepam, 16
temporalis muscle tenderness, 230
temporomandibular disc displacement
    with reduction, 232-5
    treatment, 235, 236
    without reduction (closed lock), 236
temporomandibular disorders, 228-41
    classification, 230-1
    clinical features, 229-30
    degenerative disease, 236-7, 245, 246
      surgical treatment, 247-8
    disc displacement, 245
      surgical treatment, 247
      without reduction, 243, 246
    movement limitation, 230
    muscle/joint tenderness, 230
    myofascial pain dysfunction, 231-2, 235
    noises, 230
      clicks, 230, 232, 234, 235, 236
      grating/grinding, 230, 236
    pain, 229-30
    systemic arthropathies, 237
    tumours, 250
temporomandibular joint ankylosis, 249-50
    surgical management, 250
temporomandibular joint dislocation, 248
    manual reduction, 248-9
    maxillofacial trauma, 189
    surgery for recurrence, 249
temporomandibular joint surgery, 242-52
    arthrocentesis, 245-6
    arthroscopy, 244-5
    closed manipulation for adhesions, 243-4
    complications, 251
    disc replacement/repositioning, 247
    endaural approach, 246-7
    injection into joint, 242-3
    meniscectomy (discectomy), 247
    minimally invasive techniques, 242-6
    postoperative care, 251
      mobilisation, 250
    preauricular approach, 246, 247
    recovery time, 251
    submandibular approach, 246
    total joint replacement, 247
terminology, 5
tetanus prophylaxis, 185
tetracycline, 93, 96, 203
third molars, impacted mandibular
    associated paradental cyst, 117

diagnosis, 49-50
history-taking, 46
pericoronitis, 46-7, 49, 50
preoperative assessment, 46-53
radiological assessment, 47-9, 53, 54
removal, 54-9
    anaesthesia, 50, 53
    bleeding control, 58
    bone removal, 54, 56, 59
    closure, 59
    complications, 52, 60, 60-1
    contraindications, 50, 52
    elevation, 54
    flap design, 54-6
    indications, 50
    informed consent, 52, 60
    lingual retractor placement, 54-5
    obstacles, 53-4
    path of withdrawal, 53
    perioperative drug therapy, 59
    postoperative care, 60-1
    record-keeping, 58
    referral criteria, 52
    retained fragments, 58, 60
    tooth division, 56-8
    wound debridement, 58
    spread of infection, 85-7
    surgical assessment, 53-4
    types of impaction, 52-3
third molars removal, maxillary, 61-2
    bleeding control, 62
    complications, *62*, 62
      maxillary antrum involvement, 218
    indications, 61
    surgical access, 61-2
thyroglossal duct cyst, 117, 126
TNM staging, 138-9
tobacco use
    acute necrotising sialometaplasia, 204
    implant surgery contraindication, 157
    leukoplakia aetiology, 131
    oral cancer risk, 128, 143
    stomatitis nicotina, 204
tobacco-induced melanosis, 102
toluidine blue vital staining, 131
tongue cancer, 130
    clinical presentation, 134-5
    premalignant lesions, 131
    treatment, 140-1
topical local anaesthetics, 14, 72
    abscess drainage, 90, 91
tori, 104, 107, 147
    preprosthetic removal, 153-4
total joint replacement, 247
transport of specimens, 112
traumatic bone cyst, 126
Treacher-Collins syndrome, 174
treatment planning, 4, 6, 8-9
trephine biopsy, 111

trichloroacetic acid, 47
trigeminal neuralgia, 239
triptans, 240
trismus, 7
    cervicofacial space abscess, 88
    complicating lower third molar removal, 60-1
    odontogenic infections, 86
    zygomatic fracture, 192
Trotter's syndrome, 109

ulcer, 5, 8
    malignant, 135, 136
ultrasound
    ascending bacterial sialadenitis, 202
    cysts, 118
    oral cancer metastases, 138
    salivary gland tumours, 207-8
unerupted/impacted teeth, 45-66
    autotransplantation plus surgical repositioning, 167, 168, 170-1
    causes of eruption failure, 46
    clinical assessment, 167-8
    exposure, 168
        technique, 168-70
    history-taking, 46
    indications for extraction, 167-8
    mechanical traction application, 170
    orthodontic/surgical management, 167-71

radiographic assessment, 168
    see also canines, impacted maxillary; third molars, impacted mandibular

valvular heart disease, 25, 69
varicosities, 104
venous lakes, 101
vertical subsigmoid osteotomy, 178
victim support, 197
viral papilloma (wart), 101, 103
    excisional biopsy, 109
    multiple lesions, 102
visual function, maxillofacial trauma, 190, 197

warfarin, 43
wart *see* viral papilloma
Warthin tumour, 208
Warwick-James elevator, 35, 36, 38, 55, 58, 61, 63, 120
white patches *see* leukoplakia
Whitehead's varnish, 41, 42, 111, 122

xerostomia, 212-13
    Sjögren's syndrome, 211, 212

Z-plasty fraenectomy, 150
zoledronate, 42
zygomatic fracture, 187, 189, 224
    surgical intervention, 192-3